Cardiovascular Disease in Women

Cardiovascular Disease in Women

Edited by

HUNG N WINN MD JD
David G Hall Professor of Obstetrics and Gynecology
Chairman, Department of Obstetrics, Gynecology and Women's Health
University of Missouri – Columbia School of Medicine
Columbia, MO
USA

KEVIN C DELLSPERGER MD PhD FAHA FACP FACC
Professor of Internal Medicine
Marie L Vorbeck Chair
Department of Internal Medicine
University of Missouri – Columbia School of Medicine
Columbia, MO
USA

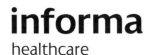

informa
healthcare

© 2006 Informa UK Ltd

First published in the United Kingdom in 2006 by Informa Healthcare Ltd, 4 Park Square,
Milton Park, Abingdon, Oxon OX14 4RN
Informa Healthcare is a trading division of Informa UK Ltd
Registered Office: 37/41 Mortimer Street, London W1T 3JH.
Registered in England and Wales Number 1072954.

Tel: +44 (0)20 7017 6000
Fax: +44 (0)20 7017 6699
Email: info.medicine@tandf.co.uk
Website: www.tandf.co.uk/medicine

Although every effort has been made to ensure that all owners of copyright material have
been acknowledged in this publication, we would be glad to acknowledge in subsequent
reprints or editions any omissions brought to our attention.

Although every effort has been made to ensure that drug doses and other information are
presented accurately in this publication, the ultimate responsibility rests with the
prescribing physician. Neither the publishers nor the authors can be held responsible for
errors or for any consequences arising from the use of information contained herein. For
detailed prescribing information or instructions on the use of any product or procedure
discussed herein, please consult the prescribing information or instructional material issued
by the manufacturer.

A CIP record for this book is available from the British Library.
Library of Congress Cataloging-in-Publication Data

Data available on application

ISBN-10: 1 84214 256 9
ISBN-13: 978 1 84214 256 1

Distributed in North and South America by
Taylor & Francis
6000 Broken Sound Parkway, NW, (Suite 300)
Boca Raton, FL 33487, USA

Within Continental USA
Tel: 1 (800) 272 7737; Fax: 1 (800) 374 3401
Outside Continental USA
Tel: (561) 994 0555; Fax: (561) 361 6018
Email: orders@crcpress.com

Distributed in the rest of the world by
Thomson Publishing Services
Cheriton House
North Way
Andover, Hampshire SP10 5BE, UK
Tel: +44 (0)1264 332424
Email: tps.tandfsalesorder@thomson.com

Composition by Scribe Design Ltd, Ashford, Kent, UK
Printed and bound in Spain by Grafos SA Arte Sobre Papel

To our wives (Lee and Linda) and children (John, Niyati, Jessica, Justin, Benjamin and David) who have made our lives meaningful.

Contents

Contributors

Kul Aggarwal MD MRCP FACC
Associate Professor of Clinical Medicine
Cardiology Division
Department of Internal Medicine
University of Missouri – Columbia
and
Chief, Cardiology Section
Harry S Truman Veterans Hospital
Columbia, MO
USA

John F Best MD
Assistant Professor of Clinical Medicine
Cardiology Division
Department of Internal Medicine
University of Missouri – Columbia
Columbia, MO
USA

Stephen A Brietzke MD
Associate Professor of Clinical Medicine
Division of Endocrinology
Department of Internal Medicine
University of Missouri – Columbia
Columbia, MO
USA

John W Cassels Jr MD
Associate Professor of Clinical Obstetrics and
Gynecology
Division of Reproductive Endocrinology and
Infertility
Department of Obstetrics, Gynecology and
Women's Health
University of Missouri – Columbia
Columbia, MO
USA

Farah Dawood-Farah MD
Fellow in Endocrinology
Department of Internal Medicine
University of Missouri – Columbia
Columbia, MO
USA

Kevin C Dellsperger MD PhD FAHA FACP
FACC
Professor of Internal Medicine
Marie L Vorbeck Chair
Professor and Chairman
Department of Internal Medicine
University of Missouri – Columbia School of
Medicine
Columbia, MO
USA

Mary L Dohrmann MD FACC
Associate Professor of Clinical Medicine
Cardiology Division
Department of Internal Medicine
University of Missouri – Columbia
Columbia, MO
USA

Greg Flaker MD FACC FACP
Brent Parker Professor of Medicine
Cardiology Division
Department of Internal Medicine
University of Missouri – Columbia
Columbia, MO
USA

David W Gardner MD
Director
Cosmopolitan International Diabetes Center
Associate Professor
University of Missouri – Columbia
Columbia, MO
USA

Punit Goel MD DM FACC
Assistant Professor
Cardiology Division
Department of Internal Medicine
University of Missouri – Columbia
and
Staff Cardiologist
Harry S Truman VA Medical Center
Columbia, MO
USA

Laura S Hillman MD
Professor
Departments of Nutritional Science and
Child Health
University of Missouri – Columbia
Columbia, MO
USA

Richard Hillman MD
Professor Emeritus
Department of Child Health
University of Missouri – Columbia
Columbia, MO
USA

Pamela S Hinton PhD
Assistant Professor
Department of Nutritional Sciences
University of Missouri – Columbia
Columbia, MO
USA

Shawn Kaser MD
Cardiology Fellow
Cardiology Division
Department of Internal Medicine
University of Missouri – Columbia
Columbia, MO
USA

James H Kerns MD MBA-HC
Assistant Professor and Clerkship Director
Division of General Obstetrics and
Gynecology
Department of Obstetrics, Gynecology and
Women's Health
University of Missouri – Columbia
Columbia, MO
USA

Uzma Khan MD
Assistant Professor
Department of Internal Medicine
University of Missouri – Columbia
Columbia, MO
USA

Saravanan Kuppuswamy MD
Cardiology Fellow
Cardiology Division
Department of Internal Medicine
University of Missouri – Columbia
Columbia, MO
USA

L Romayne Kurukulasuriya MD FACE
Assistant Professor of Medicine
Department of Internal Medicine
University of Missouri – Columbia
Columbia, MO
USA

Catherine A Peterson PhD
Assistant Professor
Department of Nutritional Sciences
University of Missouri – Columbia
Columbia, MO
USA

Maurine D Raedeke MS RD
Director
Coordinated Program in Dietetics
University of Missouri – Columbia
Columbia, MO
USA

Himal Shah MD
Cardiology Fellow
Cardiology Division
Department of Internal Medicine
University of Missouri – Columbia
Columbia, MO
USA

James R Sowers MD FACE FACP FAHA
Thomas W and Joan F Burns Missouri Chair
in Diabetology,
Director, MU Diabetes and Cardiovascular
Center,
Associate Dean for Clinical Research
and
Professor of Medicine, Physiology and
Pharmacology
Department of Internal Medicine
University of Missouri – Columbia
Columbia, MO
USA

Grace Y Sun PhD
Professor
Department of Biochemistry
University of Missouri – Columbia
Columbia, MO
USA

Lokesh Tejwani MD FACC
Assistant Professor
Cardiology Division
Department of Internal Medicine
University of Missouri – Columbia
and
Staff Cardiologist
Harry S Truman VA Medical Center
Columbia, MO
USA

Tom R Thomas PhD
Professor
Department of Nutritional Sciences
University of Missouri – Columbia
Columbia, MO
USA

Sanjeev Wasson MD
Cardiology Fellow
Division of Cardiology
Department of Internal Medicine
University of Missouri – Columbia
Columbia, MO
USA

Preface

Cardiovascular disease remains the major cause of morbidity and the most common cause of death in women. Owing to a better longevity, women constitute a greater proportion of the elderly population, however, female-specific data on pathophysiology, diagnosis and treatment are limited. This textbook addresses the cardiovascular diseases in women with emphasis on clinical practice, which focuses on common and important clinical issues affecting women mostly in the perimenopausal and postmenopausal period. We hope that the residents, fellows and practising physicians – especially those in the field of internal medicine, family medicine and obstetrics and gynecology – find this textbook a handy and useful reference. We also hope that the textbook serves as an impetus for further exploration into the causes and treatments of cardiovascular diseases in order to advance the health and well-being of women of all ages.

We would like to acknowledge the authors for their valuable contribution of expertise, knowledge and time in making this book a reality. We are indebted to our medical students, residents and fellows whose intellectual curiosity and dedication to medicine have made us better teachers in educating future compassionate and competent physicians. We are grateful to William M Crist MD, Dean of University of Missouri – Columbia School of Medicine, whose visionary leadership has inspired us to be better leaders in serving others.

Hung N Winn
Kevin C Dellsperger

1

Pathophysiology of aging

Mary L Dohrmann and Himal Shah

Introduction • Theories of aging • Cellular effects of aging • Systemic effects of aging • Effects of aging on neural regulation of the heart and arrhythmias • Effect of aging on the aortic valve • Conclusion

INTRODUCTION

The primary goal of the modern practice of medicine is preventing disease. The success of that goal in developed countries is shown in prolongation of life expectancy. The National Center for Health Statistics reports that life expectancy throughout the past century has increased from 48.3 years in 1900 to 77.3 years in 2002; a male born in 2002 will live on average 74.5 years and a female will live 79.9 years.[1] Individuals who are already aged 85 can expect to live on average an additional 6.3 years (males 5.6 years; females 6.7 years).[2] As our society ages, the dilemma of medicine becomes separating the normal aging process from preventable disease processes. The question arises whether the aging process itself can be slowed, independently of preventing those diseases which are known to accrue with age. The leading cause of death over age 65 is cardiovascular disease.[3] Understanding the pathophysiology of anticipated cardiovascular and systemic effects of aging is ultimately important in managing the elderly population. There are also specific differences in the aging process that have been identified for women compared to men that impact treatment and outcomes.

In the next 30 years there will be a boom of the elderly population due to the aging of the baby boomers, with an anticipated 20% of the population greater than age 65 by the year 2030.[4] Seventy-five percent of men and women greater than age 70 have cardiovascular disease.[5] Not only is heart disease the most common chronic disease of the elderly but also 50% of the elderly have at least two comorbid conditions.[5] Because women outlive men, the majority of the aging population will be women. Only recently have data accrued specific to diagnosing and treating women for heart disease.[6] Although the number of women enrolled in studies of treatment of coronary disease has increased over the past 40 years, gender-specific data for women continue to be underrepresented in studies of hypertension, arrhythmias, and heart failure.[7] The comorbidities of heart disease, hypertension, diabetes, and obesity add to the challenges of treatment in the aging female population. The physiologic changes of aging need to be kept in mind when treating the elderly with comorbid conditions.

THEORIES OF AGING

A variety of theories have been proposed for the mechanism of aging at the cellular level. The rate of living theory argues that stressors provoke excess energy expenditure, which in turn affects normal homeostatic mechanisms at the tissue, cellular, and molecular levels.[8] This theory argues that stress speeds aging and is supported by animal studies in which hypothalamus stimulation results in accelerated vascular smooth muscle growth.[9] The stress theory of aging proposed by Selye[10] is closely related to the endocrine theory of aging, which suggests that stress can also provoke hormonal responses that accelerate the aging process.[8] Corticosteroids, thyroxine, and growth hormone all accelerate aging at the cellular level. Spironolactone has been shown to cancel dihydrotachysterol aging effects in a rat model of progeria.[10] Loss of estrogen production at menopause is associated with an increased incidence of atherosclerosis, although estrogen replacement has not been shown to prevent atherosclerotic events.[11] Alterations of the immune system with aging have led some investigators to hypothesize the immune theory of aging; however, age-related changes in the immune system appear to be adaptive.[8]

One of the most relevant theories to senescence is cross-linking. With aging, changes in collagen elasticity in support tissues, especially vascular tissue, are explained by glycation, a random addition of glucose to collagen, which causes increased cross-linking within the collagen. Glycation of other proteins and production of advanced glycation end products also induce changes in cardiovascular tissue. Enhanced cross-linking also forms the basis of the free radical theory of aging. Reactive oxygen species (superoxide anion, hydrogen peroxide, and the hydroxyl radical) are produced by mitochondrial respiration. Superoxide is normally transformed by superoxide dismutase to hydrogen peroxide, which in turn is enzymatically changed to water through the actions of catalase and glutathione peroxidase. One negative consequence of free radicals is the production of lipid peroxides that decompose to yield aldehydes, which can cause cross-linking of amines, phospholipids, or nucleic acids.[8] Lipid peroxidation has been shown to increase with aging in human hearts.[12] The balance between generation of free radicals, antioxidant defenses (e.g. activity of catalase, superoxide dismutase, and glutathione), and repair of oxidative damage (e.g. through the action of lipases on oxidized lipids or through the action of glycosylases that excise oxidized bases in DNA) determines the progression of aging at the tissue level.[13] Cultured cardiac myocytes show increased accumulation of lipofuscin, a marker of oxidative damage, after exposure to increased levels of oxygen.[13]

Theoretically, the deleterious effects of free radicals should be counteracted by administration of antioxidants, such as β-carotene and vitamin E; however, such an effect has not been proven. The physicians' health study failed to show an effect of long-term supplementation with β-carotene on the incidence of either malignant neoplasm or cardiovascular disease.[14] Initial observational studies suggested risk reduction in cardiovascular events with chronic vitamin E supplementation.[15] More recently, the Heart Outcomes Prevention Evaluation (HOPE and HOPE-TOO) studies failed to demonstrate a reduction in cardiovascular events after prolonged use of vitamin E, and there was an increased incidence of heart failure in patients receiving long-term vitamin E at a dose of 400 IU.[16] Therefore, based on currently available information, the use of routine antioxidants in women is not advised.

CELLULAR EFFECTS OF AGING

One of the expected intracellular sites of oxidative damage is mitochondria, because it is the site of cellular respiration and oxidative phosphorylation. Reactive oxygen species are most likely to accumulate there and can damage the mitochondrial membrane, with subsequent exposure of other intracellular structures and molecules. Mitochondrial dysfunction has been demonstrated in various tissues of senescence-accelerated mouse strains, including brain, liver, and heart tissue, and has also been documented in fibroblast-like tissue cultures of these senescence-accelerated mice.[17] Similarly, antioxidative defenses have been shown to decrease with age in the senescence-accelerated mouse model.[18]

Another intracellular effect of aging seen in mitochondria is the down-regulation of genes responsible for fatty acid uptake and metabolism, with a resultant shift toward carbohydrate metabolism.[19] Calorie restriction appears to shift metabolism toward fatty acid utilization in mouse heart,[20] and also limits basal mitochondrial proton leak, thereby lowering mitochondrial energy expenditure.[19] The maximal life span of many animals is known to increase with caloric restriction, presumably by limiting oxidative stress, specifically in tissues such as brain, heart, and skeletal muscle.[21]

Vascular endothelial cell function is also altered with aging and is probably linked to the increased incidence of atherosclerosis with aging. Vascular reactivity, as measured by flow-mediated dilation in the forearms of older subjects, is diminished.[22] The rate of endothelial turnover, repair, and regeneration is linked to bone marrow-derived stem cells and endothelial progenitor cells. Endothelial progenitor cell numbers decrease with age, with no gender differential, and exhibit reduced proliferative activity in the elderly.[22] The hypothetical consequence of reduced endothelial progenitor cells is the inability to repair sites of vascular injury. The inability to repair sites of vascular injury in older patients may have implications for the success of vascular interventions, such as coronary or carotid stents. Following balloon injury, the carotid arteries of aged rats compared with adult rats showed reduced neointima formation and delay in endothelial regeneration.[23] The delay in endothelial regeneration in the aged rat model correlated with decreased endothelial nitric oxide synthase expression and could be prevented by chronic L-arginine administration.[23] It would appear that in the elderly, not only is endothelial regeneration slowed, but also the availability of the potent endothelial-derived vasodilator and platelet inhibitor, nitric oxide, is diminished. Decreased nitric oxide levels also result in increased cell death of endothelial cells in response to apoptotic stimuli such as tumor necrosis factor.[24]

Numerous other cellular alterations occur with aging. Loss of division potential, chromosomal alterations, loss of the capacity to migrate, and decreased responsiveness to growth factors have been observed in both in-vitro and in-vivo models of aging[8] and may have implications for cell renewal following injury. Aging is associated with alteration of induction of ATPase by thyroxine,[8] which suggests that aging affects ability to meet metabolic demands. Additionally, aging is associated with a decreased ability to degrade low-density lipoproteins,[8] a finding that is probably implicated in the increased incidence of atherosclerosis with aging.

Myocytes demonstrate differential changes by gender with aging. In male hearts, the total number of myocytes decrease with age and individual myocyte volume increases; in female hearts, the number and size of myocytes stay constant over the life span.[25,26] Focal myocyte apoptosis and replacement with focal areas of fibrosis occur in the male heart, and capillary density decreases with age.[25] The basis for the gender differential in myocytes has yet to be determined; however, preservation of myocardial mass with aging in the female heart may impact longevity.[26]

Changes in connective tissue and extracellular matrix are also seen with aging. The rate of total collagen synthesis declines with age, although the rate of synthesis of collagen type III and IV increases.[8] The increased production of collagen IV, fibronectin, and laminin with aging results in increased thickness of capillary basement membrane. Proportions of collagen, fibronectin, and integrin in the heart contribute to increasing stiffness of the myocardium with aging. The ratio of collagen to elastin and the ratio of endothelial to smooth muscle cells in blood vessels influences vascular compliance. Degradation of elastin and disproportionate amounts of collagen result in decreased elastic recoil in the aorta with aging.[8] Glucose cross-linking within collagen and production of advanced glycation end products contribute to vascular and myocardial stiffness. Experimental studies using thiazolium compounds in aged dogs and monkeys have been shown to break these cross-links and reduce myocardial and arterial stiffness.[27,28] Vascular stiffness may also result from impairment of blood flood in the vasa vasorum of the vessel wall. Limitation of vasa vasorum flow in dog aorta results in histologic changes similar to the human aged aorta with altered elastin and collagen-to-elastin ratio.[29]

SYSTEMIC EFFECTS OF AGING

Aging affects every organ system. Increases in body fat and decreases in total body water affect volume of distribution of fat-soluble and water-soluble medications, respectively. Presbyopia and decreasing visual acuity with aging may have important ramifications in proper self-administration of prescribed medication. Declining renal function with aging mandates adjustment of drug dosages in the elderly. Senescence also affects memory, which in turn may affect compliance with medical advice. A sedentary lifestyle, often resulting from decreased mobility due to degenerative joint disease, may mask clinical manifestations of coronary disease. The Baltimore Longitudinal Study on Aging demonstrated an increased prevalence of silent myocardial ischemia with aging in asymptomatic healthy volunteers, with 15% of subjects over age 70 having a positive stress test associated with abnormal thallium scintigraphy and which predicted future cardiovascular events.[30]

The cardiovascular system is especially vulnerable to the aging process. The increased prevalence of cardiovascular disease with age in both women and men has been documented in the Framingham Heart Study, and age is the strongest risk predictor for both genders.[31] The Women's Health and Aging Study has demonstrated that markers of systemic inflammation (C-reactive protein and interleukin-6) are predictive of 3-year mortality in women over age 65 years, although the significance of these markers was greatest for women with established cardiovascular disease.[32] Autopsy studies of octogenarians have shown that heart weight and wall thickness increase with age; calcium deposition increases in epicardial coronary arteries, aortic valvular cusps, and the mitral annulus; and fibrosis and collagen deposition increase throughout the myocardium and conduction system of the heart.[33,34] Large elastic arteries, such as the aorta and carotid arteries, show progressive wall thickening with aging. Both the Baltimore Longitudinal Study on Aging and the Cardiovascular Health Study demonstrated that the thickness of the carotid artery intimal media increased with age and was a risk factor for predicting future cardiovascular events, including stroke and myocardial infarction.[35,36] Aortic dimension also increases with aging, but the site of greatest circumference was the ascending aorta in a population with concomitant hypertension and the lower abdominal aorta in a population with a high prevalence of atherosclerosis.[37]

The decreased elasticity and compliance of the aorta and great arteries leads to an increase in systolic arterial pressure with aging and a decrease in diastolic blood pressure. In the Framingham Heart Study, systolic blood pressure rose linearly between the ages 30 and 84 years old; diastolic blood pressure rose through age 50–60, but fell thereafter.[38] Both pulse pressure and aortic pulse wave velocity increase with aging. Both parameters are measures of arterial stiffness, although the latter occurs independently of a rise in systolic blood pressure.[39] An increase in arterial stiffness, measured by any means, predicts both future occurrence of coronary heart disease and hypertension and their complications.[40–44] A widened pulse pressure is associated with progressive thickening of carotid artery intima-media, and, conversely, the observation of an increased carotid artery intimal media is associated with a widened pulse pressure.[45] It would appear that vascular stiffness and hypertension are co-dependent and lead to a perpetual cycle of vascular damage. Interestingly, indices of arterial stiffness were lower in the endurance-trained elderly volunteers compared with sedentary age-matched peers in the Baltimore Longitudinal Study on Aging.[39] A sedentary lifestyle may augment vascular stiffness, whereas physical training has cardiovascular benefits throughout life.

Myocardial stiffness also increases with aging, in part due to inherent changes in the myocardium due to changing collagen and elastin content. Increased resistance to left ventricular emptying, resulting from increased aortic stiffness and hypertension, can lead to left ventricular hypertrophy. However, left ventricular stiffening can occur independently of left ventricular hypertrophy. Echocardiographic studies in aging populations have shown progressive diastolic impairment, with a consistent decline in the ratio of early to late peak diastolic filling velocity by Doppler flow, which is independent of gender.[46,47] Resting left ventricular systolic function, as measured by ejection fraction, is preserved during aging in the absence of underlying cardiovascular disease; however, the degree of increase in left ventricular ejection fraction with exercise declines with aging.[48] Expectedly, diastolic heart failure rather than systolic failure is common in the elderly in the absence of underlying coronary or valvular disease.

EFFECTS OF AGING ON NEURAL REGULATION OF THE HEART AND ARRHYTHMIAS

Basal sympathetic nervous system activity increases with age.[48–50] Elevated levels of circulating catecholamines, due in part to deficient neuronal reuptake, leads to desensitization of the adrenergic receptors and down-regulation of adrenergic responsiveness.[50] During exercise, β-blockade results in greater reduction in exercise heart rate in young compared with older subjects; in response to β-adrenergic agonists, heart rate responsiveness is diminished in the elderly.[48] Modulation of vascular tone in response to stress, including change from supine to upright body position, is therefore deficient in the elderly. Myocardial and vascular stiffness combined with deficient autonomic modulation contribute to the sensitivity of the elderly to change in body position, with resultant risk of fall and injury due to orthostatic hypotension. Of particular note, women have less-effective baroreflex buffering than men, although both genders have declines in effective modulation with age.[50–52] Heart rate variability also decreases with age and is another marker of deficient autonomic modulation.[48]

The prevalence of various rhythm disturbances increases with age. Resting heart rate and maximum predicted heart rate for age decline with aging.[48] Sinus node dysfunction, most commonly manifest as sinus bradycardia, is not unexpected in the elderly due to decreased number of pacemaker cells and increased fibrosis in the sinus node with aging.[53] Another subset of sick sinus syndrome, alternating tachycardia–bradycardia, is also more common in the elderly.[54] Fibrosis and calcification surrounding the atrioventricular annuli contribute to the increased incidence of bundle branch block with aging.[34] The prevalence of premature atrial contractions increases with age in both men and women; short runs of supraventricular tachycardia most commonly occur with peak exercise and more frequently in men than in women.[55] Exercise-induced ventricular ectopy noted in healthy volunteers in the Baltimore Longitudinal Study on Aging was age-related in men but not women and did not imply an increased occurrence of subsequent cardiovascular events.[56] Arrhythmias, whether supraventricular or ventricular in origin, and regardless of complexity, detected by 24-hour ambulatory electrocardiographic monitoring in healthy subjects aged 60–85 years had no long-term prognostic significance.[57] The prevalence of atrial fibrillation increases with age, regardless of gender, with each decade doubling the odds of developing atrial fibrillation.[58,59] The Framingham Heart Study noted that 8.8% of individuals aged 80–89 have atrial fibrillation;[60] however, the incidence of atrial fibrillation in men aged 75–84 may be as high as 42.7 events per 1000 person-years and in age-matched women as high as 21.6 events per 1000 person-years, if self-reporting is included.[59]

EFFECT OF AGING ON THE AORTIC VALVE

Sclerosis of the aortic valve is common with advancing age and was noted in 26% of asymptomatic subjects over age 65 years and in 37% over age 75 years in the Cardiovascular Health Study.[61] Comorbid conditions that influence the likelihood of aortic valvular sclerosis are male gender, cigarette smoking, hypertension, and elevated low-density lipoproteins. Estrogen supplementation does not appear to increase the risk of aortic sclerosis.[61] Progression of aortic sclerosis to some degree of measurable aortic stenosis occurs in approximately 33% of subjects followed for 4 years,[62] although the finding of aortic sclerosis alone is associated with a 50% increased risk of cardiovascular death.[63] An elevated level of low-density lipoprotein (>130 mg/dL) influences the likelihood of progression of aortic sclerosis to aortic stenosis.[64] A recent study to prevent progression of aortic stenosis with treatment with lipid-lowering agents such as hydroxymethylglutaryl-coenzyme A reductase inhibitors, or statins, failed to show any impact on the progression of calcific aortic stenosis.[65]

CONCLUSION

The structural and functional changes expected with normal aging magnify the impact of superimposed comorbidities. Common sense suggests that primary risk factor prevention for cardiovascular disease is as important in the elderly as in younger individuals. Aging is inevitable, but successful aging is possible, and disease prevention in the elderly is plausible.

REFERENCES

1. Centers for Disease Control and Prevention. Estimated life expectancy at birth in years, by race and sex: death-registration States, 1900–28, and United States, 1929–2002. National Vital Statistic Reports 2004; 53(6): 33. accessed 12 April 2005: www.cdc.gov/nchs/data/dvs/nusr53_06t12.pdf

2. National Center for Health Statistics. Life expectancy at birth, 65 and 85 years of age, by sex and race: United States, selected years 1900–2000. Data Warehouse on Trends in Health and Aging. accessed12 April 2005: http://www.cdc.gov/nchs/agingact.htm

3. Centers for Disease Control and Prevention. Deaths and death rates for the 10 leading causes of death in specified age groups: United States, preliminary 2003. National Vital Statistic Reports 2005; 53(15): 28. accessed 12 April 2005: www.cdc.gov/nchs/data/dvs

4. Centers for Disease Control and Prevention. Healthy aging: effects of an aging population. National Center for Chronic Disease Prevention and Health Promotion. March 9, 2005. accessed 13 April 2005: http://www.cdc.gov/nccdphp/bb_aging/index.htm

5. Centers for Disease Control and Prevention. Healthy aging: preventing disease and improving quality of life among older Americans. National Center for Chronic Disease Prevention and Health Promotion. August 17, 2004. accessed 13 April 2005: http://www.cdc.gov/nccdphp/aag/aag_aging.htm

6. Schulman KA, Berlin JA, Harless W, et al. The effect of race and gender on physicians' recommendations for cardiac catheterization. N Engl J Med 1999; 340:618.

7. Harris D, Douglas P. Enrollment of women in cardiovascular clinical trials funded by the National Heart, Lung, and Blood Institute. N Engl J Med 2000; 343:475

8. Macieira-Coehlo A. Biology of Aging. Berlin: Springer-Verlag, 2003.

9. Gutstein WH, Wang CH, Wu JM, et al. Growth retardation in senescent arterial smooth muscle cells and its reversal following brain stimulation: implications for atherogenesis. Mech Ageing Dev 1991; 60:89.

10. Selye H. Stress and aging. J Am Geriatr Soc 1970; 18:669.

11. Rossouw JE, Anderson GL, Prentice RL. Risks and benefits of estrogen plus progestin in healthy postmenopausal women: principal results from the Women's Health Initiative randomized controlled trial. JAMA 2002; 288:321.

12. Miro O, Casademont J, Casals E, et al. Aging is associated with increased peroxidation in human hearts, but not with mitochondrial respiratory chain enzyme defects. Cardiovasc Res 2000; 18:623.

13. Beckman KB, Ames BN. The free radical theory of aging. Physiol Rev 1998; 78:547.

14. Omenn GS, Goodman GE, Thornquest MD, et al. Effects of a combination of beta carotene and vitamin A on lung cancer and cardiovascular disease. N Engl J Med 1996; 334:1150.

15. Gaziano JM. Vitamin E and cardiovascular disease: observational studies. Ann NY Acad Sci 2004; 1031:280.

16. Lonn E, Bosch J, Yusuf S. Effects of long-term vitamin E supplementation on cardiovascular events and cancer: a randomized controlled trial. JAMA 2005; 293:1338.

17. Hosakawa M. Mitochondrial dysfunction and an impaired response to higher oxidative states accelerate aging in SAMP strains of mice. In: Nomura Y, Takeda T, Okuma Y, eds. The Senescence-Accelerated Mouse (SAM): An Animal Model of Senescence. International Congress Series 2004; 1260:47.

18. Malhera F, Nakama Y, Ohmine N, et al. Age-related changes in the oxidation–reduction characteristics and the 8–OHdG accumulation in liver, lung, brain of SAMP1 and SAMR1. In: Nomura Y, Takeda T, Okuma Y, eds. The Senescence-Accelerated Mouse (SAM): An Animal Model of Senescence. International Congress Series 2004; 1260:259.

19. Harper M-E, Bevilacqua L, Hagopian K, et al. Aging, oxidative stress, and mitochondrial uncoupling. Acta Physiol Scand 2004; 182:321.

20. Weindruch R. Calorie restriction, gene expression and aging. In: Nomura Y, Takeda T, Okuma Y, eds. The Senescence-Accelerated Mouse (SAM): An Animal Model of Senescence. International Congress Series 2004; 1260:13.

21. Sohal RS, Weindruch R. Oxidative stress, caloric restriction, and aging. Science 1996; 273:59.

22. Heiss C, Keymel S, Niesler U, et al. Impaired progenitor cell activity in age-related endothelial cell dysfunction. J Am Coll Cardiol 2005; 45:1441.

23. Torella D, Leosco D, Indolfi C, et al. Aging exacerbates negative remodeling and impairs endothelial regeneration after balloon injury. Am J Physiol Heart Circ Physiol 2004; 287:H2850.

24. Hoffmann J, Haendeler J, Aicher A, et al. Aging enhances the sensitivity of endothelial cells toward apoptotic stimuli: important role of nitric oxide. Circ Res 2001; 89:709.

25. Anversa P, Olivetti G. Cellular basis of physiological and pathological myocardial growth. In: Page E, Fozzard HA, Solaro RJ, eds. Handbook of Physiology,

Section 2, The Cardiovascular System, Volume I: The Heart. New York: Oxford University Press; 2002.

26. Olivetti G, Giordano G, Corradi D, et al. Gender differences and aging: effects on the human heart. J Am Coll Cardiol 1995; 26:1068.

27. Asif M, Egan J, Vasan S, et al. An advanced glycation endproduct cross-link breaker can reverse age-related increase in myocardial stiffness. Proc Natl Acad Sci USA 2000; 97:2809.

28. Vaitkevicius PV, Lane M, Spurgeon H, et al. A cross-link breaker has sustained effects on arterial and ventricular properties in older rhesus monkeys. Proc Natl Acad Sci USA 2001; 98:1171.

29. Stefanadis C, Vlachopoulos C, Karayannacos P, et al. Effect of vasa vasorum flow on structure and function of the aorta in experimental animals. Circulation 1995; 91:2669.

30. Fleg JL, Gerstenblith G, Zonderman AB, et al. Prevalence and prognostic significance of exercise-induced silent myocardial ischemia detected by thallium scintigraphy and electrocardiography in asymptomatic volunteers. Circulation 1990; 81:428.

31. Wilson PW, D'Agostino RB, Levy D, et al. Prediction of coronary heart disease using risk factor categories. Circulation 1998; 97:1837.

32. Volpato S, Guralnik JM, Ferrucci L, et al. Cardiovascular disease, interleukin-6, and risk of mortality in older women: the Women's Health and Aging Study. Circulation 2001; 103:947.

33. Roberts WC. Ninety-three hearts ≥90 years of age. Am J Cardiol 1993; 71:599.

34. Shirani J, Yousefi J, Roberts WC. Major cardiac findings at necropsy in 366 American octogenarians. Am J Cardiol 1995; 75:151.

35. Nagai Y, Metter J, Earley CJ, et al. Increased carotid-artery intimal-medial thickness in asymptomatic older subjects with exercise-induced myocardial ischemia. Circulation 1998; 98:1504.

36. O'Leary DH, Polack JF, Kronmal RA, et al. Carotid-artery intima and media thickness as a risk factor for myocardial infarction and stroke in older adults: Cardiovascular Health Study Collaborative Research Group. N Engl J Med 1999; 340:14.

37. Virmani R, Avolio AP, Mergner WJ, et al. Effect of aging on aortic morphology in populations with high and low prevalence of hypertension and atherosclerosis: comparison between occidental and Chinese communities. Am J Pathol 1991; 139:1119.

38. Franklin SS, Gustin W, Wong ND, et al. Hemodynamic patterns of age-related changes in blood pressure: the Framingham Heart Study. Circulation 1997; 96:308.

39. Vaitkevicius PV, Fleg JL, Engel JH, et al. Effects of age and aerobic capacity on arterial stiffness in healthy adults. Circulation 1993; 88:1456.

40. Franklin S, Khan SA, Wong ND, et al. Is pulse pressure useful in predicting risk for coronary heart disease? The Framingham Heart Study. Circulation 1999; 100:354.

41. Liao D, Arnett DK, Tyroler HA, et al. Arterial stiffness and the development of hypertension: the ARIC Study. Hypertension 1999; 34:201.

42. Blacher J, Asmar R, Djane S, et al. Aortic pulse wave velocity as a marker of cardiovascular risk in hypertensive patient. Hypertension 1999; 33:1111.

43. Blacher J, Staessen J, Girerd X, et al. Pulse pressure not mean pressure determines cardiovascular risk in older hypertensive patients. Arch Intern Med 2000; 160:1085.

44. Glynn R, Chae C, Guralnik J, et al. Pulse pressure and mortality in older people. Arch Intern Med 2000; 160:2765.

45. Zureik M, Touboul P-J, Kopp-Bonithon C, et al. Cross-sectional and 4-year longitudinal associations between brachial pulse pressure and common carotid intima-media thickness in a general population: the EVA Study. Stroke 1999; 30:550.

46. Benjamin EJ, Levy D, Anderson KM, et al. Determinants of Doppler indexes of left ventricular diastolic function in normal subjects (the Framingham Heart Study). Am J Cardiol 1992; 70:508.

47. Gardin JM, Arnold AM, Bild DE, et al. Left ventricular diastolic filling in the elderly: The Cardiovascular Health Study. Am J Cardiol 1998; 82:345.

48. Lakatta EG, Levy D. Arterial and cardiac aging: major shareholders in cardiovascular disease enterprises. Part II: the aging heart in health: links to heart disease. Circulation 2003; 107:139.

49. Seals DR, Esler MD. Human ageing and the sympathoadrenal system. J Physiol 2000; 528:407.

50. Supiano MA, Hogikyan RV, Sidani MA, et al. Sympathetic nervous system activity and α-adrenergic responsiveness in older hypertensive humans. Am J Physiol 1999; 276:E519.

51. Jones PP, Christou DD, Jordan J, et al. Baroreflex buffering is reduced with age in healthy men. Circulation 2003; 107:1770.

52. Christou DD, Jones PP, Jordan J, et al. Women have lower tonic autonomic support of arterial blood pressure and less effective baroreflex buffering than men. Circulation 2005; 111:494.

53. Bonke FIM. The Sinus Node. The Hague: Martinus Nijhoff Medical Division; 1978.

54. Rubenstein JJ, Schulman CL, Yurchak PM, et al. Clinical spectrum of the sick sinus syndrome. Circulation 1972; 46:5.

55. Maurer MS, Shefrin EA, Fleg JL. Prevalence and prognostic significance of exercise-induced supraventricular tachycardia in apparently healthy volunteers. Am J Cardiol 1995; 75:788.

56. Busby MJ, Sherrin EA, Fleg JL. Prevalence and long-term significance of exercise-induced frequent or

repetitive ventricular ectopic beats in apparently healthy volunteers. J Am Coll Cardiol 1989; 14:1659.

57. Fleg JL, Kennedy HL. Long-term prognostic significance of ambulatory electrocardiographic findings in apparently healthy subjects ≥60 years of age. Am J Cardiol 1992; 70:748.

58. Tsang TSM, Petty GW, Barnes ME. The prevalence of atrial fibrillation in incident stroke cases and matched population controls in Rochester, Minnesota: changes over three decades. J Am Coll Cardiol 2003; 42:93.

59. Psaty BM, Manolio TA, Kuller LH, et al. Incidence of and risk factors for atrial fibrillation in older adults. Circulation 1997; 96:2455.

60. Wolf PA, Abbott RD, Kannel WB, et al. Atrial fibrillation as an independent risk factor for stroke: the Framingham Study. Stroke 1991; 22:983.

61. Stewart BF, Siscovick D, Lind BK, et al. Clinical factors associated with calcific aortic valve disease. J Am Coll Cardiol 1997; 29:630.

62. Faggiano P, Antonini-Canterin F, Erlicker A, et al. Progression of aortic valve sclerosis to aortic stenosis. Am J Cardiol 2003; 91:99.

63. Otto CM, Lind BK, Kitzman DW, et al. Association of aortic-valve sclerosis with cardiovascular mortality and morbidity in the elderly. N Engl J Med 1999; 341:142.

64. Pohle K, Mäffert R, Ropees D, et al. Progression of aortic valve calcification: association with coronary atherosclerosis and cardiovascular risk factors. Circulation 2001; 104:1927.

65. Cowell SJ, Newby DE, Prescott RJ, et al. A randomized trial of intensive lipid-lowering therapy in calcific aortic stenosis. N Engl J Med 2005; 352:2389.

2

Hypertension

James R Sowers, Uzma Khan, Farah Dawood-Farah and L Romayne Kurukulasuriya

Introduction • Essential hypertension in women • Secondary hypertension • Secondary hypertension due to renal etiology • Secondary hypertension due to adrenal–cortical causes • Other endocrine causes • Obstructive sleep apnea/hypopnea syndrome • Drugs • Coarctation of the aorta • Hypertension complicating pregnancy

INTRODUCTION

Hypertension is an important modifiable risk factor for cardiovascular disease in women. This includes essential hypertension, hypertension due to secondary causes, or hypertension associated with pregnancy. Although younger, premenopausal women have lower blood pressure (BP) than age-matched men, the prevalence of hypertension increases in older women. Depending on the clinical scenario, secondary causes should be excluded. Hypertension during pregnancy not only endangers the mother but also has serious consequences for the baby. Lifestyle modification and aggressive pharmacologic therapy is recommended in all hypertensive women to decrease morbidity and mortality. There are limited data regarding gender-specific factors contributing to pathogenesis of hypertension, as well as the effect these factors might have on treatment and complications. Further research is needed to determine the most beneficial therapeutic options for women.

ESSENTIAL HYPERTENSION IN WOMEN

Essential hypertension is defined as high BP in which secondary causes are not present. It accounts for more than 90% of all cases of hypertension and is a major modifiable cause of cardiovascular morbidity and mortality in both men and women. The Seventh Report of the Joint National Committee on Prevention, Detection, Evaluation, and Treatment of High Blood Pressure (JNC VII) defined and classified hypertension in adults aged 18 years or older. The classification is based on the mean of two or more seated BP measurements on each of two or more office visits. Prehypertension is defined as a systolic BP between 120 and 139 mmHg, or diastolic BP between 80 and 89 mmHg. Hypertension is defined as systolic BP ≥140 mmHg or diastolic BP ≥90 mmHg.[1]

A recent evaluation of hypertension trends estimated that 58.4 million people in the United States have hypertension, which is about 29% of the adult population.[2] Men in the general population have higher diastolic blood pressure than women at all ages and also have a higher prevalence of hypertension. However, menopause and advancing age tends to abolish this difference so that by age 55 years, BP is comparable between men and women, and women older than 75 years have a higher rate of hypertension than men, possibly attributable to longevity. Factors such as race and socioeconomic status also affect the prevalence, morbidity, and mortality rates of hypertension. White coat hypertension is also noted to be more common in women.

Pathophysiology

Essential hypertension is a heterogeneous disorder involving the interaction of one or more susceptibility genes with physiologic and environmental influences on blood pressure. Family studies have demonstrated associations of BP among siblings and between parents and children. This is more prominent in biological children than adopted children and in identical as opposed to non-identical twins. Genes linked with essential hypertension include angiotensin converting enzyme, angiotensinogen, α-adducin, the β_2 adrenergic receptor, angiotensin C, the G-protein β_3 binding subunit renin-binding protein, atrial natriuretic factor, and the insulin receptor. The genetic alteration responsible for essential hypertension is unknown. Up to 30 genes may be involved in hypertension, each gene contributing less than 1 mmHg in the general population.[3]

The reasons for gender differences in BP are not known. It has been suggested, but not proven, that estrogen is responsible for the lower BP in younger women. However, exogenous estrogen, particularly in the form of oral contraceptives pills, is an important cause of secondary hypertension in women, although postmenopausal hormone replacement therapy has not been associated with hypertension. Estradiol is also an antioxidant and protects against oxidative stress, which is thought to be a causative factor in endothelial dysfunction associated with hypertension. Women with essential hypertension have been reported to have a lower level of plasma hydrogen peroxide than men. Premenopausal women have also been shown to have lower levels of oxidative stress than men or postmenopausal women, which suggests a role for estrogen in lowering the levels of oxidative stress.

There is an increase in the prevalence of hypertension and cardiovascular disease in postmenopausal women, but the influence of menopause on BP is controversial. The increase in BP in postmenopausal women occurs over a number of years and has been attributed to several factors, including increases in weight, decreases in activity, and increases in alcohol intake. Studies of endothelial function using acetylcholine-induced changes in forearm blood flow demonstrate diminished endothelium-dependent vasodilatation in association with menopause, suggesting a role for endogenous estrogen in BP regulation. Clinical studies have shown that men and postmenopausal women demonstrate larger stress-induced increases in BP and higher ambulatory daytime BP than premenopausal women. A study from Finland demonstrated that women who had undergone hysterectomy with ovarian preservation had higher BP than age-matched women who had not undergone hysterectomy.[4,5] Indicating the importance of other factors contributing to postmenopausal increases in BP, plasma renin activity has been reported to be increased in some postmenopausal women. A change in the estrogen/androgen ratio, creating a relative hyperandrogenic state, may also play a role in postmenopausal hypertension, possibly by affecting the renin–angiotensin–aldosterone system (RAAS), endothelin, or oxidative stress. In support of this hypothesis, premenopausal women with polycystic ovary syndrome or virilizing tumors have elevated serum androgens and increases in BP.[6]

A significant amount of hypertension in women is attributable to obesity, although the mechanisms involved are not fully understood. Obesity is significantly more common in middle-aged women than men, and has a greater impact on BP in women than men. Obesity is accompanied by an increase in sympathetic activity, particularly in the kidney, leading to increased renin release that could contribute to hypertension. The increase in BP may also be mediated by increasing insulin resistance and hyperinsulinemia.[7]

Treatment of hypertension

The initial goal of antihypertensive therapy is to lower the diastolic blood pressure to <90 mmHg and the systolic BP to <140 mmHg, with minimal adverse effects. More aggressive BP goals are recommended for patients with diabetes mellitus and renal insufficiency.

JNC VII showed that women had a greater increase in hypertension prevalence than men from 1988 to 2000. It also showed that prevalence of hypertension was greatest in women aged 60 years or older than in any other age or sex group. Non-Hispanic black women had the greatest increase in prevalence of hypertension. Women also had lower rates of control than men, emphasizing the importance of adequate control and follow-up in this group.

Lifestyle modifications

Lifestyle modifications are generally beneficial in improving hypertension and should be used in all hypertensive patients.

Weight reduction is closely correlated with reduction in BP and appears to be the most effective of all lifestyle modifications. It also enhances the efficacy of antihypertensive drugs independent of dietary sodium restriction. Weight reduction of as little as 10 lbs (4.5 kg) reduces BP in a large proportion of overweight hypertensive patients, and is of particular importance in obese women. The Treatment of Mild Hypertension Study demonstrated that women are less likely than men to have their BP controlled with lifestyle modification alone, perhaps because they are less successful in losing weight.[8] The effects of weight reduction have not been studied extensively in women, but small clinical trials have demonstrated benefit.

Prospective trials of the effect of exercise in women are also lacking. It is recommended to increase activity for hypertensive women in the absence of unstable coronary artery disease in view of the beneficial effects of exercise on weight control, and on insulin and glucose metabolism. Studies suggest that moderate activity – such as 30 minutes of brisk walking, swimming, or bicycling 3 times per week – may lower systolic BP by 4–8 mmHg, and is more effective than strenuous exercises such as running or jogging.

Dietary recommendations for hypertensive women are similar to those for hypertensive men. Sodium restriction should be encouraged, and all patients should be encouraged to eat a diet with abundant fruits, vegetables, and low-fat dairy products to ensure adequate intake of calcium, potassium, and magnesium. Recent reports have also suggested that a higher folic acid intake may reduce the risk of high BP.[9]

More than two to three drinks of alcohol are associated with increases in BP. The effect increases with age, and is additive, but independent of the effects of obesity, oral contraceptives, and high salt intake. All hypertensive women should be advised to limit their alcohol intake. Cessation of smoking should be encouraged.

Drug therapy

The indications for drug treatment of hypertension in women are the same as in men. According to JNC VII, the goal of antihypertensive therapy is the reduction of cardiovascular and renal morbidity and mortality. The target should be a BP <140/90 mmHg in all hypertensive patients, and <130/80 mmHg in patients with diabetes or renal disease. Clinical trials have shown that several classes of drugs, including thiazide diuretics, angiotensin-converting enzyme (ACE) inhibitors, angiotensin receptor blockers (ARB), calcium channel blockers, and β-blockers will all reduce the complications of hypertension.[10]

The effects of antihypertensive therapy on the cardiovascular complications of hypertension have not been studied separately in women, but several antihypertensive drug trials have found a similar benefit in hypertensive men and women. The Women's Health Initiative showed that hypertensive women had more comorbid conditions than non-hypertensive women, and women with comorbidities were more likely to be treated pharmacologically. It also found older women, who are most at risk for cardiovascular events and strokes, were not being aggressively treated, with only 36.1% of these hypertensive women controlled. Diuretics were used by 44.3% of hypertensives as monotherapy or in combination with other drug classes, and were associated with better BP control than any of the other drug classes. As monotherapy, calcium channel blockers were used in 16%, ACE inhibitors in 14%, β-blockers in 9%, and diuretics in 14% of the hypertensive women. African-American and elderly women benefit the most from treatment, with significant reduction in cerebrovascular and cardiovascular events, and should be treated aggressively.

Although the response to antihypertensive drugs is similar in men and women, the gender-specific side-effect profile may be different. In the Treatment of Mild Hypertension Study, women who were treated with antihypertensives reported twice as many side effects as men, although the incidence of side effects in women was similar in placebo and drug-treated individuals. Biochemical responses to drugs may be gender-dependent; women are more likely to develop hyponatremia and hypokalemia associated with diuretic therapy. ACE inhibitor-induced coughing has been reported to be twice as common in women as in men.

SECONDARY HYPERTENSION

Secondary hypertension is, by definition, an elevated blood pressure ≥140/90 mmHg that is secondary to a defined etiology. Once thought to be responsible for 5% of hypertension in women, careful review of recent data suggests that the prevalence might be higher. It is important to recognize secondary causes of hypertension, especially fibromuscular dysplasia and primary hyperaldosteronism, as well as endocrine disorders that are more common in women. Early identification and treatment may ameliorate, and possibly cure the underlying cause.

Classification of secondary hypertension:

- renal
- adrenal–cortical
- adrenal–sympathetic
- other endocrine etiologies
- sleep apnea
- drugs
- coarctation of the aorta.

SECONDARY HYPERTENSION DUE TO RENAL ETIOLOGY

Renal artery stenosis

Renal vascular hypertension is defined as elevated BP associated with either unilateral or bilateral stenosis. The currently accepted limit for clinically significant renal artery stenosis (RAS) is >75% narrowing. It is a common condition, with prevalence that varies greatly from 1% in patients with mild hypertension to around 40–60% in patients ≥70 years old with refractory hypertension.[11]

Pathophysiology

The initial event in RAS is the reduction in perfusion pressure to the affected kidney, which stimulates the release of renin and activates the RAAS. High aldosterone levels cause sodium retention. The potent vasoconstrictive effect of angiotensin II and sodium retention cause hypertension. Recent studies suggest that the hypoperfusion causes oxidative stress and an increase in reactive oxygen species, which are a major player in endothelial dysfunction. This cascade of events leads to further elevation in blood pressure.[11–13]

There are three general types of renal artery stenosis.

1. Atherosclerotic renovascular disease accounts for 65–90% of cases of RAS, usually affecting men older than 50 years.
2. Fibromascular dysplasia accounts for 10–30% of cases, usually affecting women in their third and fourth decades of life.
3. Transplant renal artery stenosis, which is an atherosclerotic process that accounts for RAS in 1–23% of transplant recipients.[11]

Diagnosis

Diagnosis is suggested by the onset of hypertension before the age of 30 years, difficult-to-control hypertension, accelerated hypertension that was previously well controlled, unexplained azotemia or worsening of azotemia and hyperkalemia after starting an ACE inhibitor or an ARB, recurrent episodes of pulmonary edema, or the presence of abdominal bruits.[14]

RAS can be diagnosed by invasive and non-invasive imaging studies. The following four methods are the most commonly used to diagnose renal artery stenosis non-invasively.

- Captopril renography has a sensitivity of 85–90% and a specificity of 93–98% in detecting high-grade stenosis.
- Renal duplex ultrasonography, which is an inexpensive test. The sensitivity and specificity both approach 98%. However, this test is highly operator-dependent.

- Gadolinium-enhanced magnetic resonance imaging (MRI) has a sensitivity of 97% and a specificity of 93%.
- Spiral computed tomography (CT) angiography has a 98% sensitivity and a 94% specificity.

Invasive evaluation is limited to radiocontrast angiography. This procedure, considered the gold standard, carries the risk of contrast nephropathy in patients already manifesting azotemia.

Treatment

The treatment method depends greatly on the type of stenosis. In fibromuscular dysplasia, the treatment of choice is angioplasty, which has a high cure rate; however, restenosis occurs in 25% of cases after 1 year. On the other hand, medical treatment is preferred in atherosclerotic renal disease, with aggressive control of hypertension, lipids, hyperglycemia, and the use of antiplatelet agents.[13] Revascularization is another option; however, the likelihood of improving BP or renal function is reduced in older patients, severe atherosclerotic disease, proteinuria >1 g/day, glomerular filtration rate (GFR) <40 ml/min, more than 10 years' duration, and diabetes mellitus.[14]

Renal parenchymal hypertension

Renal parenchymal disease is a common but often unrecognized cause of hypertension. It accounts for 2.5–5% of all cases of secondary hypertension according to some authors. Chronic renal disease and systemic hypertension may coexist in two distinct settings: first, essential hypertension is an important cause of chronic renal disease; secondly, renal parenchymal disease is a well-established cause of secondary hypertension.[15]

Pathophysiology

The precise mechanism is still not fully understood. However, potential factors include sodium retention, leading to volume expansion; a digitalis-like factor that increases peripheral vascular resistance; activation of the RAAS; impaired production of the vasodilatory prostaglandins; possibly an increase in the potent vasoconstrictor endothelin; and a decrease in the vasodilator nitrous oxide.

Parenchymal kidney disease that causes hypertension can be classified as glomerular and interstitial diseases. Glomerular diseases include postinfectious glomerulonephritis, focal segmental sclerosis, renal vasculitis, diabetic nephropathy, crescentic glomerulonephritis, and systemic lupus erythematosus nephritis. Interstitial diseases include polycystic kidney disease and chronic interstitial nephritis.[15]

Diagnosis

The diagnosis of parenchymal kidney disease can be made based on the history and physical examination, family history, appropriate blood and urine testing, imaging studies, and if necessary kidney biopsy.

Treatment

The management of patients with chronic renal insufficiency prior to initiating renal replacement therapy is complex, and requires an aggressive control of BP to delay the progression of renal impairment. The target BP for this subset of patients is ≤125/75 mmHg. Sodium restriction to <2 g/day is important, along with avoidance of potassium-containing salt substitutes. Avoidance of non-steroidal anti-inflammatory drugs (NSAIDs) is another important issue. Diuretic therapy, especially loop diuretics, is a good first step to control the blood pressure. ACE inhibitors and ARBs are particularly useful in these patients, and have been proved effective in delaying the progression to end-stage renal disease. Calcium channel blockers are possibly other renoprotective agents, and can be added to ACE inhibitor therapy to achieve BP control.[15]

SECONDARY HYPERTENSION DUE TO ADRENAL–CORTICAL CAUSES

Primary hyperaldosteronism

Primary hyperaldosteronism is the most common form of secondary hypertension, with a prevalence estimated around 6–10% of patients with hypertension. The most common cause for primary hyperaldosteronism is aldosterone-producing adenoma (APA) 65%; other common causes are idiopathic bilateral adrenal hyperplasia (IHA) 30–40%, and glucocorticoid-remediable aldosteronism (GRA) 1–3%.[16]

Pathophysiology

Increased levels of aldosterone with suppressed plasma renin activity are the hallmark of these conditions, causing sodium and water retention and, subsequently, hypertension. Hypokalemia may or may not be present.

Diagnosis

Primary hyperaldosteronism should be considered in hypertensive patients with spontaneous hypokalemia, or hypokalemia associated with diuretics, refractory hypertension, family history of juvenile hypertension or cerebrovascular accident (CVA), or adrenal incidentaloma. The prevalence is similar in males and females. An aldosterone/renin ratio higher than 20, with plasma aldosterone greater than 15 ng/dl, suggests the diagnosis; however, many medications affect this test. The postural test is used to differentiate APA from IHA.

Measurement of 24-hour urinary level of 18-hydroxycortisol might help diagnosing GRA; another consideration is a 2-day dexamethasone suppression test (DST). A CT scan is used to localize APA; however, since the majority of APAs are less than 1 cm, and it is difficult to differentiate between APA and IHA on CT scans, adrenal vein sampling has became a standard.[16,17]

Treatment

Different types of primary hyperaldosteronism are treated differently. Surgery is the treatment of choice for APA, with a hypertension cure rate of 30–60%. IHA is treated medically with spironolactone and sodium restriction. Eplerenone is a good alternative, and has less antiandrogenic side effects. GRA is treated with oral glucocorticoids; however, to achieve BP control, clinicians might need to add spironolactone.[16]

Congenital adrenal hyperplasia

Congenital adrenal hyperplasia (CAH) is a group of inherited disorders caused by deficient adrenal corticosteroid biosynthesis. The most common form is 21-hydroxylase deficiency. Deficiencies in both 11β-hydroxylase and 17α-hydroxylase are associated with hypertension.[17,18]

11β-hydroxylase deficiency

This is an autosomal recessive condition with an incidence of 5–8% of all CAH. There is decreased conversion of 11-deoxycorticosterone (11-DOC) to corticosterone and 11-deoxycortisol to cortisol, which decreases the negative feedback on adrenocorticotropic hormone (ACTH). Both renin and aldosterone levels are suppressed by 11-DOC, a potent mineralocorticoid causing hypertension and hypokalemia. Virizilation occurs in females as a result of shunting into the androgen pathway. Treatment with glucocorticoid replacement therapy will achieve a reduction in 11-DOC and androgens.[17,18]

17α-hydroxylase deficiency

This is a rare condition with a prevalence of 1% of all CAH. This deficiency causes shunting into the unblocked mineralocorticoid pathway, causing hypertension and hypokalemia. Hypogonadism occurs due to a defect in the biosynthesis of both estrogen and testosterone, causing females to have primary amenorrhea and lack of development of secondary sexual characteristics. Males may have ambiguous genitalia or a female phenotype. Diagnosis is suggested by the presence of low renin, low 17β-hydroxyprogesterone, low androgens, and high 11-DOC levels. Treatment is with glucocorticoid and androgen replacement.[17,18]

Apparent mineralocorticoid excess

This syndrome is the result of impaired activity of the enzyme 11β-hydroxysteroid dehydrogenase

(11β-HSD), which normally converts cortisol to its inactive metabolite cortisone. A 10-fold increase in the ratio of cortisol to cortisone allows cortisol to bind to the mineralocorticoid receptors in the kidneys. This leads to sodium retention, hypertension, hypokalemia, and hypercalciuria. This condition is either inherited as an autosomal recessive disorder, or can be secondary to the inhibitory effects of glycyrrhetinic acid ingestion, commonly found in licorice. Demonstrating an increased ratio of urinary tetrahydrocortisol to tetrahydrocortisone can suggest the diagnosis, which can be confirmed by genetic testing.

Treatment options include high-dose steroids, spironolactone, amiloride, and hydrochlorthiazide. One report demonstrated cure after renal transplant.[17,18]

Cushing's syndrome

Endogenous Cushing's syndrome (CS) is characterized by chronic exposure to excess glucocorticoids produced by the adrenal cortex. The syndrome is ACTH-dependent (ACTH-producing pituitary adenoma, or ectopic) in 80% of cases, or ACTH-independent (adrenal adenoma, adrenal hyperplasia, or iatrogenic) in 20%. CS, in general, is four times more common in women.[19, 20]

Pathophysiology

Although cortisol and aldosterone have an equal binding affinity to mineralocorticoid receptors in the kidneys, cortisol excess overwhelms 11β-HSD and binds to the mineralocorticoid receptor. Enhanced binding and response of angiotensin II, and inhibition of nitrous oxide, are some of the other mechanisms for hypertension.[19,20]

Diagnosis

Central obesity, supraclavicular fat pad, cervical fat pad, thinned skin, purple striae, proximal muscle weakness, fatigue, acne, hirsutism, depression, and menstrual irregularities are the most common symptoms. Hypertension is seen in 80% of patients with CS, and it may be severe and lacks the physiologic nocturnal decline. A 24-hour urinary free cortisol, overnight DST, and midnight salivary cortisol are good screening tests. Low-dose DST, combined with corticotropin-releasing hormone (CRH) test, is useful to exclude pseudo Cushing state. Other tests, such as ACTH measurements, high-dose DST, pituitary MRI, and bilateral inferior petrosal sinus sampling, are useful in differentiating and localizing the source of ACTH.[20]

Treatment

Because of the high mortality associated with CS, it is crucial to recognize, diagnose, and treat it. Correcting hypercortisolism is the mainstay of treatment. Hypertension control with antihypertensive medications, before and after remission, is another important cornerstone of treatment.[19,20]

Pheochromocytoma

Pheochromocytomas are tumors of neuroectodermal origin arising from chromaffin cells of the adrenal medulla. Neuroectodermal tumors that arise in the paraganglia are termed paragangliomas. The incidence of pheochromocytomas is less than 1% of hypertensive patients, and the prevalence is equal in both genders. Approximately 10% are bilateral, extra-adrenal, familial, multiple, or malignant. In younger patients, familial causes are more likely, including MEN-2, von Hippel–Lindau, or neurofibromatosis.[21]

Pathophysiology

Many factors play a role in the pathophysiology. Sympathetic nervous system activity is enhanced and causes an increase in heart rate, vascular resistance, and subsequently BP. This mechanism is independent of the circulating catecholamines level; instead, it is caused by the increase in postganglionic norepinephrines and their effect on its receptor sites. Neuropeptide Y, which is a potent vasoconstrictor, potentiates the vasocontrictive effects of norepinephrine. Thus, hypertension in pheochromocytoma is a hyperkinetic, vasoconstrictive, hypovolemic form of hypertension.[21]

Diagnosis

Hypertension is the most common presentation in over 90% of patients. More than 90% of patients with pheochromocytoma present with two of the three symptoms in the classic triad of severe headaches, palpitations, and diaphoresis. Other symptoms include tremor, angina and MI, nausea, livedo reticularis, and mass effect from the tumor.

Patients with the following features should be screened for pheochromocytoma:

• symptoms of pheochromocytoma
• paradoxical responses to antihypertensives, especially β-blockers
• refractory hypertension
• family history of familial pheochromocytoma or a familial disorder associated with pheochromocytoma
• hypertensive paroxysms with exercise, intubation, or surgery
• adrenal incidentaloma
• idiopathic dilated cardiomyopathy.

Serum-free metanephrines have a sensitivity and specificity of >95%. The finding of plasma levels of normetanephrines <112 ng/l and metanephrines <61 ng/l virtually excludes pheochromocytoma. On the other hand, a normetanephrines level >400 ng/l or metanephrines >236 ng/l should prompt an immediate task of locating the tumor. Intermediate results should be investigated further by carrying out a clonidine suppression test or a glucagon stimulation test. Urine total metanephrines may be more useful in sporadic pheochromocytoma. Many medications interfere with the above tests, including acetaminophen, labetalol, tricyclic antidepressants, clonidine, and compazine. Imaging techniques to localize the tumor include CT scan, MRI, or an MIBG scan. An MRI is the preferred method of localizing paragangliomas.[21,22]

Treatment

Surgical excision is the treatment of choice, but unfortunately it carries a morbidity of 40% and a mortality of 2–4%. The treatment of pheochromocytoma in the preoperative period includes α-blockade and volume expansion. Traditionally, the long-acting α-blocker phenoxybenzamine has been used, but short-acting α-blockers such as prazosin, which does not cause reflex tachycardia, and calcium channel blockers such as nifedipine can also be used to control hypertension.

Mutations of *RET*, *VHL*, *SDHD*, and *SDHB* genes are present in 25% of sporadic pheochromocytomas; therefore, it is crucial to screen such patients to identify pheochromocytoma-associated syndromes that would otherwise be missed.[22]

OTHER ENDOCRINE CAUSES

Primary hyperparathyroidism

Although primary hyperparathyroidism has been associated with hypertension, the relationship is not fully understood. Studies have revealed conflicting data regarding the correction of hypertension following parathyroidectomy. The incidence of this disease is two to three times more common in women. Nifedipine reduced blood pressure in hypertensive patients with hyperparathyroidism. Hypertension may or may not remit after successful parathyroidectomy.[18,19]

Hypothyroidism

Hypothyroidism is associated with mainly diastolic hypertension. The hypertension may be due to increased vascular resistance and extracellular volume expansion. ACE inhibitors and spironolactone are effective in treating the hypertension. Correction of the hypothyroid state decreases the BP, and improves coronary insufficiency as well as heart rate variability.[18,19]

Hyperthyroidism

Hyperthyroidism causes an elevation in the systolic BP due to increased cardiac output. This increase may be due to an increased number of β-receptors in the heart, making it more sensitive to catecholamines. The disease is 10 times more common in women than it is in men.

Correction of the hyperthyroidism state leads to partial or complete resolution of hypertension. β-blockers have been used successfully to control the symptoms of hyperthyroidism, including hypertension.[18,19]

Acromegaly

Acromegaly is associated with a higher incidence of hypertension and an increase in morbidity and mortality. In these patients, hypertension is the largest independent risk factor for left ventricular hypertrophy. Hypertension tends to occur more in older women with acromegaly, who may be overweight also. Many mechanisms have been suggested to cause hypertension in acromegaly. Insulin resistance and hyperinsulinemia may induce hypertension by stimulating the sympathetic nervous system. Activation of the RAAS and suppression of atrial natriuretic peptide due to growth hormone and insulin-like growth factor-1 (IGF-1) may contribute to hypertension also. Hypertension is best treated with ACE inhibitors and spironolactone.[18,19]

OBSTRUCTIVE SLEEP APNEA/HYPOPNEA SYNDROME

Obstructive sleep apnea/hypopnea syndrome (OSAHS) is, by definition, excessive daytime sleepiness secondary to frequent episodes of apnea/hypopnea during sleep. Patients with this syndrome have higher BPs than age- and sex-matched controls. This condition is less common in premenopausal women than it is in men; however, after menopause, the prevalence is similar. About 40% of patients with resistant hypertension have detectable OSAHS.[23]

Pathophysiology

The most difficult task in understanding the link between OSAHS and hypertension is the presence of obesity in most adult patients with OSAHS, which may be an independent risk factor. The tendency is, however, to have the fat distribution mainly in the upper body, thus producing much of its effects on sleep apnea through the deposition of fat in the neck, narrowing the pharyngeal airway. In women,

neck circumference >16.5 inches (42 cm) is the strongest predictor of OSAHS.[23]

Diagnosis

If clinical suspicion is high, the diagnosis of sleep apnea is relatively easy to make by carrying out a sleep study.

Treatment

Nasal continuous positive airway pressure (CPAP) is the most effective treatment available for OSAHS. Many trials have demonstrated improvement in BP and symptoms. The degree of improvement correlates with the severity of the sleep apnea.[23]

DRUGS

Treatment with certain pharmacologic agents or chemicals can elevate BP. The mechanisms by which these drugs increase BP differ from one agent to the next. Stopping these agents, if possible, is a cornerstone in the management of hypertension.

Commonly prescribed medications such as NSAIDs and COX-2 (cyclooxygenase-2) inhibitors have been recognized to increase blood pressure by altering prostaglandin metabolism. Cyclosporine causes renal vasospasm and secondary volume expansion. Exogenous glucocorticoids in supraphysiologic doses elevate BP, but to a lesser degree than endogenous CS. Growth hormone replacement therapy in therapeutic doses can raise BP. Oral contraceptives are an important cause of hypertension in young women.[18]

Recreational drugs such as amphetamines and cocaine cause secondary hypertension by potentiating endogenous sympathetic nervous system activity. They increase cardiac output and vascular resistance. Alcohol and smoking are other causes for secondary hypertension.[18]

COARCTATION OF THE AORTA

Coarctation of the aorta accounts for about 6–8% of all congenital heart defects. It is three times less common in women; however, its prevalence is around 10% in women with Turner's syndrome.[24,25]

Pathophysiology

Coarctation of the aorta may be due to the underdevelopment of the aorta or due to the extension of the ductal tissues causing the constriction. The mechanical obstruction and activation of the RAAS result in hypertension.

Diagnosis

The difference in systolic BP between upper and lower extremities is the major clinical manifestation. If hypertension is severe, patients may present with headache, epistaxis, heart failure, intracranial hemorrhage, aortic dissection, and sometimes claudication. Diagnosis of the coarctation can be achieved accurately by non-invasive methods such as MRI and trans-esophageal echocardiography.

Treatment

Repairing the coarctation of the aorta as soon as it is diagnosed is the mainstay of treatment. Surgical repair and balloon angioplasty are the two available methods, with a tendency to favor the latter. Although BP decreases after successful repair of the coarctation, it is common to have persistent, recurrent hypertension, or disproportionate systolic hypertension with exercise.[26] Pregnant women who present with unrepaired coarctation are treated medically if their hypertension is adequately controlled; otherwise, balloon angioplasty is the treatment of choice.

HYPERTENSION COMPLICATING PREGNANCY

Hypertension (HTN) complicates 8–10% of all pregnancies and contributes significantly to maternal, fetal, and neonatal morbidity and mortality. HTN is directly responsible for 17.6% of maternal deaths in the United States. Maternal complications include cerebral hemorrhage, seizures, disseminated intravascular coagulation (DIC), and multiorgan failure. Fetal complications include prematurity, intrauterine growth retardation (IUGR), low birth weight,

and fetal death. Part of the increased neonatal mortality and morbidity is attributable to preterm delivery undertaken to prevent further deterioration of the fetus and the mother, since delivery is the definitive treatment of gestational hypertension and preeclampsia. These low birth weight infants have not only acute problems but also, more alarmingly, a long-term burden in the form of future cardiovascular risk.

Hypertension complicating pregnancy[27] is classified as chronic hypertension, gestational hypertension, preeclampsia superimposed on chronic hypertension, and preeclampsia–eclampsia.

Chronic hypertension

Chronic HTN is defined as hypertension that is present before the 20th week of gestation or persists beyond 6 weeks after delivery. Chronic hypertension can be primary or secondary.

Gestational hypertension

Gestational hypertension is defined as hypertension without proteinuria that is diagnosed for the first time between the 20th week of pregnancy and 6 weeks postpartum.

Preeclampsia superimposed on chronic hypertension

These are patients who are known to have HTN before pregnancy but develop features of preeclampsia, including proteinuria during pregnancy. Patients who have chronic HTN and proteinuria before pregnancy may have worsening proteinuria or other features of preeclampsia during pregnancy. Chronic hypertension increases the risk of superimposed preeclampsia by 25%. This group has a worse outcome for mother and fetus than de-novo preeclampsia.

Preeclampsia

Preeclampsia is characterized by hypertension that occurs after the 20th week of pregnancy and new-onset proteinuria of more than 300 mg/24 hours, >30 mg/dl, or >1+ reading on a dipstick without concomitant urinary tract infection or existing renal disease. Severe preeclampsia occurs when one of the following conditions exists: (i) systolic blood pressure ≥160 mmHg; (ii) diastolic BP ≥110 mmHg; (iii) proteinuria ≥3 g/24 hours; (iv) fetal growth restriction; or (v) maternal systemic involvement such as headache, blurred vision, abdominal pain, thrombocytopenia and elevated liver enzymes. Eclampsia is the occurrence of seizures, usually tonic clonic generalized seizure, in a woman with preeclampsia that cannot be attributed to other causes. The time between the first detection of HTN and proteinuria and the subsequent development of complications can be as short as 1–2 days.[27]

The HELLP (hemolysis, elevated liver enzymes, and low platelets) syndrome is a recognized complication of severe preeclampsia. Patients may present with right upper quadrant (RUQ) or epigastric pain, nausea, vomiting, mucosal bleeding, petechial hemorrhages, or ecchymoses. It may be associated with increased risks of maternal death (1%), pulmonary edema (8%), acute renal failure (3%), DIC (15%), abruptio placentae (9%), liver hemorrhage or failure (1%), adult respiratory distress syndrome (ARDS), sepsis, and stroke (<1%).[28]

Preeclampsia probably has immunologic components. It is more common in first pregnancies or subsequent pregnancies with new partners, extreme maternal age, daughters of preeclamptic women and pregnancies fathered by sons of preeclamptic women. Both maternal and fetal genes appear to play a role in the syndrome.[29]

Pathophysiology

Preeclampsia is a syndrome with both maternal and fetal manifestations. The maternal disease is characterized by vasospasm, activation of the coagulation system, and disturbances in volume and BP control. Oxidative stress and inflammatory response may also be important in the pathophysiology of preeclampsia. The pathologic changes of this disease are ischemic in nature and affect the placenta, kidney, liver, and brain. It appears that reduced placental perfusion due to abnormalities in vascular remodeling of spiral arteries, as well as atherosis causing occlusion of decidual vessels, may lead to preeclampsia. In multiple gestations, a relative reduction in placental perfusion due to large placentae may contribute to the increased risk of preeclampsia.[29]

In preeclampsia, vasoconstriction, microthrombi, and reduced plasma volume secondary to loss of fluid, as well as accelerated loss of proteins from the intravascular compartment, leads to decreased blood flow to essential organs. Hemorrhage and necrosis can occur in the liver. In the heart, subendocardial necrosis can occur similar to that seen in hypovolemic shock. Renal biopsy in preeclamptic women shows glomeruloendotheliosis, a lesion consisting of enlargement of the glomerulus caused by hypertrophy of the endothelial cells. This is a unique lesion not seen in any other form of hypertension. The vasoconstriction is not attributable to increased endogenous pressors, but rather to an increased sensitivity to them. Activation of the coagulation cascade and platelet activation leads to increased platelet turnover, and DIC, although consumption of procoagulants sufficient to be detected by standard testing occurs in only 10% of preeclamptic women.[29]

Loss of anti-inflammatory regulation by peroxisome proliferator-activated receptors (PPARs) may be an initiating factor in the maternal syndrome of preeclampsia. PPAR activity is decreased significantly in women months before the onset of preeclampsia. Inflammatory cytokines tumor necrosis factor-α (TNF-α) and interleukin-1 (IL-1) levels are elevated in preeclampsia. Reduced levels of PPAR activators would result in increased levels of inflammatory cytokines that in turn results in decreased PPAR activation seen in preeclampsia pregnancy compared with normal pregnancy. The loss of PPAR activation in preeclampsia may account for the widespread increase in inflammatory cytokines and endothelial cell activation seen in preeclampsia. Maternal PPAR activity may be a good early diagnostic marker of preeclampsia and may also be a potential therapeutic target.[30]

High serum levels of soluble fms-like tyrosine kinase 1 (sFlt1), an angiogenic protein, and low levels of placental growth factor (PlGF), a proangiogenic factor, may predict development of preeclampsia. PlGF is readily filtered into urine, whereas sFlt1 is too large to be filtered. Decreased urinary PlGF at mid gestation is strongly associated with subsequent development of preeclampsia.[31]

Many features of insulin resistance have been associated with new-onset hypertension of pregnancy. These include hypertension, hyperinsulinemia, glucose intolerance, obesity, dyslipidemia, elevated leptin, TNF-α, tissue plasminogen activator inhibitor-1 (PAI-1), and testosterone. The presence of these features may be associated with a higher risk for cardiovascular disease later in life. Interventions to reduce insulin resistance may reduce the risk of hypertension during pregnancy, as well as later cardiovascular complications.[32]

Treatment

There is no consensus that antihypertensive drugs improve maternal or fetal outcome in mild to moderate hypertension. However, severe hypertension, with BP >170/110 mmHg, should be treated because it increases maternal risk of liver and kidney failure, cerebrovascular hemorrhage, and seizures. Fetal compromise or demise may occur due to vasoconstriction causing reduction in the blood supply across the placenta and placental abruption. Even though complete or partial bed rest is commonly recommended for women with gestational HTN and preeclampsia, there is no evidence to show that it improves pregnancy outcome. Out of all the antihypertensives available, only a few have been used in pregnancy, and only some are considered safe to be used during pregnancy.

Centrally acting alpha agonists

Methyldopa, a short-acting agent with a broad safety margin, is the most commonly used antihypertensive during pregnancy. Methyldopa has some peripheral action to stimulate α_2-receptors, which decrease sympathetic tone and arterial blood pressure.[33] In a study of 195 children born to hypertensive women on methyldopa treatment during pregnancy, it has been shown that at 7.5 years there was no adverse outcome compared with control.

β-blockers

β-blockers act both on the peripheral vasculature and the heart. Atenolol has been shown to decrease the incidence of severe hypertension, preeclampsia, proteinuria, and the number of hospital admissions and preterm delivery. Follow-up of 120 children at 1 year of age following the use of atenolol in the last trimester of pregnancy showed no adverse effects on development compared with placebo. There is decreased incidence of respiratory distress syndrome (RDS) in neonates but β-blockers may be associated with increases in small-for-gestational-age infants and fetal bradycardia. Atenolol taken in the first trimester of pregnancy was associated with low birth weight, but it did not cause the same effect in the second trimester.[34]

Labetalol is a commonly used antihypertensive for acute severe HTN or chronic HTN. It is a combined α- and β-blocker that decreases systemic vascular resistance with little effect on cardiac output. It has been shown to be more effective than methyldopa in the control of moderate to severe hypertension. Mild transient hypotension may occur in the neonate.[33–36]

Calcium channel blockers

Nifedipine has been used for patients with moderate to severe hypertension. One study of 94 exposed pregnancies recorded no adverse perinatal impact, as reflected by infant development at 18 months.[30] Nifedipine has been shown to be effective in acute hypertensive emergencies in pregnancy with similar efficacy to hydralazine.

Vasodilators

Hydralazine has been used either as primary or additional therapy in the management of severe hypertension or preeclampsia. It acts directly on arterial smooth muscles to cause vasodilatation and subsequent reduction in peripheral resistance. Chronic use of hydralazine has been reported to lead rarely to a neonatal lupus-like syndrome with thrombocytopenia.

Sodium nitroprusside is a potent vasodilator of both arterial and venous smooth muscle. It can be used for the treatment of hypertensive crises during pregnancy. Higher infusion rates for longer periods can cause fetal cyanide poisoning, so it is only used when another agent is not efficacious or when a hypertensive crisis occurs postpartum.[33–36]

Diuretics

A meta-analysis involving more than 7000 patients found no significant risk with diuretic use during pregnancy. There is a theoretical concern that its antepartum use might reduce plasma volume and cause placental insufficiency.[33] Thiazide diuretics increase serum uric acid levels and render its measurement useless for the diagnosis of superimposed preeclampsia. Furosemide is used in mothers with heart failure.

ACE inhibitors and ARBs

ACE inhibitors and ARBs are contraindicated in pregnancy, particularly in the second and third trimester. The main fetal abnormalities recorded are oligohydramnios, calvarial and pulmonary hypoplasia, renal dysfunction, and increased rates of fetal/neonatal death. In a study of 18 mothers who were taking ACE inhibitors at the time of conception, careful follow up of babies revealed no congenital abnormalities. No congenital abnormalities have been found in three children of mothers who were exposed to ARBs before 18 weeks.[36]

Treatment of chronic and gestational hypertension

Most patients can continue their antihypertensive medications if BP is adequately controlled, unless the medications are contraindicated in pregnancy. Treatment is usually started once diastolic pressures are consistently greater than 95–100 mmHg, with treatment targets to reduce BPs to <90 mmHg. Continued close monitoring of BP levels, and maternal and fetal investigations are paramount.

Treatment of preeclampsia

The main aims of treating preeclampsia are to avoid the complications of severe HTN, to avoid the development of eclampsia, and to prolong the pregnancy to allow fetal maturation, particularly the respiratory system. Treatment may be started when diastolic BP >90 mmHg, especially in the presence of other abnormal symptoms. Severe hypertension, defined as BP >170/110 mmHg, requires aggressive treatment and close patient monitoring. Care must be taken not to lower BP too much and too quickly, as reduced placental perfusion can have serious fetal consequences. The definitive treatment of preeclampsia is delivery of the fetus and placenta despite the high risks of neonatal mortality. If delivery is necessary between 24 and 34 weeks of gestation, the fetuses could benefit from maternal administration of betamethasone 48 hours prior to delivery. Management of preeclampsia before 23 weeks of gestation or after 34 weeks of gestation is individualized depending on the clinical situations.[35]

Treatment of eclampsia

Eclampsia is a medical emergency. The main risks arise from maternal and fetal hypoxia, aspiration of gastric contents, and trauma. Close monitoring of maternal BP, oxygenation status, airway, fetal heart rate, and uterine activity, is essential. Uterine bleeding may indicate abruptio placentae. Seizures should be treated with magnesium sulfate, and the patient monitored closely for worsening neurologic status, airway compromise, cardiovascular status, and urine output. Magnesium sulfate significantly reduces the recurrence of seizures, reduces maternal mortality, and, compared with phenytoin, reduces neonatal morbidity. Magnesium sulfate should be given during labor and at least 24 hours postpartum.[35]

Postpartum follow-up

If the hypertension was pregnancy-induced, BP usually normalizes by 6 weeks after delivery. Some patients with severe hypertension or preeclampsia during the intrapartum period may require continued parenteral antihypertensive therapy. Hydralazine has been found to be more effective in reducing BP in these patients than methyldopa in the first 24 hours after delivery.

Chronic hypertension should be adequately treated and drugs to treat should be chosen depending on the mother's plans on lactation and future pregnancies. Patients with preeclampsia will have a higher risk of hypertension in subsequent pregnancies. Some patients may develop severe hypertension or preeclampsia for the first-time postpartum.

Possible prophylactic treatment

At present, no effective therapy has been consistently demonstrated to reduce the risk of preeclampsia. A meta-analysis showed that calcium supplementation reduced the risk of preeclampsia compared with placebo in very high-risk patients. Use of antiplatelet drugs, mainly aspirin, has been shown to be associated with a 15% reduction in the risk of preeclampsia, an 8% reduction in preterm birth, and a 14% reduction in fetal and neonatal death compared with placebo. Vitamins C and E have also been shown to reduce rates of preeclampsia in patients with abnormal uterine Doppler studies, although no change in perinatal outcome has been seen.[37,38]

REFERENCES

1. Chobarian AV, Bakris GL, Black HR, et al. The Seventh Report of the Joint National Committee on Prevention, Detection, Evaluation, and Treatment of High Blood Pressure: the JNC 7 report. JAMA 2003; 289:2560.

2. Hajjar I, Kotchen TA. Trends in prevalence, awareness, treatment and control of hypertension in the United States, 1988–2000. JAMA 2003; 290(2):199.

3. Luft FC. Molecular genetics of human hypertension. J Hypertens 1998; 16:1871.

4. Reckelhoff JF. Sex steroids, cardiovascular disease, and hypertension. Unanswered questions and some speculations. Hypertension 2005; 45:170.

5. August P, Oparil S. Hypertension in women. J Clin Endocrinol Metab 1999; 84(6):1862.

6. Luoto R, Kaprio J, Reunanen A, Rutanenen EM. Cardiovascular morbidity in relation to ovarian function after hysterectomy. Obstet Gynecol 1995; 85:515.

7. Reckelhoff J, Fortepiani L. Novel mechanisms responsible for postmenopausal hypertension. Hypertension 2004; 43:918.

8. Sowers JR. Diabetes in the elderly and in women: cardiovascular risks. Cardiol Clin 2004; 22(4):541.

9. Forman JP, Rimm EB, Stampfer MJ, Curhan GC. Folate intake and the risk of incident hypertension among US women. JAMA 2005; 293(3):320.

10. Lewis CI, Grandits GA, Flack J, McDonald R, Elmer PJ. Efficacy and tolerance of antihypertensive treatment in men and women with stage one diastolic hypertension. Arch Intern Med 1996; 156:377.

11. Salifu MO, Haria DM, Badero O, Aytug S, McFarlane SI. Challenges in the diagnosis and management of renal artery stenosis. Curr Hypertens Rep 2005; 7(3):219.

12. Textor S. Managing renal arterial disease and hypertension. Curr Opin Cardiol 2003; 18:260.

13. Vaziri N. Roles of oxidative stress and antioxidant therapy in chronic kidney disease and hypertension. Curr Opin Nephrol Hypertens 2004; 13:93.

14. Radermacher J, Haller H. The right diagnostic work-up: investigating renal and renovascular disorders. J Hypertens 2003; 21(S):S19.

15. Preston R. Renal parenchymal hypertension: current concepts of pathogenesis and management. Arch Intern Med 1996; 156(6): 602.

16. Khan U, Gomez-Sanchez E. Primary aldosteronism-evolving concepts in diagnosing and treatment. Curr Opin Endocrinol Metab 2004; 11(3):153.

17. Cappricchione A, Winer N, Sowers JR. Adrenocortical Hypertension. Curr Urol Rep 2006; 7(1):73.

18. Stewart PM. The adrenal cortex. In: Larsen PR, Kronenberg HM, Melmed S, Polonsky KS, eds. Williams Textbook of Endocrinology, 10th edn. Philadelphia: WB Saunders 2003: 491.

19. Cappricchione A, Sowers J. Hypertension, endocrine. Encycloped Endocr Dis 2004; 2:592.

20. Arnaldi G. Diagnosing and complications of Cushing's syndrome: a consensus statement. J Clin Endocrinol Metab 2003; 88(12):5593.

21. Bravo E, Tagle R. Pheochromocytoma: state-of-the-art and future prospects. Endocr Rev 2003; 24(4):539.

22. Eisenhofer G, Goldstein DS, Walther MM, et al. Biochemical diagnosis of pheochromocytoma: how to distinguish true- from false-positive test results. J Clin Endocrinol Metab 2003; 88(6):2656.

23. Robinson G. Obstructive sleep apnea/hypopnea syndrome and hypertension. Thorax 2004; 59:1089.

24. Gotzsche CO, Krag-Olsen B, Nielsen J, Sorensen KE, Kristensen BO. Prevalence of cardiovascular malformations and association with karyotypes in Turner's syndrome. Arch Dis Child 1994; 71:433.

25. Brickner M, Hillis LD, Lange RA. Congenital heart disease in adults. N Engl J Med 2000; 342:334.

26. Clarkson PM, Nicholson MR, Barratt-Boyes BG, Neutze JM, Whitlock RM. Results after repair of coarctation of the aorta beyond infancy: a 10 to 28 year follow-up with particular reference to late systemic hypertension. Am J Cardiol 1983; 51:1481.

27. Anonymous Report of the National High Blood Pressure Education Program Working Group on High Blood Pressure in Pregnancy. Am J Obstet Gynecol 2000; 183(1):s1.

28. Sibai BM. Diagnosis, controversies and management of the syndrome of hemolysis, elevated liver enzymes and low platelet count. Obstet Gynecol 2004; 105(5 Pt 1):981.

29. Roberts JM, Pearson G, Culter J, Lindheimer MD. Summary of the NHLBI Working Group on Research on Hypertension during Pregnancy. Hypertension 2003; 41:437.

30. Waite LL, Louie RE, Taylor NT. Circulating activators of peroxisome proliferator activated receptors are reduced in preeclamptic pregnancy. J Clin Endocrinol Metab 2005; 90:620.

31. Levine RJ, Thadhani R, Qian C, Lam C, et al. Urinary placental growth factor and risk of preeclampsia. JAMA 2005; 293:77.

32. Seely EW, Solomon CG. Insulin resistance and its potential role in pregnancy-induced hypertension. J Clin Endocrinol Metab 2003; 88(6):2393.

33. Barrilleaux PS, Martin Jr JN. Hypertension therapy during pregnancy. Clin Obstet Gynecol 2002; 45(1):22.

34. Montan S. Drugs used in hypertensive disease in pregnancy. Curr Opin Obstet Gynecol 2004; 16(2):111.

35. Sibai BM. Diagnosis and management of gestational hypertension and preeclampsia. Obstet Gynecol 2003; 102(1):181.

36. Chung NA, Beevers DG, Lip GY. Management of hypertension in pregnancy. Am J Cardiovasc Drugs 2001; 1(14):253.

37. Vainio M, Riutta A, Koisto AM, Maenpaa J. Prostacyclin and thromboxane A and the effect of low dose ASA in pregnancies at high risk of hypertensive disorders. Acta Obstet Gynaecol Scand 2004; 83(12):1119.

38. Atallah AN, Hofmeyr GJ, Duley L. Calcium supplementation during pregnancy for preventing hypertensive disorders and related problems. Cochrane Database Syst Rev 2004; Volume 4.

3

Ischemic heart disease

Sanjeev Wasson and Lokesh Tejwani

Introduction • Epidemiology • Clinical presentation of ischemic heart disease in women • Diagnosis • Management of ischemic heart disease in women • Prevention • Prognosis • Summary

INTRODUCTION

Ischemic heart disease (IHD) is the leading cause of mortality in women in the United States.[1] About 500 000 women die of cardiovascular disease (CVD) every year, which is more than the number of CVD deaths in men or the combined mortality each year from all other causes (Figure 3.1). Although the incidence of myocardial infarction (MI) in premenopausal women is lower, women statistically have a worse prognosis after diagnosis and the mortality related to IHD is higher in women compared with men. In addition, the incidence of MI increases exponentially after the menopause. Women also differ in underlying pathophysiology, presentation, and risk–benefit profiles with current therapeutic modalities.

EPIDEMIOLOGY

Prevalence

Overall, 13.7 million people in the United States suffer from IHD (MI or angina). The National Health and Nutrition Surveys (NHANES) reported an increasing prevalence of IHD in women with age, from 5% at ages 40–49 years, to 8% at 50–59 years, 11% at 60–69 years, and 14% at 70–79 years. The corresponding prevalence in men was substantially higher.[2]

Incidence

Demographics

According to the National Center for Health Statistics, 1 in 9 women between the ages of 45 and 64 develop symptoms of some form of cardiovascular disease. The ratio climbs to 1 in 3 women after age 65. Although women have a greater life expectancy than men and tend to develop coronary artery disease (CAD) 10–20 years later than men, the burden of CAD in women is high, with a lifetime risk >20%. The Framingham Study[3] demonstrated that the lifetime risk of developing IHD increases with age, from 32% in women aged 40 years and 24%

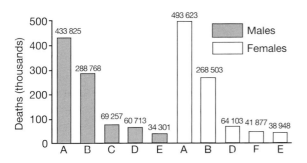

A Total CVD (preliminary) D Chronic lower respiratory diseases
B Cancer E Diabetes mellitus
C Accidents F Alzheimer's disease

Figure 3.1 Leading causes of death in men and women in the United States (2002). CVD, cardiovascular disease.

in women aged 70 years. The incidence of total coronary events in women lags behind men by 10 years. The incidence and severity of coronary disease increase abruptly after menopause, with rates three times those of women of the same age who remain premenopausal.[3] The initial presentation of coronary disease in women under age 75 is more likely to be angina pectoris than MI. Angina in women is mostly uncomplicated (80%), whereas it often occurs after an MI in men (66%).

Temporal trends

Recent data have shown a significant decline in overall incidence of IHD,[4] more pronounced in women ≥65 years of age. The incidence of ST elevation MI (STEMI) and Q-wave MI has also decreased over time. In contrast, the incidence of a non-ST elevation MI (NSTEMI) has increased from 45% in 1994 to 63% in 1999.[5] However, the overall incidence of MI has not changed significantly.

IHD mortality

Mortality rates are higher in men than in women (three times higher between the ages of 25 and 34, and 1.6 times between the ages of 75 and 84) and in blacks than in whites. However, by age 65, the number of deaths from IHD in women surpasses deaths in men by 11%. The incidence of IHD and the case fatality rate have declined in both men and women. This has resulted in a decline of overall mortality rates for IHD by 63% in men (331 to 121 per 100 000) and by 60% in women (166 to 67 per 100 000) in the United States (Figure 3.2).[6] About 45% of this decline in IHD mortality is due to improved medical therapies and 55% is due to risk factor modifications, especially smoking cessation.

Risk factors

Table 3.1 describes a spectrum of cardiovascular risk factors in women.[1] Below age 65, all the major risk factors (e.g. hypertension, dyslipidemia, diabetes mellitus, smoking) impact significantly on the rate of development of

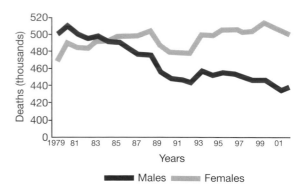

Figure 3.2 Cardiovascular mortality trends for males and females in the United States (1979–2002). Source: CDC/NCHS.

coronary and peripheral artery disease. Above age 65, the serum total cholesterol predicts less well than the total/HDL (high-density lipoprotein) cholesterol ratio. The HERS trial has also demonstrated that yearly cardiovascular morbidity and mortality increase in proportion to the number of risk factors.[7] The Framingham Risk Algorithm for sex-specific quantitative risk assessment is applicable for both the white and black population, although it may overestimate risk among some other populations, e.g.

Table 3.1 Risk factors for cardiovascular disease in women

Modifiable	1. Dyslipidemia
	2. Diabetes
	3. Hypertension
	4. Cigarette smoking
	5. Obesity
	6. Sedentary lifestyle
	7. Poor nutrition
Non-modifiable	Older age
	Positive family history of heart disease
Recently identified	1. Abnormal circulating levels of lipoprotein (a)
	2. Homocysteine
	3. C-reactive protein
	4. Serum amyloid A
	5. Intercellular adhesion molecule-1
	6. Interleukin-6

Hispanic persons in Puerto Rico. This algorithm can be used for matching the intensity of treatment to absolute risk.

Dyslipidemia

For men, elevated low-density lipoprotein cholesterol (LDL-C) is perhaps the most important risk indicator for the development of IHD. For women, on the other hand, lowered HDL-C and elevated triglycerides are notable independent risk factors. The Lipid Research Clinic's follow-up study found that low HDL-C was the most significant predictor of death from IHD in women after adjusting for age.[8] The relation between hypertriglyceridemia and CAD appears to be stronger in women, especially diabetics. Plasma triglyceride levels are directly related to plasma very low-density lipoprotein cholesterol (VLDL-C) concentration, which, also, is a more important risk marker for women than for men. Oral estrogen administration leads to elevation of plasma triglyceride levels. This effect can be eliminated by transdermal application, since it bypasses the hepatic first-pass metabolism of estrogen.

Premenopausal women have more favorable lipoprotein profiles than men, which is reflected in a lower burden of atherosclerotic disease. At the time of menopause, lipoprotein profiles undergo adverse changes, including increases in total and LDL-C, decreases in HDL_2, and shift in LDL particle size toward smaller, denser particles. Women with premature CAD tend to have low HDL rather than high LDL, smaller average LDL particle size and LDL pattern B, and higher levels of lipoprotein(a), apolipoprotein B, and A-1.[9] Lipoprotein(a) is a glycoprotein that is associated with apoprotein B, and it exaggerates atherogenesis by increasing the deposition of LDL in the arterial wall, as well as by inhibiting thrombolysis. In addition, lipoprotein(a) is an antiplasminogen, which accounts for its inhibition of thrombolysis. Estrogen treatment lowers lipoprotein(a) levels and, somewhat paradoxically, so does androgen treatment. Many clinical trials of lipid-lowering therapy have shown conclusively a more significant reduction in coronary events, although similar survival benefit, among

women as compared with men. Other prognostic risk factors for IHD – in addition to conventional risk factors such as family history, diabetes mellitus, smoking (relative risk (RR) = 2.4 for 1.4 cigarettes/day)[10] and hypertension – are also more prevalent in women.

Diabetes

The risk of IHD in women with diabetes is three- to seven-fold higher than in women without diabetes. The corresponding risk for men with diabetes is two- to three-fold higher. This sex-based difference may be explained by the negative impact of diabetes on both lipid markers and blood pressure in women. Women with diabetes have greater elevations of triglycerides and LDL-C and lower levels of HDL-C than men with diabetes.

Obesity

Large, prospective cohort studies in women have shown a positive correlation between obesity and coronary artery disease.[11] The Nurses' Health Study showed that women carry a two-fold risk in the mild to moderate overweight category and a three-fold risk in the heaviest category for IHD compared with lean women.[12] Obesity, more specifically abdominal or central obesity (waist–hip ratio of above 0.9), is associated with an increased cardiac mortality.[12] Based on the Nurses' Health Study (Table 3.2),[12] the recommended target body mass index (BMI) is 18.5–24.9 kg/m^2 (less than 110% of

---

Table 3.2 Body mass index and risk of ischemic heart disease

BMI (kg/m^2)	Adjusted RR for CAD
21–22.9	1.19
23–24.9	1.46
25–28.9 (overweight but not obese)	2.06
≥29	3.56

BMI, body mass index; RR, relative risk; CAD, coronary heart disease.

desirable body weight) and a waist circumference of <35 inches (91.5 cm). Increased cardiac mortality has been noted in women with weight cycling (repeated weight loss and weight gain) (RR = 1.67) presumably due to a significant decrease in HDL-C concentration with each cycle.[13] Obesity is associated with elevated C-reactive protein, particularly in women.

Hypertension

Hypertension has been correlated with the increased risk of stroke and IHD in women. A study of almost 14 000 women in Holland showed a two- to three-fold increase in cardiovascular deaths in patients with systolic blood pressure ≥185 mmHg as compared to women with a systolic blood pressure ≤135 mmHg.[14] Reduction in hypertension substantially affects the incidence of IHD in men and women. Clinical trials for antihypertensive therapies have not shown any gender differences in blood pressure response and outcomes so far.

Smoking

Smoking predisposes to accelerated atherosclerosis and vascular thrombosis. It is responsible for more than 60% of coronary events in middle-aged women, and they are at six- to nine-fold increased risk for IHD compared with non-smokers. This risk decreases over time, to 50% after the first year of smoking cessation and even more thereafter. Although the smoking rates in women have declined since the 1960s, they are decreasing at a slower rate than the smoking rates in men.[11]

Chronic renal disease

The National Kidney Foundation and the American College of Cardiology/American Heart Association (ACA/AHA) Task Force have recommended that chronic kidney disease be considered a CAD risk equivalent in both men and women.[15] The Atherosclerosis Risk in Communities (ARIC) study has shown a 5% higher cardiovascular risk for every 10 ml/min/1.73 m² decrease in the glomerular filtration rate (GFR).[16]

Nutrition

The Nurses' Health Study has estimated a 42% decline in the IHD risk by replacement of only 5% of saturated fat with unsaturated fats, and a 53% decline by replacing 2% of transunsaturated fat with unhydrogenated, unsaturated fat.[17] The IHD risk in females can be reduced by more intake of fruits, vegetables, legumes, fish, poultry, and whole grains (prudent diet, median fiber intake = 26 g/day) and lesser intake of red and processed meats, sweets, fried foods, and refined grains (adjusted RR for total CVD and myocardial infarction 0.79 and 0.68, respectively).[17,18] Although decline in cardiovascular mortality was seen in women who consumed less than 18 drinks per week, heavier drinking (more than 18 drinks per week) was associated with an increased mortality from breast cancer and cirrhosis in women.

Metabolic syndrome

Both NHANES III (odds ratio (OR) = 2.2)[19] and the Women's Ischemia Syndrome Evaluation (WISE) study[13] have clearly shown a significant increase in the subsequent risk of death (94 vs 98%) or major cardiovascular events (88 vs 94%) in women with metabolic syndrome (Table 3.3).[20]

Sedentary lifestyle

Sedentary lifestyle is more prevalent in women and there is an incremental benefit with increasing intensity and frequency of exercise.[21] The

---

Table 3.3 Clinical identification of metabolic syndrome in women

Risk factor	Defining level
Abdominal obesity	Waist circumference >88 cm (>35 inches)
Triglycerides	≥150 mg/dl
HDL cholesterol	<50 mg/dl
Blood pressure	≥130/85 mmHg
Fasting glucose	≥110 mg/dl

HDL, high-density lipoprotein.

risk of IHD can be reduced by up to 75% in women who exercise regularly.

Hormone levels

Contrary to earlier beliefs, the Women's Health Initiative (WHI) and the HERS trials[22,23] have suggested that postmenopausal hormonal status is not a significant risk factor and estrogen–progestin replacement has no cardioprotective effect and may even have harmful effects, including stroke, breast cancer, and thromboembolic events. As a result, the American Heart Association has recommended against initiating postmenopausal hormones for the secondary prevention of cardiovascular disease. Limited data from the Framingham Heart Study and the NHEFS study suggested a higher rate of IHD in multigravid women with six or more pregnancies,[24] probably related to their high-risk lifestyle.

Oral contraceptives

The combination of oral contraceptives use and smoking in women over the age of 35 is related to increased risk of MI, hypertension, and ischemic stroke.

Genes

Gender differences in gene regulation are most likely responsible for differences with respect to risk factors, disease manifestations, and response to treatment and patient outcomes, ultimately which may be explained by the nuclear estrogen receptors present in cardiac myocytes of both men and women.

Inflammatory markers

Several inflammatory markers, including C-reactive protein (CRP), serum amyloid A, interleukin-6, elevated plasma fibrinogen concentration ($\geq$2.6 g/l)[25] and procoagulant factor V Leiden levels, especially in smokers, are independent risk factors for CVD among women. In men, high sensitivity CRP was the strongest non-lipid predictor of cardiovascular risk, whereas in women, high sensitivity CRP

was the strongest risk predictor overall. However, there is lack of strong evidence in support of CRP as a target of therapies. Recently, a statin trial has shown better clinical outcomes with lowering of CRP levels.[26]

Additional risk factors for IHD includes low bone density at menopause,[27] related to extent of estrogen exposure; hyperhomocysteinemia,[28] due to low intake of folate (<400 µg/day) and vitamin B_6 (<3 mg/day); microalbuminuria independent of diabetes and hypertension;[29] and lower socioeconomic status and psychosocial stress.[30]

Silent MIs

Two risk factors, hypertension and diabetes mellitus, are associated with an increased tendency toward unrecognized silent MIs. The infarction is unrecognized in 48% of women and 32% of men, among patients with moderate to severe hypertension (>160/95 mmHg).[31] However, diabetes is a risk factor for silent MI in men only. Diabetic women in the Framingham Study and in the HERS trial were less likely to have unrecognized MIs.[31]

In summary, low levels of HDL-C, elevated triglyceride levels, and diabetes have more of an impact on the risk picture for women than for men. The metabolic syndrome (also known as insulin resistance or syndrome X) is highly associated with IHD risk in women, especially in middle age.

Risk stratification

Clinical assessment for risk of coronary disease in women can be undertaken by determining the presence and severity of traditional and measurable risk factors using the Framingham risk score for women (Table 3.4) and the spectrum of risk with concomitant clinical diagnoses (Table 3.5).[32]

CLINICAL PRESENTATION OF ISCHEMIC HEART DISEASE IN WOMEN

Although there are many similarities, women differ from men in both disease presentation and prognosis for IHD. Women presenting with

Table 3.4 Framingham point score for estimation of 10-year risk in women[32]

Age	Points				
20–34	–7				
35–39	–3				
40–44	0				
45–49	3				
50–54	6				
55–59	8				
60–64	10				
65–69	12				
70–74	14				
75–79	16				

Total cholesterol (mg/dl)	Age 20–39	Age 40–49	Age 50–59	Age 60–69	Age 70–79
<160	0	0	0	0	0
160–199	4	3	2	1	1
200–239	8	6	4	2	1
240–279	11	8	5	3	2
≥280	13	10	7	4	2

Smoking					
Non-smoker	0	0	0	0	0
Smoker	9	7	4	2	1

HDL (mg/dl)	Points
≥ 60	–1
50–59	0
40–49	1
<40	2

Systolic BP (mmHg)	Untreated	Treated
<120	0	0
120–129	1	3
130–139	2	4
140–159	3	5
≥160	4	6

Total points	10-year risk (%)
<9	<1
9	1
10	1
11	1
12	1
13	2
14	2
15	3
16	4
17	5
18	6
19	8
20	11
21	14
22	17
23	22
24	27
≥25	≥30

Table 3.5 Spectrum of IHD risk in women

Risk group	Framingham absolute 10-year IHD risk	Additional clinical features determining risk level
High risk	>20%	Established IHD Carotid artery disease (symptomatic or asymptomatic with >50% stenosis) Peripheral artery disease Abdominal aortic aneurysm Diabetes mellitus Chronic renal disease
Intermediate risk	10–20%	Subclinical cardio-vascular disease (e.g. coronary calcification) Metabolic syndrome Multiple risk factors Markedly elevated levels of a single risk factor First-degree relatives with early-onset (<55 years in men and <65 years in women) atherosclerotic CVD
Low risk	<10%	May include women with multiple risk factors, metabolic syndrome, or one or no risk factors
Optimal risk	<10%	Optimal levels of risk factors and heart-healthy lifestyle

IHD, ischemic heart disease; CVD, cardiovascular disease.

IHD or MI are generally 6–10 years older than men.[33] While assessing women, symptoms of angina are usually considered diagnostically unreliable. The initial presentation in women is mostly atypical chest pain rather than a well-defined cardiovascular event such as MI,[33] with lower prevalence of significant coronary disease among such women.

Psychosocial factors significantly influence the emergency care provided to women with

Table 3.6 Frequency of presentation of acute myocardial infarction in women

Symptoms on presentation	Frequency (%)
Shortness of breath	58
Weakness	55
Fatigue	43
Chest pain	30
Sleep disturbance	48

new-onset chest pain. Women are approached and diagnosed less aggressively than men, with low likelihood of receiving an electrocardiogram, cardiac monitoring, cardiac enzyme measurements, or cardiology consult. About 41–46% of silent Q-wave infarctions[31] go unrecognized due to atypical presentation and absence of prodromal chest pain (43%) in women. Women with MI are more likely to experience back pain, nausea, vomiting, and dyspnea associated with chest discomfort, whereas men are more likely to have concomitant diaphoresis. Women present more frequently with crackles, tachycardia, and higher killip-class and conduction abnormalities. Table 3.6 summarizes the usual frequency of presentation of acute MI in women.[34]

The GUSTO IIb trial pointed out that women were less likely to present with STEMI (27 vs 37% for men).[35] Women with a NSTEMI are less likely to have elevated cardiac enzymes and more likely to have elevated CRP and BNP (brain natriuretic peptide) levels than men.[36] Although women with unstable angina have a lower risk for death (RR = 0.81) or cardiac event (RR = 0.83), the outcome did not differ between men and women with NSTEMI.

Women presenting with chest pain, on angiographic evaluation, have more commonly normal coronary arteries (41 vs 8% in men).[37] Similarly, women with unstable angina or NSTEMI also have more commonly normal coronary vessels or non-critical coronary artery disease (≤50–60% stenosis) (17 vs 9% in men).[37] Lower prevalence of significant coronary disease in these patients could be due to clot lysis, coronary vasospasm, or microvascular disease.

Spontaneous coronary dissection, although a rare cause of sudden cardiac death and acute coronary syndromes, is more prevalent in younger women (mean age 39 years) during the peripartum period (incidence of 25–31%).[38] Such women usually lack any previous cardiac history or IHD risk factors. Although its exact etiology is not known, an inflammatory response of the adventitia and periarteritis is usually seen. High hemodynamic stress or hormonal effects on the arterial wall during the peripartum period have been implicated as possible etiologies.[38] Such patients should be considered for emergent coronary angiography and percutaneous coronary intervention (PCI) or coronary artery bypass grafting (CABG). Management of 30 such patients in a review included CABG in 14, primary PCI in 4, thrombolysis in 7, and medical management without reperfusion or revascularization in 5 patients.[38]

Symptomatic heart failure develops more frequently in women with IHD than men, partly due to greater frequency of diastolic dysfunction (see Chapter 4 for more details). Sudden cardiac death (SCD) is less frequent in women with IHD,[39] being one-half that of men with IHD, and a higher proportion of sudden deaths occurs in women without any previous history of IHD (63 vs 44% in men). The absolute risk of mortality and SCD in women with heart failure was only one-third that of men (see Chapter 4 for more details).

DIAGNOSIS

Stress testing for the diagnosis of coronary heart disease in women

Diagnosing IHD in the woman is challenging, as there are several issues related to diagnostic testing that put women at a disadvantage. There is evidence that diagnostic testing is underused in women. Also, there is relative lack of data validating diagnostic accuracy of these tests, due to underrepresentation of women in clinical trials, which has led to sketchy data on diagnostic accuracy of most non-invasive tests. The initial evaluation of patients presenting with chest pain and suspected CAD often includes some form of stress testing. The choice of stress test is determined by several factors that take into account the patient's ability to exercise and the ability of the test to detect ischemic changes. Coronary angiography, the 'gold standard' for diagnosing CAD, is an invasive test that is appropriate as an initial diagnostic study in only a minority of patients.

Stress test results must be interpreted in light of the pretest likelihood of IHD, which determines the accuracy of the test. Several variables determine pretest probability of CAD. These include age, gender, and the characteristics of the chest pain.[40] Women more commonly have atypical angina or non-ischemic chest pain (28 vs 55% in a review of over 3100 patients).[40] Based on clinical parameters, the pretest probability of CAD can vary between 1 and 94%:

- A low pretest probability of CAD (5%) lowers the positive predictive value of an abnormal test (using a sensitivity and specificity of 50 and 90%, respectively) to <25%, thereby increasing the chances of a false-positive result in such patients.
- On the other hand, a high pretest probability of CAD (90%) increases the positive predictive value of a test. In such a group of patients, the non-invasive test will be less sensitive, thereby increasing chances of it being a false-negative result.
- Lastly, patients with an intermediate pretest probability of CAD (50%) are the ones to benefit the most from non-invasive testing, with a positive predictive value of 83% and a negative predictive value of 36%.

Exercise electrocardiographic testing

Treadmill exercise testing has a lower sensitivity and specificity (61 and 70%, respectively),[41] and therefore lower positive and negative predictive values in women compared with men. Several factors have been cited for lower predictive values in women than in men: suboptimal performance due to comorbid conditions; a lower prevalence of IHD in women; and a much higher incidence of false-positive ST depression on electrocardiography

(ECG) during stress,[41] which is explained by a higher incidence of mitral valve prolapse (MVP) and the cardiac syndrome X in women. Also, unlike men, exercise-induced ST depression does not increase the probability of cardiovascular death in women.[41] Duke treadmill scoring, although improving the diagnostic accuracy of the test, has a limited value for predicting short-term (2-year) mortality.

Stress myocardial perfusion imaging

Myocardial perfusion imaging (MPI), when added to stress testing, greatly increases diagnostic accuracy. MPI can be combined exercise or pharmacologic stress (using dipyridamole, adenosine, or dobutamine) in patients who are unable to exercise sufficiently. Perfusion defects have both diagnostic and prognostic significance. Syndrome X, which is characterized by chest pain in women with normal coronary arteries and is most likely due to microvascular disease, can be associated with perfusion defects on MPI.[42]

Stress testing with MPI is most useful in women at intermediate risk of IHD, those with an abnormal resting ECG, or those with a prior false-positive stress test. Addition of imaging to stress improves specificity and provides an excellent (>99%) negative predictive value for excluding IHD.[42] Most initial studies utilized standard perfusion imaging with thallium (Tl)-201 as the radiotracer.[43] However, recently, Tc-99 is being used increasingly. In women, use of Tl-201 is more often associated with attenuation artifacts mimicking fixed or reversible perfusion defects (up to 11%)[43] and the use of a Tc-99 radiotracer,[44] attenuation correction techniques, and breast markers have improved interpretation of such defects. Abnormal SPECT (single-photon emission computed tomography) imaging for diagnosis of occlusive CAD (>50% stenosis) has an overall sensitivity of 91–93% and a specificity of 70–78%.[44] In contrast to exercise stress echo, MPI is equally effective in women and men for diagnosing significant coronary artery disease.[45] MPI was found to discriminate between low and high risk more effectively in women than in men.[44]

Stress echocardiography

Stress echocardiography has been studied in several trials involving women with chest pain, although less extensively than MPI. A meta-analysis showed overall sensitivity and specificity of 86 and 79%, respectively. Addition of echo imaging to the exercise stress test added significantly to the specificity and accuracy of the test.[45] Exercise echocardiography in women is cost-effective for diagnosis of CAD, maintaining a sensitivity of 81% (higher for multivessel CAD, i.e. 89%) and a specificity of 86%.[46] The overall accuracy is lower in women than in men, largely due to a greater prevalence of single-vessel CAD in women as well as abnormal ECG at baseline.[47] In addition, women, in general, achieve a lower exercise workload. Exercise should be the preferred form of stress, because it provides prognostic information in addition to the patient's symptoms during exercise and the hemodynamic response.

MANAGEMENT OF ISCHEMIC HEART DISEASE IN WOMEN

Women are underrepresented in randomized clinical trials for the management of coronary syndromes. The ACC/AHA Task Force recommends similar treatment for women and men with unstable angina or NSTEMI.[48]

Medical therapy

Women are less likely than men to receive standard medications for IHD, including thrombolytic drugs, aspirin, heparin, β-blockers, and nitroglycerin.[49] The HERS trials showed no evidence of cardioprotection with hormone replacement therapy; hence, they are not recommended for women with CAD.[23]

Aspirin

Antiplatelet Trialists' Collaboration showed that aspirin is beneficial for secondary prevention in women with IHD[50] and may provide similar benefit for primary prevention in women with at least one risk factor. Beneficial effects of β-adrenergic blockers, angiotensin-converting enzyme (ACE) inhibitors,[51] and statins[52] in women after MI is well demonstrated in clinical trials. The HOPE trial demonstrated that ACE inhibitors improve the incidence of MI or stroke, as well as cardiovascular mortality in women with IHD.[51] In patients who cannot tolerate ACE inhibitor due to cough, an angiotensin receptor blocker can be substituted. The 4S (Scandinavian Simvastatin Survival Study with simvastatin), CARE (Cholesterol and Recurrent Events with pravastatin) trial, and the Heart Protection Study (HPS) showed similar significant reduction in major cardiovascular events and mortality with statins in women,[52] with the number needed to treat being 31 for women and 27 for men. Recently, the PROVE IT-TIMI 22 trial showed a more marked benefit of atorvastatin (80 mg/day) in women with an acute coronary syndrome (ACS) in terms of significant reduction in all-cause mortality, MI, unstable angina, revascularization, or stroke with atorvastatin.[26]

Non-ST elevation acute coronary syndrome

Gender is not an independent predictor of outcome after an uncomplicated MI. The ACC/AHA Task Force recommended similar management of men and women with unstable angina or NSTEMI, including indications for aspirin, clopidogrel, glycoprotein (GP) IIb/IIIa inhibitors, and non-invasive and invasive testing.[49] It is well known that early invasive strategy with revascularization improves outcome of men with a non-ST elevation acute coronary syndrome; however the data in women are not so clear. The FRISC II and RITA 3 trials[53,54] with low-risk women have favored early invasive therapy only in men, and TACTICS-TIMI 18 and other prospective studies have shown similar benefits in men and women.[36] Women who underwent PCI in TACTICS-TIMI 18 had a significantly higher risk of major bleeding (8.3 vs 2.9%).[36] Women undergoing CABG had a higher mortality rate in FRISC II[53] as compared with TACTICS-TIMI 18,[36] mostly related to comorbidity.

ST elevation MI

Thrombolytic therapy is usually underutilized and delayed, even in eligible women. Studies have shown a higher rate of mortality and recurrent MI in women receiving thrombolysis compared with men,[55] primarily related to the differences in their baseline characteristics, such as age, diabetes mellitus, hypertension, and prior heart failure. Bleeding risk is modestly increased in women receiving thrombolysis. Benefits of thrombolytic therapy outweigh moderate bleeding risk in menstruating women and, therefore, they should not be excluded from thrombolytic therapy.

Primary PCI

The PAMI trial suggested that primary angioplasty was more beneficial in women compared with thrombolysis.[55] Other studies have shown similar procedural success rates and long-term 1 year survival among both sexes, but significantly higher in-hospital mortality in the early postcatheterization period among women undergoing primary PCI or percutaneous transluminal coronary angioplasty (PTCA) without stenting.[56]

Cardiogenic shock

Left ventricular failure is the most common etiology for cardiogenic shock in both genders. Women had a significantly higher incidence of mechanical complications (ventricular septal rupture or acute severe mitral regurgitation) as a cause of cardiogenic shock (19 vs 10.6% in men) in the SHOCK trial registry.[57]

Invasive procedures

In spite of there being a greater burden of risk factors in women, some studies have shown a possible gender bias and less likelihood of use of cardiac catheterization procedures in women with equivocal indications.[58] However, the Nationwide Independent Sample in the United States report showed similar access to percutaneous interventions in both men and women with strong indications for catheterization.[59]

Cardiac catheterization

Women who are referred for PCI are more likely to be older than men, and more likely to

have a history of heart failure and unstable angina, but less likely to have suffered an MI. They are also more likely to have comorbid hypertension, hyperlipidemia, and diabetes. Initial procedural success rates and both short- and long-term outcomes of PCI have improved in women despite being older and having a greater risk burden than men.

Coronary artery stenting

Coronary artery stenting is obviously superior to PTCA alone. However, there are conflicting data on outcomes after PCI in women. The Healthcare Cost and Utilization Project showed higher mortality among women with an MI (4 vs 2% for men, adjusted OR = 1.47) and without an MI (1.1 vs 0.5%, adjusted OR = 1.65).[60] Women also had a higher CABG rate. On the other hand, the National Cardiovascular Network Database showed similar procedural mortality, but a higher incidence of stroke, vascular complications, and repeat in-hospital revascularization in women. Higher in-hospital mortality in women could be accounted for by their smaller coronary arteries, by virtue of their smaller body surface area.[61]

Bypass surgery

Women are also less likely to undergo CABG. Women undergoing CABG are at increased risk for procedural complications (new neurologic event, heart failure, perioperative infarction, and hemorrhage), graft failure,[61] and in-hospital mortality at 30 days. This may be explained by the older age, greater burden of coronary risk factors and comorbidities, and smaller body size with consequent smaller coronary artery size in women. Neurologic complications occur less frequently in both men and women undergoing 'off-pump' CABG.[62] After undergoing CABG, women are more likely to have recurrent angina and poor quality of life than men. However, long-term survival after 1 year of CABG is similar in both men and women.[63]

Cardiac rehabilitation in women

Cardiac rehabilitation is an important component in recovery from a coronary event; women

Table 3.7 Clinical recommendations

Lifestyle interventions

Cigarette smoking
Consistently encourage women not to smoke and to avoid environmental tobacco. (Class I, Level B)$_{Gl=1}$

Physical activity
Consistently encourage women to accumulate a minimum of 30 minutes of moderate-intensity physical activity (e.g. brisk walking) on most, and preferably all, days of the week. (Class I, Level B)$_{Gl=1}$

Cardiac rehabilitation
Women with a recent acute coronary syndrome or coronary intervention, new-onset or chronic angina should participate in a comprehensive risk-reduction regimen, such as cardiac rehabilitation or a physician-guided home- or community-based program. (Class I, Level B)$_{Gl=2}$

Heart-healthy diet
Consistently encourage an overall healthy eating pattern that includes intake of a variety of fruits, vegetables, grains, low-fat or non-fat dairy products, fish, legumes, and sources of protein low in saturated fat (e.g. poultry, lean meats, plant sources). Limit saturated fat intake to <10% of calories, limit cholesterol intake to <300 mg/day, and limit intake of *trans* fatty acids. (Class I, Level B)$_{Gl=1}$

Weight maintenance/reduction
Consistently encourage weight maintenance/reduction through an appropriate balance of physical activity, caloric intake, and formal behavioral programs when indicated to maintain/achieve a BMI between 18.5 and 24.9 kg/m^2 and a waist circumference <35 inches. (Class I, Level B)$_{Gl=1}$

Psychosocial factors
Women with CVD should be evaluated for depression and referred/treated when indicated. (Class IIa, Level B)$_{Gl=2}$

Omega 3 fatty acids
As an adjunct to diet, omega 3 fatty acid supplementation may be considered in high-risk[a] women. (Class IIb, Level B)$_{Gl=2}$

Folic acid
As an adjunct to diet, folic acid supplementation may be considered in high-risk[a] women (except after revascularization procedure) if a higher-than-normal level of homocysteine has been detected. (Class IIb, Level B)$_{Gl=2}$

Major risk factor interventions

Blood pressure − lifestyle
Encourage an optimal blood pressure of <120/80 mmHg through lifestyle approaches. (Class I, Level B)$_{Gl=1}$

Blood pressure − drugs
Pharmacotherapy is indicated when blood pressure is ≥140/90 mmHg or an even lower blood pressure in the setting of blood pressure-related target-organ damage or diabetes. Thiazide diuretics should be part of the drug regimen for most patients unless contraindicated. (Class I, Level A)$_{Gl=1}$

Lipid, lipoproteins
Optimal levels of lipids and lipoproteins in women are LDL-C <100 mg/dl, HDL-C >50 mg/dl, triglycerides <150 mg/dl, and non-HDL-C (total cholesterol − HDL cholesterol) <130 mg/dl and should be encouraged through lifestyle approaches. (Class I, Level B)$_{Gl=1}$

Lipids − diet therapy
In high-risk women or when LDL-C is elevated, saturated fat intake should be reduced to <7% of calories, cholesterol to <200 mg/day, and *trans* fatty acid intake should be reduced. (Class I, Level B)$_{Gl=1}$

Lipids − pharmacotherapy − high risk[a]
Initiate LDL-C-lowering therapy (preferably a statin) simultaneously with lifestyle therapy in high-risk women with LDL-C ≥100 mg/dl (Class I, Level A)$_{Gl=1}$, and initiate statin therapy in high-risk women with an LDL-C <100 mg/dl unless contraindicated (Class 1, Level B)$_{Gl=1}$.

 Initiate niacin[d] or fibrate therapy when HDL-C is low, or non-HDL-C elevated in high-risk women. (Class I, Level B)$_{Gl=1}$

continued

Table 3.7 Clinical recommendations – *continued*

Lipids – pharmacotherapy – intermediate risk[b]
Initiate LDL-C-lowering therapy (preferably a statin) if LDL-C level is ≥130 mg/dl on lifestyle therapy (Class I, Level A), or niacin[d] or fibrate therapy when HDL-C is low or non-HDL-C elevated after LDL-C goal is reached. (Class I, Level B)[GI=1]

Lipids – pharmacotherapy – lower risk[c]
Consider LDL-C-lowering therapy in low-risk women with 0 or 1 risk factor when LDL-C level is ≥190 mg/dl or if multiple risk factors are present when LDL-C is ≥160 mg/dl (Class IIa, Level B) or niacin[d] or fibrate therapy when HDL-C is low or non-HDL-C elevated after LDL-C goal is reached. (Class IIa, Level B)[GI=1]

Diabetes
Lifestyle and pharmacotherapy should be used to achieve near normal HbA$_{1C}$ (<7%) in women with diabetes. (Class I, Level B)[GI=1]

Preventive drug interventions

Aspirin – high risk[a]
Aspirin therapy (75–162 mg), or clopidogrel if patient is intolerant to aspirin, should be used in high-risk women unless contraindicated. (Class I, Level A)[GI=1]

Aspirin – intermediate risk[b]
Consider aspirin therapy (75–162 mg) in intermediate-risk women as long as blood pressure is controlled and benefit is likely to outweigh risk of gastrointestinal side effects. (Class IIa, Level B)[GI=2]

β-Blockers
β-Blockers should be used indefinitely in all women who have had a myocardial infarction or who have chronic ischemic syndromes unless contraindicated. (Class I, Level A)[GI=1]

ACE inhibitors
ACE inhibitors should be used (unless contraindicated) in high-risk[a] women. (Class I, Level A)[GI=1]

ARBs
ARBs should be used in high-risk[a] women with clinical evidence of heart failure or an ejection fraction <40% who are intolerant to ACE inhibitors. (Class I, Level B)[GI=1]

Atrial fibrillation/stroke prevention

Warfarin – atrial fibrillation
Among women with chronic or paroxysmal atrial fibrillation, warfarin should be used to maintain the INR at 2.0–3.0 unless the woman is considered to be at low risk for stroke (<1%/year) or high risk of bleeding. (Class I, Level A)[GI=1]

Aspirin – atrial fibrillation
Aspirin (325 mg) should be used in women with chronic or paroxysmal atrial fibrillation with a contraindication to warfarin or at low risk for stroke (<1%/year). (Class I, Level A)[GI=1]

Class III interventions

Hormone therapy
Combined estrogen plus progestin hormone therapy should not be initiated to prevent CVD in postmenopausal women. (Class III, Level A)
    Combined estrogen plus progestin hormone therapy should not be continued to prevent CVD in postmenopausal women. (Class III, Level C)
    Other forms of menopausal hormone therapy (e.g. unopposed estrogen) should not be initiated or continued to prevent CVD in postmenopausal women pending the results of ongoing trials. (Class III, Level C)

Antioxidant supplements
Antioxidant vitamin supplements should not be used to prevent CVD pending the results of ongoing trials. (Class III, Level A)[GI=1]

continued

Table 3.7 Clinical recommendations – *continued*

Aspirin – lower risk[c]
Routine use of aspirin in lower-risk women is not recommended pending the results of ongoing trials. (Class III, Level B)[GI=2]

GI, generalizability index; LDL-C, low density lipoprotein cholesterol; HDL-C, high-density lipoprotein cholesterol; ACE, angiotensin-converting enzyme; ARB, angiotensin receptor blocker; BMI, body mass index; CAD, coronary artery disease; CVD, cardiovascular disease; INR, international normalized ratio.
[a]High risk is defined as CAD or risk equivalent, or global risk >20%.
[b]Intermediate risk is defined as global risk 10–20%.
[c]Lower risk is defined as global risk <10%.
[d]Dietary supplement niacin must not be used as a substitute for prescription niacin, and over-the-counter niacin should only be used if approved and monitored by a physician.

---

are 20% less likely to be enrolled in such programs.[64] Barriers to cardiac rehabilitation participation among women included lack of physicians' referral; a concomitant illness such as diabetes, arthritis, or osteoporosis; transportation problems; inconvenient timing; and depressive and anxiety symptoms. Postevent recovery is also slower in women, with delayed return to work and more psychosomatic disorders.

PREVENTION

Because IHD is often fatal and nearly two-thirds of women who die suddenly have no previously recognized symptoms, it is essential to prevent IHD. The 2004 AHA guidelines have grouped clinical recommendations for the prevention of CVD in women into several major categories. Table 3.4 illustrates a spectrum of CVD, showing risk groups defined by their absolute probability of having a coronary event in 10 years according to the Framingham Risk Score for women.[65]

Clinical recommendations

Evidence-based recommendations for the prevention of CVD in women are listed in Tables 3.7–3.9.[65] Each recommendation is accompanied by the strength of recommendation, level of evidence to support it, and the generalizability index (Table 3.10). The strength of the recommendation is based not only on the

---

Table 3.8. CVD prevention strategies for clinical practice

1. Assess and stratify women into high-, intermediate-, lower-, or optimal-risk categories.
2. Lifestyle approaches (smoking cessation, regular exercise, weight management, and heart-healthy diet) to prevent CVD are Class I recommendations for all women and a top priority in clinical practice.
3. Other CVD risk-reducing interventions should be prioritized on the basis of strength of recommendation (Class I > Class IIa > Class IIb) and within each class of recommendation on the basis of the level of evidence, with the exception of lifestyle, which is a top priority for all women (A>B>C).
4. Highest priority for risk intervention in clinical practice is based on risk stratification: (high risk > intermediate risk > lower risk > optimal risk).
5. Avoid interventions designated as Class III.

CVD, cardiovascular disease.

---

level of evidence to support a clinical recommendation but also on factors such as feasibility of conducting randomized controlled trials in women. Recommendations are grouped in the following categories: lifestyle interventions; major risk factor interventions; atrial fibrillation/stroke prevention; preventive drug interventions; and a Class III category, where routine intervention for cardiovascular disease prevention is not recommended.

Table 3.9. Priorities for prevention in practice according to risk group

High-risk women (>20% risk)
Class I recommendations:
- Smoking cessation
- Physical activity/cardiac rehabilitation
- Diet therapy
- Weight maintenance/reduction
- Blood pressure control
- Lipid control/statin therapy
- Aspirin therapy
- β-blocker therapy
- ACE inhibitor therapy (ARBs if contraindicated)
- Glycemic control in diabetics

Class IIa recommendation:
- Evaluate/treat depression

Class IIb recommendations:
- Omega 3 fatty acid supplementation
- Folic acid supplementation

Intermediate-risk women (10–20% risk)
Class I recommendations:
- Smoking cessation
- Physical activity
- Heart-healthy diet
- Weight maintenance/reduction
- Blood pressure control
- Lipid control

Class IIa recommendation:
- Aspirin therapy

Lower-risk women (<10% risk)
Class I recommendations:
- Smoking cessation
- Physical activity
- Heart-healthy diet
- Weight maintenance/reduction
- Treat individual CVD risk factors as indicated

Stroke prevention among women with atrial fibrillation
Class I recommendations:
High-intermediate risk of stroke
- Warfarin therapy
Low risk of stroke (<1%/year) or contraindication to warfarin
- Aspirin therapy

ACE, angiotensin-converting enzyme; ARB, angiotensin receptor blocker; CVD, cardiovascular disease.

Table 3.10. Classification and levels of evidence for cardiovascular disease prevention in women

Parameter	Strength of recommendation
Classification	
Class I	Intervention is useful and effective
Class IIa	Weight of evidence/opinion is in favor of usefulness/efficacy
Class IIb	Usefulness/efficacy is less well established by evidence/opinion
Class III	Intervention is not useful/effective and may be harmful
Level of evidence	
A	Sufficient evidence from multiple randomized trials
B	Limited evidence from a single randomized trial or other non-randomized studies
C	Based on expert opinion, case studies, or standard of care
Generalizability index	
1	Very likely that the results generalize to women
2	Somewhat likely that the results generalize to women
3	Unlikely that the results generalize to women
0	Unable to project whether the results generalize to women

PROGNOSIS

The prognosis for women with IHD is less favorable than it is for men, secondary to delay in diagnosis. Although the mean age of death due to myocardial infarction is lower for men than for women, by age 65, the number of cardiovascular deaths in women exceeds by 11% that in men. Case fatality rates in the 1-year post-MI period are also higher in women than in men. Although the number of deaths caused by IHD has been decreasing in men, this trend has yet to be seen in women.

Morbidity

In the Framingham Study, after 6 years following a recognized MI,[66] 33% of women had recurrent recognized MI, 30% of women had heart failure, and 13% of women had stroke. The age-adjusted mortality rate for MI and heart failure was similar in men and women after unrecognized MIs, but risk ratios were higher in women than men for all events except stroke. The risk of developing congestive heart failure (CHF) in the 10 years after an MI is higher in women than in men.

Short-term mortality

Most of the studies report higher in-hospital and 30-day mortality after MI in women compared with men.[53,54] This effect is primarily seen in younger women and progressively declines with age, with equivalent outcomes in the elderly. The worse outcome in women is largely related to increased age and greater comorbidity. This was illustrated in the ISIS-3 trial, which involved 9600 women and 26 480 men with a suspected STEMI.[67] The unadjusted OR for death within the first 35 days among women compared with men was 1.73; however, women were significantly older than men and after adjustment for age and other baseline characteristics, the OR was 1.14, which was still significant. The excess in major non-fatal clinical events in women was reduced by a similar degree after adjustment. Another factor that may explain the higher short-term mortality in women is a difference in the proportion of men and women who survive to reach the hospital. This was examined in a population-based study of 201 114 patients with a first myocardial infarction.[68] Women, who were on average 7 years older than men, were more likely than men to reach the hospital. When deaths before hospitalization were included, the 30-day mortality was lower in women than men (adjusted OR = 0.9).

Long-term mortality

Similar principles apply to long-term outcomes. Women with an MI have a higher long-term mortality after MI than men,[69] which is higher in black women compared with white women. The difference between women and men tends to disappear when the results are adjusted for age (women tend to be older) and other risk factors.[69] However, there may be true differences at specific patient ages. This was demonstrated in a report of 6826 patients who survived hospitalization for an acute MI.[70] Compared with men of similar age at 2-year

follow-up, women under age 60 had a higher mortality, women between the ages of 60 and 69 had a similar outcome, and women ≥70 had a lower mortality. Coronary mortality is also increased in women, compared with men, with diabetes mellitus.[71] Why this might occur is not known.

Non-ST elevation acute coronary syndrome (ACS)

The above data were derived from studies of women with STEMI and all infarctions (both ST elevation and non-ST elevation). Several studies have specifically evaluated the outcomes in women with a non-ST elevation ACS (unstable angina or non-ST elevation [non-Q wave] MI). Despite more comorbidities, such women have a similar[72] or better outcome than men.[69]

Mortality trends

Improvement in medical care has led to decreasing in-hospital and long-term mortality rates following MI. The ARIC study[73] showed a decline in the in-hospital mortality in women by 9.8% per year, more significantly in white women, and in overall mortality in women by 6.1% per year. The National Registry of Myocardial Infarction (NRMI) 1, 2, and 3[5] have also shown similar declining trends for in-hospital mortality after an acute MI. The Framingham Study illustrated improving IHD survival trends[74] from the time period of 1950–1969 to the subsequent decades of 1970–1979 (hazards ratio = 0.69) and 1980–1989 (hazards ratio = 0.48). However, most of the improvement in survival after acute MI has occurred in patients with an STEMI, with no significant decrease in mortality rates following an NSTEMI. In-hospital or 6-month mortality rates in FRISC II and TACTICS-TIMI 18 were not significantly reduced.[36,53] After STEMI and non-STEMI, higher in-hospital and 30-day mortality rates have been shown in patients not enrolled in clinical trials like the GRACE registry[75] and the Euro Heart Survey review.[76] In most studies, patients with an NSTEMI have a similar or even worse long-term outcome than those with a STEMI.[35]

Risk scores

Many risk scores have been developed to assess short- and long-term outcomes after MI. The most widely used risk scores are the TIMI risk scores for both STEMI and NSTEMI to predict 14–30-day mortality,[77,78] and the GISSI risk index to estimate 4-year mortality.[79]

Sudden cardiac death

There is a clear relationship between SCD and IHD. The SCD risk in women with IHD is one-half that in men, and its incidence lags behind men by more than 10 years.[80] MI confers twice the SCD risk as angina in both the sexes.[80]

SUMMARY

There is an urgent need for comprehensive health policy initiatives designed to equalize access to care across all women. Future policy solutions should include:

- education campaigns to increase physician awareness of current race and sex disparities in the use of cardiovascular tests and therapies
- programs to improve communication between physicians and patients across race and sex
- comprehensive efforts to determine whether patients have received indicated tests and therapies and mechanisms for rectifying deficiencies.

Timely prevention and minimization of risk factors through education, medication, and lifestyle modification are essential to altering current ischemic mortality and morbidity trends in women.

REFERENCES

1. Mosca L, Manson JE, Sutherland SE, et al. Cardiovascular disease in women. A statement for healthcare professionals from the American Heart Association. Circulation 1997; 96:2468.

2. American Heart Association. Heart and Stroke Facts Statistics 2003 Update. Dallas, Texas: American Heart Association; 2002.

3. Gordon T, Kannel WB, Hjortland MC, McNamara PM. Menopause and coronary heart disease. The Framingham Study. Ann Intern Med 1978; 89:157.

4. Arciero TJ, Jacobsen SJ, Reeder GS, et al. Temporal trends in the incidence of coronary disease. Am J Med 2004; 117:228.

5. Rogers WJ, Canto JG, Lambrew CT, et al. Temporal trends in the treatment of over 1.5 million patients with myocardial infarction in the US from 1990 through 1999: the National Registry of Myocardial Infarction 1, 2 and 3. J Am Coll Cardiol 2000; 36:2056.

6. Levi F, Lucchini F, Negri E, La Vecchia C. Trends in mortality from cardiovascular and cerebrovascular diseases in Europe and other areas of the world. Heart 2002; 88:119.

7. Vittinghoff E, Shlipak MG, Varosy PD, et al. Risk factors and secondary prevention in women with heart disease: the Heart and Estrogen/progestin Replacement Study. Ann Intern Med 2003; 138:81.

8. Jacobs DR, Mebane IL, Bangdiwala SI, Criqui MH, Tyroler HA. High density lipoprotein cholesterol as a predictor of cardiovascular disease mortality in men and women: the follow-up study of the Lipid Research Clinics Prevalence Study. Am J Epidemiol 1990;131:32.

9. Kamigaki AS, Siscovick DS, Schwartz SM, et al. Low density lipoprotein particle size and risk of early-onset myocardial infarction in women. Am J Epidemiol 2001; 153:939.

10. Willett WC, Green A, Stampfer MJ, et al. Relative and absolute excess risks of coronary heart disease among women who smoke cigarettes. N Engl J Med 1987; 317:1303.

11. Rich-Edwards JW, Manson JE, Hennekens CH, Buring JE. The primary prevention of coronary heart disease in women. N Engl J Med 1995; 332:1758.

12. Manson JE, Willet WC, Stampfer MJ, et al. Body weight and mortality among women. N Engl J Med 1995; 333:677.

13. Olson MB, Kelsey SF, Bittner V, et al. Weight cycling and high-density lipoprotein cholesterol in women: evidence of an adverse effect: a report from the NHLBI-sponsored WISE study. Women's Ischemia Syndrome Evaluation Study Group. J Am Coll Cardiol 2000; 36:1565.

14. van der Giezen AM, Schopman-Geurts van Kessel JG, Schouten EG, et al. Systolic blood pressure and cardiovascular mortality among 13,740 Dutch women. Prev Med 1990; 19:456.

15. K/DOQI clinical practice guidelines for chronic kidney disease: evaluation, classification and stratification. Am J Kidney Dis 2002; 39:S1.

16. Manjunath G, Tighiouart H, Ibrahim H, et al. Level of kidney function as a risk factor for atherosclerotic

cardiovascular outcomes in the community. J Am Coll Cardiol 2003; 41:47.

17. Fung TT, Willett WC, Stampfer MJ, et al. Dietary patterns and the risk of coronary heart disease in women. Arch Intern Med 2001; 161:1857.

18. Liu S, Buring JE, Sesso HD, et al. A prospective study of dietary fiber intake and risk of cardiovascular disease among women. J Am Coll Cardiol 2002; 39:49.

19. Ninomiya JK, L'Italien G, Criqui MH, et al. Association of the metabolic syndrome with history of myocardial infarction and stroke in the Third National Health and Nutrition Examination Survey. Circulation 2004; 109:42.

20. Summary of the Third Report of the National Cholesterol Education Program (NCEP) Expert Panel on Detection, Evaluation, and Treatment of High Blood Cholesterol in Adults (Adult Treatment Panel III). NIH Publication No. 02–5215, Sept 2002.

21. Lee IM, Rexrode KM, Cook NR, et al. Physical activity and coronary heart disease in women: is 'no pain, no gain' passe? JAMA 2001; 285:1447.

22. Rossouw JE, Anderson GL, Prentice RL, et al. Risks and benefits of estrogen plus progestin in healthy postmenopausal women: principal results from the Women's Health Initiative randomized controlled trial. JAMA 2002; 288:321.

23. Grady D, Herrington D, Bittner V, et al. Cardiovascular disease outcomes during 6.8 years of hormone therapy: Heart and Estrogen/progestin Replacement Study follow-up (HERS II). JAMA 2002; 288:49.

24. Ness RB, Harris T, Cobb J, et al. Number of pregnancies and the subsequent risk of cardiovascular disease. N Engl J Med 1993; 328:1528.

25. Ridker PM, Hennekens CH, Buring JE, Rifai N. C-reactive protein and other markers of inflammation in the prediction of cardiovascular disease in women. N Engl J Med 2000; 342:836.

26. Cannon CP, Braunwald E, McCabe CH, et al. Intensive versus moderate lipid lowering with statins after acute coronary syndromes. N Engl J Med 2004; 350:1495.

27. von der Recke P, Hansen MA, Hassager C. The association between low bone mass at the menopause and cardiovascular mortality. Am J Med 1999; 106:273.

28. Ridker PM, Manson JE, Buring JE. Homocysteine and risk of cardiovascular disease among postmenopausal women. JAMA 1999; 281:1817.

29. Roest M, Banga JD, Janssen WM, et al. Excessive urinary albumin levels are associated with future cardiovascular mortality in postmenopausal women. Circulation 2001; 103:3057.

30. Haynes SG, Czajkowski SM. Psychosocial and environmental correlates of heart disease. In: Douglas PS, ed. Cardiovascular Health and Disease in Women. Philadelphia: WB Saunders; 1993: 269.

31. Shlipak MG, Elmouchi DA, Herrington DM, et al. The incidence of unrecognized myocardial infarction in women with coronary heart disease. Ann Intern Med 2001; 134:1043.

32. Wilson PW, D'Agostino RB, Levy D, et al. Prediction of coronary heart disease using risk factor categories. Circulation 1998; 97:1837.

33. Lerner DJ, Kannel WB. Patterns of coronary heart disease morbidity and mortality in the sexes: 26-year follow-up of the Framingham population. Am Heart J 1986; 111:383.

34. McSweeney JC, Cody M, O'Sullivan P, et al. Women's early warning symptoms of acute myocardial infarction. Circulation 2003; 108:2619.

35. Armstrong PW, Fu Y, Chang W-C, et al. for the GUSTO-IIb Investigators. Acute coronary syndromes in the GUSTO-IIb trial: prognostic insights and impact of recurrent ischemia. Circulation 1998; 98:1860.

36. Wiviott SD, Cannon CP, Morrow DA, et al. Differential expression of cardiac biomarkers by gender in patients with unstable angina/non-ST-elevation myocardial infarction: a TACTICS-TIMI 18 (Treat Angina with Aggrastat and determine Cost of Therapy with an Invasive or Conservative Strategy – Thrombolysis In Myocardial Infarction 18) substudy. Circulation 2004; 109:580.

37. Roe MT, Harrington RA, Prosper DM, et al. Clinical and therapeutic profile of patients presenting with acute coronary syndromes who do not have significant coronary artery disease. The Platelet Glycoprotein IIb/IIIa in Unstable Angina: Receptor Suppression Using Integrilin Therapy (PURSUIT) Trial Investigators. Circulation 2000; 102:1101.

38. Leone F, Macchiusi A, Ricci R, Cerquetani E, Reynaud M. Acute myocardial infarction from spontaneous coronary artery dissection: a case report and review of the literature. Cardiol Rev 2004; 12:3.

39. Kim C, Fahrenbruch CE, Cobb LA, Eisenberg MS. Out-of-hospital cardiac arrest in men and women. Circulation 2001; 104:2699.

40. Alexander KP, Shaw LJ, Delong ER, et al. Value of exercise treadmill testing in women. J Am Coll Cardiol 1998; 32:1657.

41. Mora S, Redberg RF, Cui Y, et al. Ability of exercise testing to predict cardiovascular and all-cause death in asymptomatic women: a 20-year follow-up of the Lipid Research Clinics prevalence study. JAMA 2003; 290:1600.

42. Mieres JH, Shaw LJ, Hendel RC, et al; Writing Group on Perfusion Imaging in Women. American Society of Nuclear Cardiology consensus statement: Task Force on Women and Coronary Artery Disease – the role of myocardial perfusion imaging in the clinical evaluation of coronary artery disease in women. J Nucl Cardiol 2003; 10:95.

43. Goodgold HM, Rehder JG, Samuels LD, Chaitman BR. Improved interpretation of exercise thallium-201 scintigraphy in women: characterization of breast attenuation artifacts. Radiology 1987; 165:361.

44. Amanullah AM, Berman DS, Hachamovitch R, et al. Identification of severe or extensive coronary artery disease in women by adenosine technetium-99m sestamibi SPECT. Am J Cardiol 1997; 80:132.

45. Williams MJ, Marwick TH, O'Gorman D, Foale RA. Comparison of exercise echocardiography with an exercise score to diagnose coronary artery disease in women. Am J Cardiol 1994; 74:435.

46. Cheitlin MD, Armstrong WF, Aurigemma GP, et al. ACC/AHA/ASE 2003 guideline update for the clinical application of echocardiography: summary article: a report of the American College of Cardiology/American Heart Association Task Force on Practice Guidelines (ACC/AHA/ASE Committee to Update the 1997 Guidelines for the Clinical Application of Echocardiography). Circulation 2003; 108:1146.

47. Lewis JF, Lin L, McGorray S, et al. Dobutamine stress echocardiography in women with chest pain. Pilot phase data from the National Heart, Lung and Blood Institute Women's Ischemia Syndrome Evaluation (WISE). J Am Coll Cardiol 1999; 33:1462.

48. Braunwald E, Antman E, Beasley J, et al. ACC/AHA 2002 guideline update for the management of patients with unstable angina and non-ST-segment elevation myocardial infarction – summary article. A report of the American College of Cardiology/American Heart Association task force on practice guidelines (Committee on the Management of Patients With Unstable Angina). J Am Coll Cardiol 2002; 40:1366.

49. Gan SC, Beaver SK, Houck PM, et al. Treatment of acute myocardial infarction and 30-day mortality among women and men. N Engl J Med 2000; 343:8.

50. Collaborative overview of randomised trials of antiplatelet therapy I: Prevention of death, myocardial infarction, and stroke by prolonged antiplatelet therapy in various categories of patients. Antiplatelet Trialists' Collaboration [published erratum appears in BMJ 1994; 308:1540]. BMJ 1994; 308:81.

51. Lonn E, Roccaforte R, Yi Q, et al. Effect of long-term therapy with ramipril in high-risk women. J Am Coll Cardiol 2002; 40:693.

52. LaRosa JC, He J, Vupputuri S. Effect of statins on risk of coronary disease: a meta-analysis of randomized controlled trials. JAMA 1999; 282:2340.

53. Lagerqvist B, Safstrom K, Stahle E, et al. Is early invasive treatment of unstable coronary artery disease equally effective for both women and men? FRISC II Study Group Investigators. J Am Coll Cardiol 2001; 38:41.

54. Fox K, Poole-Wilson P, Henderson R, et al. Interventional versus conservative treatment for patients with unstable angina or non-ST-elevation myocardial infarction: the British Heart Foundation RITA 3 randomised trial. Lancet 2002; 360:743.

55. Stone GW, Grines CL, Browne KF, et al. A comparison of in-hospital outcome in men versus women treated by either thrombolytic therapy or primary coronary angioplasty for acute myocardial infarction. Am J Cardiol 1995; 75:987.

56. Vakili BA, Kaplan RC, Brown DL. Sex-based differences in early mortality of patients undergoing primary angioplasty for first acute myocardial infarction. Circulation 2001; 104:3034.

57. Wong SC, Sleeper LA, Monrad ES, et al, for the SHOCK Investigators. Absence of gender differences in clinical outcomes in patients with cardiogenic shock complicating acute myocardial infarction. A report from the SHOCK trial Registry. J Am Coll Cardiol 2001; 38:1395.

58. Rathore SS, Wang Y, Radford MJ, et al. Sex differences in cardiac catheterization after acute myocardial infarction: the role of procedure appropriateness. Ann Intern Med 2002; 137:487.

59. Bertoni AG, Bonds DE, Lovato J, et al. Sex disparities in procedure use for acute myocardial infarction in the United States, 1995 to 2001. Am Heart J 2004; 147:1054.

60. Watanabe CT, Maynard C, Ritchie JL. Comparison of short-term outcomes following coronary artery stenting in men versus women. Am J Cardiol 2001; 88:848.

61. Jacobs AK. Coronary revascularization in women in 2003: sex revisited. Circulation 2003; 107:375.

62. Capdeville M, Chamogeogarkis T, Lee JH. Effect of gender on outcomes of beating heart operations. Ann Thorac Surg 2001; 72:S1022.

63. Jacobs AK, Kelsey SF, Brooks MM, et al. Better outcome for women compared with men undergoing coronary revascularization: a report from the bypass angioplasty revascularization investigation (BARI). Circulation 1998; 98:1279.

64. Ades PA, Waldmann ML, Polk DM, et al. Referral patterns and exercise responses in the rehabilitation of female coronary patients aged greater than 62. Am J Cardiol 1992; 69:1422.

65. Mosca L, Appel LJ, Benjamin EJ, et al. Evidence-based guidelines for cardiovascular disease prevention in women. Circulation 2004; 109:672.

66. Thom TJ, Kannel WB, Silbershatz S, et al. Incidence, prevalence, and mortality of cardiovascular diseases in the United States. In: Alexander RW, Schlant RC, Fuster V, Roberts R, eds. Hurst's The Heart, 9th edn. New York: McGraw-Hill; 1998: 3.

67. Boersma E, Harrington RA, Moliterno DJ, et al. Platelet glycoprotein IIb/IIIa inhibitors in acute coronary

syndromes: a meta-analysis of all major randomised clinical trials. Lancet 2002; 359:189.

68. MacIntyre K, Stewart S, Capewell S, et al. Gender and survival: a population-based study of 201,114 men and women following a first acute myocardial infarction. J Am Coll Cardiol 2001; 38:729.

69. Chang WC, Kaul P, Westerhout CM, et al. Impact of sex on long-term mortality from acute myocardial infarction vs unstable angina. Arch Intern Med 2003; 163:2476.

70. Vaccarino V, Krumholz HM, Yarzebski J, et al. Sex differences in 2-year mortality after hospital discharge for myocardial infarction. Ann Intern Med 2001; 134:173.

71. Barrett-Connor EL, Cohn BA, Wingard DL, Edelstein SL. Why is diabetes mellitus a stronger risk factor for fatal ischemic heart disease in women than in men? JAMA 1991; 265:627.

72. Hochman JS, McCabe CH, Stone PH, et al, for the TIMI Investigators. Outcome and profile of women and men presenting with acute coronary syndrome: a report from TIMI IIIB. J Am Coll Cardiol 1997; 30:141.

73. Rosamond WD, Chambless LE, Folsom AR, et al. Trends in the incidence of myocardial infarction and in mortality due to coronary heart disease, 1987 to 1994. N Engl J Med 1998; 339:861.

74. Guidry UC, Evans JC, Larson MG, et al. Temporal trends in event rates after Q-wave myocardial infarction: The Framingham Heart Study. Circulation 1999; 100:2054.

75. Steg P, Goldberg R, Gore J, et al. Baseline characteristics, management practices, and in-hospital outcomes of patients hospitalized with acute coronary syndromes in the Global Registry of Acute Coronary Events (GRACE). Am J Cardiol 2002; 90:358.

76. Hasdai D, Behar S, Wallentin L, et al. A prospective survey of the characteristics, treatments and outcomes of patients with acute coronary syndromes in Europe and the Mediterranean basin. The Euro Heart Survey of Acute Coronary Syndromes (Euro Heart Survey ACS). Eur Heart J 2002; 23:1190.

77. Morrow DA, Antman EM, Charlesworth A, et al. TIMI risk score for ST-elevation myocardial infarction: a convenient, bedside, clinical score for risk assessment at presentation: an intravenous nPA for treatment of infarcting myocardium early II trial substudy. Circulation 2000; 102:2031.

78. Antman EM, Cohen M, Bernink PJ, et al. The TIMI risk score for unstable angina/non-ST elevation MI: a method for prognostication and therapeutic decision making. JAMA 2000; 284:835.

79. Marchioli R, Avanzini F, Barzi F, et al; GISSI-Prevenzione Investigators. Assessment of absolute risk of death after myocardial infarction by use of multiple-risk-factor assessment equations; GISSI-Prevenzione mortality risk chart. Eur Heart J 2001; 22:2085.

80. Kannel WB. Sudden coronary death in women. Am Heart J 1998; 136:205.

4

Cardiomyopathy

John F Best and Shawn Kaser

Introduction • Pathophysiology • Gender differences in heart failure • Peripartum cardiomyopathy • Cardiomyopathy of the middle-aged female • Cardiomyopathy of the elderly female • Preventive strategies • Mechanical and surgical intervention • Summary

INTRODUCTION

The clinical syndrome of heart failure is the final outcome for a myriad of diseases that affect the heart. Nearly 5 million Americans have heart failure today and it is responsible for 20% of all admissions among patients older than age 65.[1] Almost half of the patients in the United States with heart failure are women and, among persons older than 70 years, the incidence of heart failure is much higher in women than men.[2]

PATHOPHYSIOLOGY

Heart failure is a pathophysiologic state in which the heart is unable to pump blood at a rate commensurate with the requirements of the metabolizing tissues, or can do so only at elevated filling pressure. Heart failure can result from any structural or functional cardiac disorder that impairs the ability of the ventricle to fill with or eject blood, including disorders of the pericardium, myocardium, endocardium, great vessels, or impairment of left ventricular (LV) systolic or diastolic function. The clinical manifestations of heart failure are dyspnea, fatigue, limited exercise tolerance, fluid retention, and eventually pulmonary congestion and peripheral edema. Heart failure is not equivalent to cardiomyopathy or to LV dysfunction. These terms describe possible structural reasons for the development of heart failure. Instead,

heart failure is a clinical syndrome that is characterized by specific signs and symptoms. There is no one diagnostic test for heart failure. A variety of clinical tools are available to the clinician to help in the diagnosis of heart failure. These include physical examination, chest X-ray, and echocardiography. Recently, brain natriuretic peptide (BNP) has been found to be elevated in both acute and chronic heart failure. This polypeptide is released from ventricular myocytes in response to stretch and acts as a vasodilator as well as a natriuretic factor. It is a helpful tool in the diagnosis of heart failure, but is by no means specific. Elevations in BNP are commonly seen in patients with renal failure, ascites, primary pulmonary hypertension, and other states of fluid overload. The diagnosis of heart failure, therefore, is based on a careful history and physical examination.

To determine the best course of therapy, physicians often assess heart failure according to the New York Heart Association (NYHA) functional classification system (Table 4.1). This system relates symptoms to everyday activities and the patient's quality of life and helps to assess response to treatments. It is important to note that classification methods are limited, as symptoms may not relate to the actual severity of the condition and in part are related to the patient's own perception and may not indicate chances for survival. For example, patients may complain of breathlessness after exercise and

Table 4.1 New York Heart Association (NYHA) functional classification

Class	Patient symptoms
Class I (mild)	No limitation of physical activity. Ordinary physical activity does not cause undue fatigue, palpitation, or dyspnea (shortness of breath)
Class II (mild)	Slight limitation of physical activity. Comfortable at rest, but ordinary physical activity results in fatigue, palpitation, or dyspnea
Class III (moderate)	Marked limitation of physical activity. Comfortable at rest, but less than ordinary activity causes fatigue, palpitation, or dyspnea
Class IV (severe)	Unable to carry out any physical activity without discomfort. Symptoms of cardiac insufficiency at rest. If any physical activity is undertaken, discomfort is increased

Table 4.2 ACC/AHA stages of heart failure progression

Stage	Description	Examples
A	Patients at risk of developing heart failure	Hypertension, coronary artery disease, diabetes mellitus, chemotherapy, alcohol, family history
B	Patients with structural heart disease without heart failure	Prior myocardial infarction, asymptomatic valvular disease, left ventricular hypertrophy
C	Patients with structural heart disease with heart failure	Dyspnea or fatigue due to decreased left ventricular systolic dysfunction
D	Patients with marked structural heart disease and marked symptoms of heart failure	Patients requiring frequent hospitalizations, awaiting transplant

have only mild heart abnormalities. However, some patients do not report fatigue or shortness of breath after physical activity and yet may have severe heart abnormalities.

The evolution and progression of heart failure can be appropriately characterized by the four stages outlined by the Heart Failure Society (Table 4.2).[3] This staging system recognizes that heart failure, like coronary artery disease, has established risk factors and structural prerequisites, and unlike the NYHA functional class, has specific treatments targeted at each stage that can reduce the morbidity and mortality of heart failure.

GENDER DIFFERENCES IN HEART FAILURE

The current literature suggests there may be significant gender differences in heart failure.

These differences include etiologies of heart failure, risk factors for the development of heart failure, and even prognosis in heart failure. Hypertension is a stronger risk factor for the development of heart failure in women than men. In the Framingham Study, hypertension conferred a two-fold excess risk of developing heart failure in men and a three-fold risk in women.[4] This observation has been duplicated and could be a difference in cardiac response to pressure overload. Although the incidence of myocardial infarction (MI) is lower in women than in men, women who sustain an MI are more likely to develop heart failure.

The National Health and Nutrition Examination Survey Epidemiological Follow-Up Study examined more than 13 000 men and women without evidence of congestive heart failure (CHF) at baseline and followed them for an average of 19 years. In this study, African-American women had a higher incidence of heart failure than white women. Cigarette smoking was a stronger risk factor for women than for men, conferring a 45% higher risk of heart failure in men and an 88% risk in women.[5]

Discrepancies exist in the early literature regarding gender-based differences in survival for patients with heart failure. Several studies have shown a better prognosis for women than for men with symptomatic heart failure. In the Framingham Study – prior to ACE (angiotensin-converting enzyme) inhibitor and β-blocker use – the prognosis for women after the diagnosis of heart failure was better than for men despite an older age at presentation.[6,7] It should be noted that echocardiographic estimation of LV systolic function was not routinely obtained in this study, and therefore the heart failure population probably represented a heterogeneous group with differing physiologic causes of heart failure.

In distinction to the Framingham data, the Studies of Left Ventricular Dysfunction (SOLVD) Trial registry reported a poorer outcome in women than men presenting with symptomatic heart failure.[8,9] Women were older than men at study entry but had equivalent depression of systolic function. The conflicting results between these studies could reflect the inclusion of patients with heart failure with preserved LV systolic function in the Framingham cohort and the probable inclusion of a greater percentage of women with ischemic heart disease in the SOLVD trial.

Although some of this gender-based survival advantage has been ascribed to the lesser prevalence of ischemic heart disease in women, mortality has been shown to be lower for women with heart failure in several large clinical trials after adjustment for differences in baseline variables. In the Metoprolol CR/XL Randomized Intervention Trial in Congestive Heart Failure study, the relative risk for total mortality in the placebo arm was significantly lower for women as compared with men, regardless of heart failure etiology.[10]

The University of North Carolina database provides valuable information on the relationship among gender, etiology, and survival in patients with symptomatic heart failure.[11] A study of 557 patients (380 men and 177 women) with symptomatic heart failure, predominantly non-ischemic in origin (68%), and severe LV dysfunction with a mean left ventricular ejection fraction (LVEF) of 25%, revealed a better survival in women compared with men when heart failure was the result of non-ischemic cause. Although baseline LVEF was higher in women than in men with non-ischemic heart failure, the mortality in women remained lower after adjustment for this variable. In contrast, the relative risk of death was similar for the subset of men and women with ischemic heart disease as the primary cause of heart failure.

PERIPARTUM CARDIOMYOPATHY

Etiology

Multiple studies have attempted to elucidate a distinct etiology of peripartum cardiomyopathy; however, the cause remains unknown. There is some evidence that cytokines may play a role in the pathogenesis and progression of cardiomyopathy and heart failure.[12] Other investigators have proposed an immunologic response to a fetal antigen as a potential etiology.[13,14] Familial clustering of peripartum cardiomyopathy has been observed, so a genetic etiology cannot be excluded.[15] During pregnancy, there is a significant increase in blood volume and cardiac output, which results in LV remodeling and transient hypertrophy. Although these changes normally reverse after delivery, it is possible that there is an exaggerated decrease in LV systolic function in women who develop peripartum cardiomyopathy.

A number of studies evaluating endomyocardial biopsies in patients with peripartum cardiomyopathy have implicated myocarditis as a possible cause based on inflammatory cell infiltration within the myocardium.[16,17] However, insufficient sample sizes have precluded statistical significance in these studies. Additionally, one retrospective review of endomyocardial biopsy specimens found a lower incidence of myocarditis that was comparable to that found in an age- and sex-matched control population undergoing transplantation

---

Table 4.3 Risk factors for peripartum cardiomyopathy

1. Age >30 years[36–38]
2. Multiparity
3. Women of African descent[39]
4. Pregnancy with multiple fetuses[40]
5. History of preeclampsia, eclampsia, or postpartum hypertension
6. Long-term (>4 weeks) oral tocolytic therapy with β-adrenergic agonists[41]
7. Association with maternal cocaine abuse or selenium deficiency[42–45]

---

for idiopathic dilated cardiomyopathy.[18] The reason for this discrepancy was unclear. It was suggested that the time of biopsy in relation to the onset of symptoms may be factor.[16,18]

Although the etiology remains unclear, a number of potential risk factors have been identified (Table 4.3). However, clinicians should remember that the disease can occur in women without these risk factors.

Clinical presentation

Peripartum cardiomyopathy usually presents during the first 4–5 months postpartum and is rarely seen before 36 weeks of gestation. This time of onset is in contrast to patients with underlying cardiac disease (e.g. ischemic, valvular, or myopathic) who tend to develop symptoms of heart failure during the second trimester of gestation, coinciding with the greatest hemodynamic burden of the gravid state. Patients may complain of dyspnea, cough, orthopnea, paroxysmal nocturnal dyspnea, and hemoptysis. Fatigue, chest discomfort, or abdominal pain may confuse the initial evaluation due to the occurrence of similar symptoms during normal pregnancy.[19]

Diagnosis

The diagnosis is based upon the following established clinical criteria:[19]

- the development of heart failure in the last month of pregnancy or within 5 months after delivery

- the absence of a determinable cause for the heart failure
- the absence of demonstrable heart disease before the last month of pregnancy.

In addition to fulfilling these clinical criteria, other conditions which may lead to heart failure in the puerperium (which include infectious, toxic, or metabolic disorders, and underlying ischemic or valvular heart disease) should be carefully excluded before the diagnosis of peripartum cardiomyopathy is considered. The diagnostic work-up should include an electrocardiogram (ECG), chest X-ray, and echocardiography. Other studies such as cardiac catheterization, endomyocardial biopsy, and viral serologies may be considered in selected cases to exclude other potential etiologies.

ECG findings include sinus tachycardia (or rarely, atrial fibrillation), non-specific ST- and T-wave abnormalities and voltage abnormalities. The chest X-ray typically shows enlargement of the cardiac silhouette, with evidence of pulmonary venous congestion and/or interstitial edema with or without pleural effusions. The echocardiogram and Doppler usually reveal LV enlargement with significant global reduction in overall performance without left ventricular hypertrophy (LVH). The echocardiographic threshold of LV enlargement and dysfunction necessary to diagnose peripartum cardiomyopathy has been debated. The following definition, based upon a 1992 NHLBI workshop definition for idiopathic dilated cardiomyopathy, was proposed: LVEF <45% and LV end-diastolic dimension >2.7 cm/m^2.[20,21] Other echocardiographic findings may include regional wall motion abnormalities, left atrial enlargement, mitral and tricuspid regurgitation, and small pericardial effusion.

Right heart catheterization should be considered for patients who present in the antepartum period if optimization of hemodynamics is necessary for a safe delivery. In addition, postpartum patients who do not respond adequately to initial empiric therapy may benefit from a more complete assessment of their hemodynamic state. Left heart catheterization with coronary angiography should be considered on an individual basis. It is most important in patients with significant risk factors for coronary artery disease. Endomyocardial biopsy is not currently recommended for the routine evaluation or diagnosis of peripartum cardiomyopathy because of its lack of clinical utility.

Treatment

Treatment is similar to that for other types of heart failure. The combination of diuretics and sodium restriction to remove excess fluid, β-blockers, and afterload reduction to improve long-term survival forms the cornerstone of therapy. However, concerns regarding the adverse consequences of these therapies for the mother, fetus, or breast-feeding infant can complicate the management of these patients. Diuretics can be used if sodium restriction alone is insufficient, although a bleeding diathesis and hyponatremia have been reported in infants born to mothers taking thiazide diuretics during pregnancy.

There is clear evidence of benefit from β-blockers, such as carvedilol and metoprolol, in patients with heart failure. β-Blockers can delay progression of myocardial dysfunction in patients with idiopathic dilated cardiomyopathy and possibly those with peripartum cardiomyopathy.[12] β Blockers are generally safe and effective during pregnancy, although there may be an increased rate of fetal growth retardation when they are administered. Occasional cases of neonatal apnea, hypotension, bradycardia, and hypoglycemia have also been reported. Infants born to mothers treated with these medications should be observed for 72–96 hours after parturition. β-Blockers are not associated with an increased risk of congenital anomalies.

Nitrates are generally not recommended during pregnancy. ACE inhibitors are absolutely contraindicated, particularly prepartum, when they may be associated with adverse fetal renal effects and an increase in neonatal mortality. Hydralazine is thought to be a safe vasodilator both antepartum and in the postpartum period for the newborn who is breast-feeding.

Patients with peripartum cardiomyopathy are highly predisposed to thromboembolic phenomena due to both the hypercoagulable state of pregnancy and stasis of blood in the left ventricle secondary to severe LV dysfunction. Clinicians may be faced with the consideration of anticoagulants in these patients. This decision is based on the degree of LV dilation, the severity of LV function, and the presence of atrial fibrillation. Warfarin is classified by the Food and Drug Administration (FDA) as a class D agent. Class D agents cross the placenta and are associated with teratogenic effects. Thus, warfarin cannot be routinely recommended, and there is a preference toward heparin in the antepartum period. The partial thromboplastin time (PTT) should be maintained at 1.5–2.0 × control. Either heparin or warfarin may be used safely in the postpartum period. Since neither drug is secreted into breast milk, the infant is therefore not at risk of an anticoagulated state.

Prognosis

The prognosis in women with peripartum cardiomyopathy has largely been based upon reports of small series of patients which suggest that, similar to other forms of congestive heart failure, LV size and the severity of LV dysfunction at the time of presentation are important determinants of outcome.[22,23] Deterioration has been associated with the several characteristics outlined in Table 4.4. Most hearts that are destined to recover normal function probably do so within 6 months from the time of diagnosis.[12,19] Mortality estimates for patients with peripartum cardiomyopathy in the United

---

Table 4.4 Risk factors for clinical deterioration in peripartum cardiomyopathy

1. Older patients (age ≥30 years)
2. Higher parity (≥3 pregnancies)
3. Later onset of symptoms following pregnancy (≥7.6 weeks)
4. Higher echocardiographic left ventricular end-diastolic dimensions (≥7.0 cm) at presentation
5. Higher mean pulmonary arterial (≥38 mmHg)
6. Pulmonary arterial wedge pressures ≥24 mmHg
7. Conduction defects on the surface electrocardiogram at presentation

States range from 25 to 50%; most deaths occur within the first 3 months postpartum.[12,19] Death is usually caused by progressive pump failure, arrhythmias, or thromboembolic events.

Future pregnancy

The general consensus among most experts is that patients with peripartum cardiomyopathy and persistent LV dysfunction are at extremely high risk of complications and death with subsequent pregnancies.[24] Thus, these patients should be advised to avoid pregnancy. The data have been conflicting in patients with peripartum cardiomyopathy in whom LV function recovers, but these women also appear to have some risk for recurrence.[24] In one survey of 28 patients who had normalization of LV function after the initial episode, subsequent pregnancy was associated with a reduction in LVEF and the development of heart failure symptoms during the pregnancy in 6 patients.[24] Therefore, some women who recover LV function after an initial episode of peripartum cardiomyopathy are at risk in subsequent pregnancy. These women should be counseled about the potential risks prior to pregnancy, and carefully monitored for signs of ventricular dysfunction should they choose to become pregnant again.

CARDIOMYOPATHY OF THE MIDDLE-AGED FEMALE

The cardiomyopathy of middle-aged women can generally be attributed to ischemic, dilated, infectious, or toxin-induced etiologies. Other etiologies are less common in the middle-aged female.

Ischemic cardiomyopathy

Coronary atherosclerosis is the most common cause of cardiomyopathy in the United States, constituting 50–75% of patients with heart failure. Most patients with ischemic cardiomyopathy have known atherosclerotic coronary artery disease. However, it is not uncommon for previously undiagnosed coronary artery disease to present initially with heart failure. By some accounts, ischemic cardiomyopathy may

explain as many as 24% of otherwise unexplained cases of idiopathic dilated cardiomyopathy. These observations, along with the potential reversibility of ischemic/hibernating myocardium, underlie the rationale for performing angiography in most patients with heart failure of uncertain etiology.

The cardiomyopathy secondary to coronary artery disease is usually related to MI and ventricular remodeling. Myocyte death from prolonged ischemia results in scar tissue and subsequently leads to systolic heart failure. The end result is an irreversible myocardial dysfunction. However, ischemic/hibernating myocardium may contribute to the decline in myocardial function.[25,26] Hibernating myocardium is ischemic dysfunctional myocardium that remains viable; in such patients, LV function may improve markedly, and even normalize, following successful revascularization. One meta-analysis involving more than 3000 patients (mean ejection fraction 32%) with documented viability reported a significant 80% reduction in annual mortality with revascularization.[25] There was a direct relationship between the severity of LV dysfunction and the magnitude of benefit. In contrast, there was no difference in outcome with revascularization or medical therapy in patients without viability. Without evidence of prior MI or hibernating myocardium, the presence of asymptomatic coronary artery disease in patients with dilated cardiomyopathy does not prove causality.

Dilated cardiomyopathy

The other common cause of cardiomyopathy in the middle-aged female population is dilated cardiomyopathy. Dilated cardiomyopathy is currently responsible for approximately 10 000 deaths and 46 000 hospitalizations each year in the United States, and is the primary indication for cardiac transplantation. Dilated cardiomyopathy is characterized by dilation and impaired contraction of one or both ventricles.[27] Affected patients have impaired systolic function and may or may not develop overt heart failure. The presenting manifestations can include, among other common heart failure symptoms, atrial and/or ventricular arrhythmias, and sudden

Table 4.5 Causes of dilated cardiomyopathy	
Etiology	*Percent*
Idiopathic	50
Myocarditis	9
Ischemic heart disease	7
Infiltrative disease	5
Peripartum cardiomyopathy	4
Hypertension	4
HIV infection	4
Connective tissue disease	3
Substance abuse	3
Doxorubicin	1
Other	10

death can occur at any stage of the disease. Most patients present between the ages of 20 and 60 years, but dilated cardiomyopathy can occur in children and the elderly.[27]

Dilated cardiomyopathy can be caused by a variety of disorders, including myocarditis, ischemia, hypertension, infiltrative processes, and substance abuse among others (Table 4.5).[28] Often, however, no etiology can be found and the cardiomyopathy is deemed idiopathic.

Infectious cardiomyopathy

A variety of infectious organisms can lead to myocarditis and dilated cardiomyopathy. Viral infection is the most common cause of myocarditis and has been implicated in the development of dilated cardiomyopathy. Viruses known to involve the myocardium include coxsackievirus, influenza virus, adenovirus, echovirus, cytomegalovirus, human immunodeficiency virus (HIV), and Epstein–Barr virus (EBV). The initial immune response limits the degree of viremia early during infection and protects against myocarditis. If, however, this response is insufficient, the virus may not be eliminated and myocyte injury may ensue via one or both of two mechanisms:

- direct cytotoxicity via receptor-mediated entry of the virus into cardiac myocytes
- an adverse autoimmune response induced by persisting viral genomic fragments that

may not be capable of replicating as intact virus.

Heart disease associated with HIV infection is being recognized with increasing frequency.[29] The proposed mechanisms of cardiac damage include drug toxicity, secondary infection, myocardial damage by HIV itself, and an autoimmune process induced by HIV itself or in association with other cardiotropic viruses such as coxsackievirus, cytomegalovirus, or EBV.[29]

Chagas' disease, caused by the protozoan *Trypanosoma cruzi*, is the leading cause of dilated cardiomyopathy in Central and South America. It is characterized clinically by an acute myocarditis, cardiac enlargement, tachycardia, and non-specific ECG abnormalities including right bundle branch block and premature ventricular contractions. Patients can develop LV apical aneurysms that are pathognomonic for this disease.

Cardiac involvement with Lyme disease is usually manifested as a conduction abnormality. Cardiac muscle dysfunction can also occur; it is often self-limited and mild, leading to transient cardiomegaly or pericardial effusion on echocardiogram or chest X-ray. Occasionally, patients develop symptomatic myocarditis and dilated cardiomyopathy.

Toxins

Excessive alcohol can result in myocardial dysfunction, although the pathogenesis and factors that determine patient susceptibility are still poorly understood. Alcohol is believed to be toxic to cardiac myocytes via oxygen-derived free radical damage and defects in cardiac protein synthesis. The risk of developing alcoholic cardiomyopathy is related to both mean daily alcohol intake and the duration of drinking. The typical findings in patients with alcoholic dilated cardiomyopathy are LV dilatation, with reduced ejection fraction. More advanced cases have biventricular failure. Abstinence can lead to an improvement in cardiac function if the disease is diagnosed early.

The use of cocaine is associated with cardiomyopathy, but the relationship is less well understood than that between cocaine and coronary ischemia. Cardiomegaly with unexplained heart failure in a young person should raise the possibility of cocaine abuse. Possible mechanisms include a direct toxic effect, cocaine-induced hyperadrenergic state, and, in parenteral cocaine abusers, an infectious cardiomyopathy. Abstinence usually leads to complete reversal of the myocardial dysfunction.

A number of medications are associated with cardiomyopathy, and discontinuation of the implicated drug may result in significant improvement. Anthracycline-induced cardiomyopathy has been the most extensively studied. It usually appears in patients treated with adriamycin at a dose greater than 400 mg/m^2. Other chemotherapeutic agents appear to be idiosyncratic or not entirely dose-related.

Tachycardia-mediated cardiomyopathy

A cardiomyopathy has been reported in patients with chronic supraventricular tachycardias, including atrial fibrillation, atrioventricular nodal reentry, and preexcitation syndromes with ventricular rates of 130–200 beats/min.[30,31] The mechanism of myocardial dysfunction in this setting is not clear. Several mechanisms based on tachycardia-induced cardiomyopathy models in animals have been proposed. These include myocardial energy depletion, ischemia, abnormalities of calcium handling, and myocyte and extracellular matrix remodeling. However, conclusive evidence to favor any of these mechanisms has not been forthcoming. Among the changes that have been observed are a reduction in myocyte contractility, abnormalities in myocardial architecture, and a decrease in calcium responsiveness. LV dysfunction can occur without dilatation. The rate of the tachycardia appears to correlate with the degree of LV dysfunction. Definitive treatment of the arrhythmia results in complete reversal of the myocardial dysfunction, generally within 3 months.

Obstructive sleep apnea

Sleep disturbances, including obstructive and non-obstructive sleep apnea, can contribute to the impairment of LV dysfunction. A history of snoring, daytime somnolence, and obesity should alert the clinician to the diagnosis. Effective therapy, as with nasal continuous positive airway pressure during sleep, can lead to a significant improvement in LV dysfunction.[32]

Endocrine dysfunction

Thyroid dysfunction, excess sympathetic activity in pheochromocytoma, and, rarely, Cushing's syndrome and growth hormone excess or deficiency can cause cardiac dysfunction, which can usually be reversed by correction of the endocrine disorder.[33]

Other

Among patients with idiopathic dilated cardiomyopathy, it is estimated that approximately 25% have familial disease. The mode of inheritance is usually autosomal dominant, although autosomal recessive, X-linked, and mitochondrial inheritance have also been described. Dilated cardiomyopathy may be a common and important component of a number of inherited disorders, including hereditary hemochromatosis, a number of neuromuscular diseases, and the hereditary sideroblastic anemias. Dilated cardiomyopathy can also be a manifestation of various other disease processes such as systemic lupus erythematosus, sarcoidosis, celiac disease, or even nutritional deficiencies such as thiamine and L-carnitine.

Treatment of ischemic and dilated cardiomyopathy

Treatment of heart failure due to systolic dysfunction is aimed at interrupting the pathophysiologic mechanisms that are stimulated in heart failure (Figure 4.1). ACE inhibitors and angiotensin receptor blockers interfere with the renin–angiotensin–aldosterone system, resulting in peripheral vasodilation and decreased afterload. These medications may also affect LV remodeling, LVH, and renal blood flow. Aldosterone is increased in heart failure and results in sodium retention and potassium excretion. Aldosterone has been implicated in

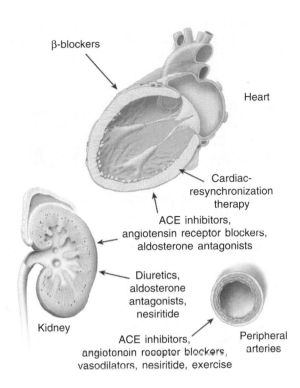

β-blockers

Heart

Cardiac-
resynchronization
therapy

ACE inhibitors,
angiotensin receptor blockers,
aldosterone antagonists

Diuretics,
aldosterone
antagonists,
nesiritide

Kidney

ACE inhibitors,
angiotensin receptor blockers,
vasodilators, nesiritide, exercise

Peripheral
arteries

Figure 4.1 Treatment of heart failure due to systolic dysfunction.

the pathophysiology of myocardial fibrosis during chronic exposure. Aldosterone antagonists such as spironolactone counteract these mechanisms and have been shown to decrease mortality in patients with Class II and III heart failure as demonstrated by the RALES trial. β-Blockers inhibit the sympathetic nervous system, which is activated in heart failure. They slow heart rate, decrease blood pressure, and have beneficial direct effects on the myocardium. MERIT-HF and COMET have established the mortality benefit of β-blockers in patients with heart failure secondary to systolic dysfunction. More recently, the A-HeFT study established a role for the combination of hydralazine/nitrates in African-American patients with systolic dysfunction (Table 4.6).

CARDIOMYOPATHY OF THE ELDERLY FEMALE

The most common cause of heart failure in elderly women is heart failure with preserved

LV systolic function, commonly referred to as diastolic dysfunction. Diastolic dysfunction refers to cardiac dysfunction in which LV filling is abnormal and is accompanied by elevated filling pressures.[34] Among patients who have heart failure, as many as 40–60% have normal systolic function.[34,35] In such patients, diastolic dysfunction is the presumed cause of the heart failure, which can be confirmed by objective measures.[34,36,37] The prevalence of diastolic dysfunction as the cause of heart failure increases with age.[34] A greater proportion of women than men have heart failure with preserved LV systolic function[38,39] (Table 4.7). The major causes[34] of isolated diastolic dysfunction include:

- chronic hypertension with LV hypertrophy[40]
- hypertensive hypertrophic cardiomyopathy in the elderly
- hypertrophic cardiomyopathy
- aortic stenosis with a normal LVEF
- ischemic heart disease
- restrictive cardiomyopathy, which can be idiopathic or caused by infiltrative diseases of the heart.

Relaxation of the contracted myocardium occurs at the onset of diastole. The rapid pressure decay and the concomitant relaxation and elastic recoil of the left ventricle produce a suction effect that augments the left atrial-to-left ventricular pressure gradient, thereby promoting diastolic filling. During the later phases of diastole, the normal left ventricle is composed of completely relaxed myocytes and is very compliant and easily distensible, offering minimal resistance to LV filling over a normal volume range. As a result, LV filling can normally be accomplished by very low filling pressures in the left atrium and pulmonary veins, preserving a low pulmonary capillary pressure (<12 mmHg). The contribution of atrial contraction is relatively small.

Loss of normal LV diastolic relaxation and distensibility, due to either structural (e.g. LVH) or functional (e.g. ischemia) causes, impairs LV filling. This results in increases in LV diastolic, left atrial, and pulmonary venous and

Table 4.6 Targeted doses for heart failure treatment

Therapy	Target dose	Reference
β-Blockers		
Carvedilol	37.5–44 mg/day	1, 3
Metoprolol	150 mg/day	2, 3
ACE inhibitors		
Quinapril	40 mg/day	3
Captopril	50 mg tid	3, 4
Lisinopril	40 mg/day	3
Enalapril	10 mg bid	3, 5
Angiotensin receptor blockers (ARBs)		
Losartan	50 mg/day	6
Valsartan	160 mg/day	7
Candesartan	32 mg/day	8
Aldosterone antagonist		
Aldactone	25 mg/day	9
Other		
Hydralazine + nitrate	titrate to 100 mg tid isosorbide dinitrate 40 mg tid or qid or isosorbide mononitrate 40–120 mg/day	10

1. Packer M, Bristow M, Cohn JN, et al. The effect of carvedilol on morbidity and mortality in patients with chronic heart failure. U.S. Carvedilol Heart Failure Study Group. N Engl J Med 1996; 334(21):1349.
2. Effect of metoprolol CR/XL in chronic heart failure. Metoprolol CR/XL Randomised Intervention Trial in Congestive Heart Failure (MERIT-HF). Lancet 1999; 353(9169):2001.
3. Hunt SA, Baker DW, Chin MH, et al. ACC/AHA guidelines for the evaluation and management of chronic heart failure in the adult: executive summary. J Am Coll Cardiol 2001; 38:2101.
4. Pfeffer MA, Braunwald E, Moye LA, et al. Effect of captopril on mortality and morbidity in patients with left ventricular dysfunction after myocardial infarction. Results of the survival and ventricular enlargement trial. The SAVE Investigators. N Engl J Med 1992; 327(10):669.
5. Effect of enalapril on survival in patients with reduced left ventricular ejection fractions and congestive heart failure. The SOLVD Investigators. N Engl J Med 1991; 325(5):293, and N Engl J Med 1992; 327(10):685.
6. Pitt B, Poole-Wilson PA, Segal R, et al. Effect of losartan compared with captopril on mortality in patients with symptomatic heart failure: randomised trial – the Losartan Heart Failure Survival Study ELITE II. Lancet 2000; 355(9215):1582.
7. Cohn JN, Tognoni G. A randomized trial of the angiotensin-receptor blocker valsartan in chronic heart failure. N Engl J Med 2001; 345(23):1667.
8. Granger CB, McMurray JJ, Yusuf S, et al. Effects of candesartan in patients with chronic heart failure and reduced left-ventricular systolic function intolerant to angiotensin-converting-enzyme inhibitors: the CHARM-Alternative trial. Lancet 2003; 362(9386):772.
9. Pitt B, Zannad F, Remme WJ, et al. The effect of spironolactone on morbidity and mortality in patients with severe heart failure. Randomized Aldactone Evaluation Study Investigators. N Engl J Med 1999; 341(10):709.
10. Cohn JN, Archibald DG, Ziesche S, et al. Effect of vasodilator therapy on mortality in chronic congestive heart failure. Results of a Veterans Administration Cooperative Study. N Engl J Med 1986; 314(24):1547.

pulmonary capillary pressures. The net effect is a relative shift of LV filling to the later part of diastole, with a greater dependence on atrial contraction. This analysis of diastolic heart failure is accepted by most experts in the field,[34] although it is challenged by some.[41]

Patients with diastolic dysfunction have particular difficulty in tolerating certain types of hemodynamic stress. They tolerate atrial fibrillation poorly, since the loss of atrial contraction can dramatically reduce left atrial emptying, LV filling, and LV stroke volume. They do not tolerate tachycardia well, since the increase in heart rate shortens the duration of diastole and truncates the important late phase of diastolic filling. Elevations in systemic blood pressure, especially the abrupt, severe, or refractory elevations often seen with renovas-

Table 4.7 Characteristics of patients with diastolic heart failure and patients with systolic heart failure

Characteristic	Diastolic heart failure	Systolic heart failure
Age	Elderly	All ages
Sex	More often female	More often male
LVEF	Preserved	Depressed
LV cavity size	Usually normal	Usually dilated
LVH on ECG	Usually present	Sometimes present
Chest X-ray	Congestion with or without cardiomegaly	Congestion and cardiomegaly
Gallop rhythm present	Fourth heart sound	Third heart sound
Coexisting conditions:		
Hypertension	+++	++
Diabetes mellitus	+++	++
Previous MI	+	+++
Obesity	+++	+
Chronic lung disease	++	−
Sleep apnea	++	−
Long-term dialysis	++	−
Atrial fibrillation	+	−

ECG, electrocardiography; LV, left ventricle; LVEF, left ventricular ejection fraction; LVH, left ventricular hypertrophy; MI, myocardial infarction.

cular hypertension, increase LV wall stress, which can worsen myocardial relaxation in patients with diastolic dysfunction. The acute induction or worsening of diastolic dysfunction by ischemia raises left atrial and therefore pulmonary venous pressure. This explains why many patients with coronary artery disease have respiratory symptoms with their anginal pain, including wheezing, shortness of breath, and overt pulmonary edema. These respiratory symptoms can occur in the absence of anginal pain and are often referred to as 'anginal equivalents.' Episodes of hemodynamic decompensation may result in pulmonary congestion or edema severe enough to be life-threatening. This phenomenon is referred to as flash pulmonary edema.

The diagnosis of diastolic dysfunction is often made, or presumed, in patients who have symptoms of heart failure and a normal LVEF by echocardiography. It is important to consider possible mimics of diastolic dysfunction. Among patients who have intact LV systolic function, symptoms suggestive of heart failure (such as shortness of breath, ankle edema, or paroxysmal nocturnal dyspnea) may be due to disorders such as obesity, lung disease, poorly controlled atrial fibrillation, and occult coronary ischemia.

Echocardiography can demonstrate that the LVEF and LV volume are normal in a patient with heart failure. It can also identify many of the causes of heart failure with intact LV function. These including LVH, regional wall motion abnormalities due to ischemic heart disease, constrictive pericarditis, severe mitral regurgitation, amyloidosis, hemochromatosis, or sarcoidosis. The distinction among causes of diastolic dysfunction, whether by echocardiography or by other means, is important, because some are responsive to specific therapies directed at the underlying disease.

Doppler echocardiography is an effective method of establishing the presence of abnormalities in diastolic function.[34,36,42] In patients with impaired relaxation, assessment of mitral valve inflow velocity may demonstrate diminished early diastolic filling velocity, manifested by an abnormally low E wave, and increased late diastolic filling, manifested by an increased A wave; as a result, the E/A ratio is less than 1.[34] In contrast, patients with reduced LV compliance have a restrictive pattern, which is associated with an increased E/A ratio. In addition to mitral valve inflow Doppler, tissue Doppler imaging and measurement of pulmonary vein blood flow velocity may also be helpful.

The plasma concentration of BNP is increased in patients with asymptomatic and symptomatic LV systolic dysfunction and can be used for both diagnosis and prognosis. Plasma BNP is also elevated in patients with diastolic dysfunction, but cannot be used to distinguish diastolic from systolic dysfunction.[43]

Treatment

The treatment of heart failure due to diastolic dysfunction remains empiric, since trial data are limited. Guidelines for treatment of patients with heart failure due to diastolic dysfunction were published in 2001 by an ACC/AHA Task Force.[44] It was concluded that the weight of evidence supported only four modalities:

- control of systolic and diastolic hypertension
- control of ventricular rate in patients with atrial fibrillation
- control of pulmonary congestion and peripheral edema with diuretics
- coronary revascularization in patients with coronary artery disease in whom ischemia is judged to have an adverse effect on diastolic function.

An important caveat is that the patient who has LV diastolic dysfunction with a small, stiff LV chamber is particularly susceptible to excessive preload reduction, which can lead sequentially to underfilling of the left ventricle, a fall in cardiac output, and hypotension. In patients with severe LVH due to hypertension or hypertrophic cardiomyopathy (HCM), excessive preload reduction can also create a dynamic subaortic outflow obstruction.

For these reasons, the administration of diuretics or venodilators such as nitrates, dihydropyridine calcium channel blockers, and ACE inhibitors must be performed with caution. Careful attention is required for

symptoms of ventricular underfilling such as weakness, dizziness, near syncope, and syncope.

The choice of medications in patients with diastolic dysfunction is determined by two factors. First, the major goal is to treat specific underlying processes such as hypertension or symptomatic coronary artery disease. Combined therapy may be warranted since hypertrophied hearts are more sensitive to the deleterious effects of ischemia on LV relaxation than non-hypertrophied hearts.[45] The second goal is to evaluate the possibility of beneficial drug effect on the pathophysiology of diastolic dysfunction.

LV filling in diastolic dysfunction occurs primarily in late diastole and is therefore more dependent than normal hearts on atrial contraction. Tachycardia is also deleterious by shortening the time of diastole. For these reasons, restoration and maintenance of sinus rhythm is preferred when atrial fibrillation occurs in patients with diastolic dysfunction. When this cannot be achieved, rate control becomes important. β-Blockers and calcium channel blockers are the usual first-line agents. A combination of these drugs may be required to achieve adequate heart rate control. It is important to measure heart rate during moderate exercise and not to base heart rate control solely on values obtained in the resting state. An important component of the management of atrial fibrillation, regardless of whether rhythm control or rate control is chosen, is anticoagulation to prevent systemic embolization.

β-Blockers have a variety of beneficial effects in patients with diastolic dysfunction, including slowing the heart rate (which increases the time available for both LV filling and coronary flow, particularly during exercise), reducing myocardial oxygen demand, and, by lowering the blood pressure, causing regression of LVH. Slowing the heart rate is particularly important in the treatment of pulmonary congestion due to ischemic diastolic dysfunction and, as noted above, in patients in atrial fibrillation. β-Blockers may also directly improve diastolic function in patients with idiopathic dilated cardiomyopathy and those with an acute MI; both are settings in which β-blockers are recommended because they improve survival.[46] Slowing of the heart rate may contribute to this effect by providing more time for calcium exit from myocytes, thereby reversing the cellular calcium overload characteristic of diastolic dysfunction.

Exercise conditioning

During exercise in healthy individuals, diastolic function is enhanced so that LV input remains precisely matched to LV output, despite the shortened duration of diastole resulting from the associated tachycardia. This is achieved in the normal left ventricle by a rapid and marked decrease in intraventricular pressure during early diastole, thereby creating a greater LV 'suction' effect, which enhances the transmitral pressure gradient without increasing left atrial pressure and compromising pulmonary function. This mechanism is lost in patients with diastolic dysfunction; as a result, dyspnea with exertion is often their most common complaint.

Long-term exercise training produces physiologic cardiac hypertrophy with enhanced diastolic function. Experimental animal studies suggest that exercise conditioning has the potential to reverse the diastolic dysfunction of pathologic LVH or aging.[47] It is not known if exercise training is beneficial in patients with diastolic dysfunction. Any exercise training program for the potential treatment of diastolic dysfunction should be based upon dynamic isotonic exercise, not static exercise, since the latter causes changes in cardiac geometry similar to those of hypertensive LVH.

PREVENTIVE STRATEGIES

As heart failure has become an epidemic, focus should be on prevention of heart failure as well as the treatment of established heart failure. The Heart Outcomes Prevention Evaluation (HOPE) trial was a large, randomized, placebo-controlled trial that evaluated the ACE inhibitor ramipril in high-risk patients without clinical heart failure or known decrease in LV systolic dysfunction. All participants in the trial were 55 years or older, had established vascular disease (involving the coronary, cerebral, or peripheral circulation) or diabetes mellitus plus one additional cardiovascular risk factor (elevated total cholesterol, low high-density lipoprotein cholesterol, hypertension, known microalbuminuria, or current cigarette smoking) and thus were considered high risk for the development of CHF.

The primary end point of the HOPE trial was a composite of MI, stroke, and cardiovascular death. Among women in this study, the primary end-point incidence was reduced 23%.[48] The risk of stroke declined 36%, and the risk of cardiovascular death saw a 38% reduction. Additionally, there was a trend toward decreased incidence of MI, heart failure, and all-cause mortality. The beneficial effects of ACE inhibitor therapy were additive to other medications with known cardioprotective effects or favorable actions on cardiovascular risk factors, including β-blockers (taken by 34% of women in the HOPE trial), aspirin or other antiplatelet agents (taken by 64% of enrollees), and cholesterol-lowering agents (initially taken by 30% increasing to 50% by the end of the study). The magnitude of the observed benefit for ACE inhibition was similar in men and women.

At baseline, women were slightly older than men and were more likely to have a history of peripheral arterial disease, hypertension, diabetes mellitus, and hypercholesterolemia. They were less likely to have a history of coronary artery disease, previous MI, angina pectoris, or prior revascularization procedure. Overall, men had worse outcomes when compared with women. This outcome difference persisted after adjustment for differences in baseline characteristics.

MECHANICAL AND SURGICAL INTERVENTION

Recent studies have demonstrated that mechanical interventions have additional benefits for the heart failure patient. Biventricular pacing (a left lateral venous lead in concert with the standard right ventricular lead) has led to improved symmetry of contractions, improved treadmill times, improved Minnesota Life Scale Scores, improved ejection fractions, and also decreased mitral insufficiency. Candidates are patients with low ejection fractions, i.e. below

35%, and a QRS duration that is wide (>0.12 seconds). The evidence for these findings is strongly supported by the MIRACLE trial. In addition, there are other trials currently underway looking at long-term outcomes such as RESTORE.

In addition, patients with cardiomyopathy and low ejection fractions of less than 30% are at high risk for sudden cardiac death. This is particularly seen in NYHA Class II and Class III patients. Recent trials have shown improved survival in patients with ejection fractions under 35% who have prophylactic defibrillators placed in comparison with standard treatment or amiodarone antiarrhythmic therapy.

Transplantation remains an option for Class IV patients who fail to respond to medical therapy. Survival rates post transplant are reportedly 80–90% at 1 year, 65–80% at 5 years, and 40% in 12 years. Women represent 20% of the heart transplant recipients and have an increased risk of rejection and a higher mortality rate at 1 year when compared with men.[49]

SUMMARY

In general, women with heart failure tend to be older, are more likely to have diabetes,[50] are less likely to have ischemic etiologies of heart failure, and are more likely to have heart failure related to hypertension and valvular disease,[50] and heart failure from diastolic dysfunction occurs more often in women.[51] Women have been underrepresented in major heart failure trials, in part due to the age limits and systolic causes that are examined in those trials. Women therefore pose a treatment challenge because they present with heart failure at an older age, have a different comorbidity profile, and often present with a greater degree of diastolic dysfunction than men;[50,52] therefore they constitute a population that significantly deviates from those found in large clinical trials.[53] Gender-specific differences in myocardial adaptations to physiologic stress may play a role in these clinical variations, which emphasizes the importance of addressing future trials to evaluate therapies specifically for women.[50] We cannot assume results in men can be generalized to women.

REFERENCES

1. American Heart Association. 2000 Heart and Stroke Statistical Update. Available at http://www.americanheart.org/statistics/index.html.
2. Luchi R, Taffet G, Teasdale T. Congestive heart failure in the elderly. J Am Geriatr Soc 1991; 39:810.
3. Hunt SA, Baker DW, Chin ML, et al. ACC/AHA guidelines for the evaluation and management of chronic heart failure in the adult – executive summary. J Am Coll Cardiol 2001; 38:2101.
4. Levy D, Larsen MG, Vasan RS, et al. The progression from hypertension to congestive heart failure. JAMA 1996; 275:1557.
5. He J, Ogden LG, Bazzano LA, et al. Risk factors for congestive heart failure in US men and women. NHANES I epidemiology follow-up study. Arch Intern Med 2001; 161:996.
6. McKee P, Castelli W, McNamara P, et al. Natural history of congestive heart failure: the Framingham Study. N Engl J Med 1971; 285:1441.
7. Ho K, Anderson K, Kannel W, et al. Survival after onset of congestive heart failure in the Framingham Heart Study subjects. Circulation 1993; 88:107.
8. The SOLVD Investigators. Effects of enalapril on survival in patients with reduced left ventricular ejection fraction and congestive heart failure. N Engl J Med 1991; 325:293.
9. Bourassa MG, Gurne O, Bangdiwala SI, et al. Natural history and patterns of current practice in heart failure. J Am Coll Cardiol 1993; 22(Suppl A):14A.
10. Ghali JK, Pina IL, Gottleib SS, et al. Metoprolol CR/XL in female patients with heart failure. Analysis of the experience in Metoprolol Extended-Release Randomized Intervention Trial in Heart Failure (MERIT-HF). Circulation 2002; 105:1585.
11. Adams KF Jr, Dunlap SH, Sueta CA, et al. Relation between gender, etiology and survival in patients with symptomatic heart failure. J Am Coll Cardiol 1996; 28:1781.
12. Sliwa K, Skudicky D, Bergemann A, et al. Peripartum cardiomyopathy: analysis of clinical outcome, left ventricular function, plasma levels of cytokines and Fas/APO-1. J Am Coll Cardiol 2000; 35:701.
13. Pearson GD, Veille JC, Rahimtoola S, et al. Peripartum cardiomyopathy: National Heart, Lung, and Blood Institute and Office of Rare Diseases (National Institutes of Health) workshop recommendations and review. JAMA 2000; 283:1183.
14. Cenac A, Beaufils H, Soumana I, et al. Absence of humoral autoimmunity in peripartum cardiomyopathy. A comparative study in Niger. Int J Cardiol 1990; 26:49.
15. Pearl W. Familial occurrence of peripartum cardiomyopathy. Am Heart J 1995; 129:421.

16. Midei MG, DeMent SH, Feldman AM, et al. Peripartum myocarditis and cardiomyopathy. Circulation 1990; 81:922.

17. O'Connell JB, Costanzo-Nordin MR, Subramanian R, et al. Peripartum cardiomyopathy: clinical, hemodynamic, histologic and prognostic characteristics. J Am Coll Cardiol 1986; 8:52.

18. Rizeq MN, Rickenbacher PR, Fowler MB, et al. Incidence of myocarditis in peripartum cardiomyopathy. Am J Cardiol 1994; 74:474.

19. Demakis JG, Rahimtoola SH, Sutton GC, et al. Natural course of peripartum cardiomyopathy. Circulation 1971; 44:1053.

20. Manolio TA, Baughman KL, Rodeheffer R, et al. Prevalence and etiology of idiopathic dilated cardiomyopathy (summary of a National Heart, Lung and Blood Institute workshop). Am J Cardiol 1992; 69:1458.

21. Hibbard JU, Lindheimer M, Lang RM. A modified definition for peripartum cardiomyopathy and prognosis based on echocardiography. Obstet Gynecol 1999; 94:311.

22. Hadjimiltiades S, Panidis IP, Segal BL, Iskandrian AS. Recovery of left ventricular function in peripartum cardiomyopathy. Am Heart J 1986; 112:1097.

23. Felker GM, Jaeger CJ, Klodas E, et al. Myocarditis and long-term survival in peripartum cardiomyopathy. Am Heart J 2000; 140:785.

24. Elkayam U, Tummala PP, Rao K, et al. Maternal and fetal outcomes of subsequent pregnancies in women with peripartum cardiomyopathy. N Engl J Med 2001; 344:1567.

25. Allman KC, Shaw LJ, Hachamovitch R, Udelson JE. Myocardial viability testing and impact of revascularization on prognosis in patients with coronary artery disease and left ventricular dysfunction: a meta-analysis. J Am Coll Cardiol 2002; 39:1151.

26. Elefteriades JA, Tolis G Jr, Levi E, et al. Coronary artery bypass grafting in severe left ventricular dysfunction: excellent survival and improved EF and functional state. J Am Coll Cardiol 1993; 22:1411.

27. Dec GW, Fuster,V. Idiopathic dilated cardiomyopathy. N Engl J Med 1994; 331:1564.

28. Felker GM, Thompson RE, Hare JM, et al. Underlying causes and long-term survival in patients with initially unexplained cardiomyopathy. N Engl J Med 2000; 342(15):1077.

29. Barbaro G, Di Lorenzo G, Grisorio B, et al. Incidence of dilated cardiomyopathy and detection of HIV in myocardial cells of HIV-positive patients. N Engl J Med 1998; 339:1093.

30. Corey WA, Markel ML, Hoit BD, Walsh RA. Regression of a dilated cardiomyopathy after radiofrequency ablation of incessant supraventricular tachycardia. Am Heart J 1993; 126:1469.

31. Packer DL, Bardy GH, Worley SJ, et al. Tachycardia-induced cardiomyopathy: A reversible form of left ventricular dysfunction. Am J Cardiol 1986; 57:563.

32. Malone S, Liu PP, Holloway R, et al. Obstructive sleep apnea in patients with dilated cardiomyopathy: Effects of continuous positive airway pressure. Lancet 1991; 338:1480.

33. Kantharia BK, Hanno RB, Battaglia J. Reversible dilated cardiomyopathy: an unusual case of thyrotoxicosis. Am Heart J 1995; 129:1030.

34. Zile MR, Brutsaert DL. New concepts in diastolic dysfunction and diastolic heart failure: Part I: diagnosis, prognosis, and measurements of diastolic function. Circulation 2002; 105:1387.

35. Banerjee P, Banerjee T, Khand A, et al. Diastolic heart failure: neglected or misdiagnosed? J Am Coll Cardiol 2002; 39:138.

36. Zile MR, Gaasch WH, Carroll JD, et al. Heart failure with a normal ejection fraction: is measurement of diastolic function necessary to make the diagnosis of diastolic heart failure? Circulation 2001; 104:779.

37. Zile MR, Baicu CF, Gaasch WH. Diastolic heart failure – abnormalities in active relaxation and passive stiffness of the left ventricle. N Engl J Med 2004; 350:1953.

38. Masoudi FA, Havranek EP, Smith G, et al. Gender, age, and heart failure with preserved left ventricular systolic function. J Am Coll Cardiol 2003; 41:217.

39. Kitzman DW, Gardin JM, Gottdiener JS. Importance of heart failure with preserved systolic function in patients > or =65 years of age. Am J Cardiol 2001; 87:413.

40. Vasan RS, Levy D. The role of hypertension in the pathogenesis of heart failure. A clinical mechanistic overview. Arch Intern Med 1996; 156:1789.

41. Burkhoff D, Maurer MS, Packer M. Heart failure with a normal ejection fraction: is it really a disorder of diastolic function? Circulation 2003; 107:656.

42. Cohen GI, Pietrolungo JF, Thomas JD, et al. A practical guide to assessment of ventricular diastolic function using Doppler echocardiography. J Am Coll Cardiol 1996; 27:1753.

43. Maisel AS, Koon J, Krishnaswamy P, et al. Utility of B-natriuretic peptide as a rapid, point-of-care test for screening patients undergoing echocardiography to determine left ventricular dysfunction. Am Heart J 2001; 141:367.

44. Hunt SA, Baker DW, Chin MH, et al. ACC/AHA guidelines for the evaluation and management of chronic heart failure in the adult: executive summary. A report of the American College of Cardiology/ American Heart Association task force on practice guidelines (committee to revise the 1995 guidelines for the evaluation and management of heart failure) developed in collaboration with the International

Society for Heart and Lung Transplantation endorsed by the Heart Failure Society of America. J Am Coll Cardiol 2001; 38:2101.

45. Eberli FR, Apstein CS, Ngoy S, Lorell BH. Exacerbation of left ventricular ischemic diastolic dysfunction by pressure-overload hypertrophy. Modification by specific inhibition of cardiac angiotensin converting enzyme. Circ Res 1992; 70:931.

46. Andersson B, Caidahl K, di Lenarada A, et al. Changes in early and late diastolic filling patterns induced by long-term adrenergic β-blockade in patients with idiopathic dilated cardiomyopathy. Circulation 1996; 94:673.

47. Brenner DA, Apstein CS, Saupe KW. Exercise training attenuates age-associated diastolic dysfunction in rats. Circulation 2001; 104:221.

48. The Heart Outcomes Prevention Evaluation Study Investigators. Effects of an angiotensin-converting-enzyme inhibitor, ramipril, on cardiovascular events in high-risk patients. N Engl J Med 2000; 342:145.

49. Wechsler ME, Giardina EV, Sciacca RR, et al. Valvular heart disease/cardiac transplantation: increased early mortality in women undergoing cardiac transplantation. Circulation 1995; 91(4):1029.

50. Lorell BH, Stevenson LW. Congestive heart failure. In: Wilansky S, Willerson JT, eds. Heart Disease in Women. Philadelphia: Elsevier Science; 2002: 311.

51. Tendera M. Aging and heart failure: the place of ACE inhibitors in heart failure with preserved systolic function. Eur Heart J 2000; 2 (Suppl I):I8.

52. Richardson LG, Rocks M. Women and heart failure. Heart Lung 2001; 30:87.

53. Heiat A, Gross CP, Krumholz HM. Representation of the elderly, women, and minorities in heart failure clinical trials. Arch Intern Med 2002; 162:1682.

5

Valvular heart disease

Punit Goel and Kul Aggarwal

Introduction • Mitral stenosis • Mitral regurgitation • Mitral valve prolapse • Aortic stenosis • Aortic regurgitation • Tricuspid valve disease • Pulmonic valve disease • Prosthetic heart valves • Pregnancy and valvular heart disease • Valvular heart disease associated with 'collagen' or rheumatic disorders • Endocarditis

INTRODUCTION

Valvular heart disease is an important cause of cardiovascular morbidity and mortality. Recent advances in the evaluation and management of this group of disorders have resulted in improved patient outcomes. Many of the valvular problems are equally common among men and women, but several are more common in women. These include mitral stenosis (MS), mitral valve prolapse (MVP) syndrome, and valvular heart diseases associated with collagen vascular disorders such as systemic lupus erythematosus (SLE). Cardiomyopathies are often associated with mitral and tricuspid regurgitation and will not be further discussed in this section. Pregnancy places additional hemodynamic burden, and patients with MS, pulmonary hypertension and severe aortic stenosis (AS) and those with prosthetic heart valves have increased fetal and maternal morbidity and mortality. Cardiovascular drugs also pose potential hazards in pregnancy. Treatment of advanced valvular disease is generally surgical but severe mitral stenosis and pulmonic stenosis can be treated by balloon valvuloplasty.

MITRAL STENOSIS

Etiology and pathology

Two-thirds of all patients with MS are female.[1] Rheumatic fever is the predominant cause of MS in 99% of mitral valves excised during mitral valve replacement. Approximately 25% of patients with rheumatic heart disease have pure MS and 40% have combined MS and mitral regurgitation (MR). Rheumatic fever causes fusion of the components of the mitral apparatus, leading to a funnel-shaped deformity of the valve with a 'fish mouth' or button hole-shaped mitral orifice.[2] Rare causes of MS include congenital, malignant carcinoid, SLE, rheumatoid arthritis, and certain storage disorders. Chronic hypercalcemia from various causes leads to calcium deposition in the valvular cusps and fibrous skeleton of heart. Calcification of mitral annulus usually causes regurgitation; however, MS may result if leaflet or subvalvular involvement is extensive. Conditions which cause obstruction to left atrial (LA) outflow and simulate MS include LA tumors, ball valve thrombus, infective endocarditis with large vegetations, and cor triatriatum.

Pathophysiology

In normal adults the mitral valve orifice area is 4–6 cm^2. MS is considered to be mild when the valve area is <2 cm^2 and critical when it is <1 cm^2. In critical MS, a mean left atrial pressure of approximately 25 mmHg is required to maintain adequate forward cardiac output at rest.[3] High LA pressure leads to pulmonary venous hypertension manifesting as dyspnea, initially on exertion and subsequently at rest. The pressure gradient across the mitral valve depends upon valve area and flow across the valve. The flow across the valve in turn depends upon heart rate and cardiac output. Increase in heart rate leads to increase in flow and disproportionate decrease in diastolic period during which mitral flow occurs. This leads to further elevation of LA pressure and gradients across the mitral valve, with worsening of symptoms. Conditions which decrease diastolic flow period (atrial fibrillation with fast ventricular response) or cause increased flow across the mitral valve (pregnancy, anemia, hyperthyroidism) increase transvalvular gradients.

High LA pressure leads to pulmonary hypertension due to passive backward transmission of pressure, pulmonary arteriolar constriction, and obliterative changes in pulmonary vasculature. High pulmonary pressure results in right-sided heart failure. Combination of high LA pressure, mitral valve disease, and atrial inflammation causes structural changes in the atrial wall, leading to the onset of atrial fibrillation.[4]

Clinical features

The interval between initial rheumatic fever and development of symptoms due to MS is generally about two decades; however, rapid progression has been found in younger patients in developing countries. Patients with mild MS may be asymptomatic. Exertional dyspnea is the main initial symptom due to pulmonary venous congestion and interstitial edema. It may be associated with cough and wheezing and may progress to orthopnea and pulmonary edema. Systemic embolization from thrombus in LA appendage may be a presenting feature in patients with even mild MS. Hemoptysis results from rupture of pulmonary bronchial venous connection due to venous hypertension and is usually not fatal. Chest pain occurs in 10% of cases and may be secondary to pulmonary hypertension or associated coronary artery disease. Infective endocarditis is rare in pure MS but is not uncommon in combined MS and MR.

On examination, the systemic arterial pressure is normal or mildly reduced, the pulse may be irregular due to atrial fibrillation, and

jugular venous pressure may be elevated due to right-heart failure. On cardiac auscultation, the first heart sound is accentuated due to delayed closure of the mitral valve. The second heart sound may be accentuated due to pulmonary hypertension. A low-pitched diastolic murmur is audible at apex. The length of murmur correlates with MS severity. A pansystolic murmur may be audible along the left lower sternal border due to tricuspid regurgitation secondary to pulmonary hypertension.

Laboratory evaluation

An electrocardiogram (ECG) during sinus rhythm may reveal P-wave abnormalities suggestive of atrial enlargement. Right ventricular hypertrophy due to pulmonary hypertension leads to right-axis deviation. A chest X-ray reveals straightening of the left heart border, dilatation of the upper lobe pulmonary veins, and displacement of the esophagus due to enlarged LA.

The echocardiogram is the most useful test for assessment of MS. It demonstrates thickened, calcified, stenotic valves with poor leaflet separation in diastole (Figure 5.1), cardiac chamber sizes, and ventricular function. A transesophageal echocardiogram is more sensitive in detecting LA appendage thrombus.

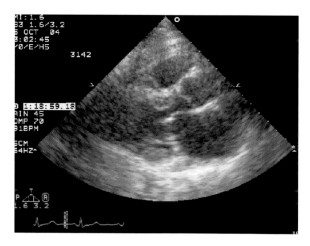

Figure 5.1 Transthoracic echocardiogram in a parasternal long-axis view demonstrating thickened leaflets of the mitral valve with restricted opening in a patient with mitral stenosis.

Doppler echocardiography provides assessment of MS severity and estimation of pulmonary hypertension. Cardiac catheterization and angiography is not usually necessary in decision-making in young patients with typical findings for severe MS by clinical examination and echocardiography.[5] It may be useful to clarify the issue when discrepancy exists between clinical and echocardiographic findings, in assessing associated valvular lesions and in patients with possible coronary stenosis.

Treatment

Patients with rheumatic mitral valve disease need chronic penicillin prophylaxis for rheumatic fever[6] and prophylaxis for infective endocarditis.[7] Symptomatic patients may benefit from salt restriction and oral diuretics. Digoxin and β-blockers reduce ventricular rate in atrial fibrillation and reduce gradients across the mitral valve with improvement in symptoms. Chronic oral anticoagulation is indicated for patients with atrial fibrillation or a history of prior embolization. Conversion to sinus rhythm may be considered in patients with recent-onset atrial fibrillation not associated with a severely dilated LA.

Mitral valvotomy is indicated in symptomatic patients with mitral valve area $<1.0 \text{ cm}^2/\text{m}^2$ body surface area in the absence of significant MR. It can be performed percutaneously or surgically. Valvotomy improves symptoms and hemodynamics, with improvement in survival. Valvotomy is not indicated in asymptomatic patients, regardless of MS severity unless recurrent systemic embolization has occurred. In pregnant patients, valvotomy (surgical or percutaneous) may be carried out if pulmonary congestion occurs despite intensive medical therapy.[8] Symptomatic patients with significant MR usually require valve replacement.

MITRAL REGURGITATION

Etiology and pathology

The mitral valve is a complex structure composed of the mitral valve annulus, leaflets, chordae tendineae, and papillary muscles. Structural or functional abnormalities of any of these components could lead to MR.[9] The leading causes of MR include MVP, ischemic heart disease, rheumatic heart disease (RHD), infective endocarditis, cardiomyopathy, and annular calcification. Uncommon causes include carcinoid, appetite-suppressant medications, collagen vascular disorders, trauma, and hypereosinophilic syndrome. Unlike MS, predominant MR due to RHD is more common in men, whereas MR secondary to annular calcification is more common in women.

Pathophysiology

The presence of MR provides an additional receiving chamber for left ventricular (LV) emptying with low impedance compared with the aorta, leading to enhanced ventricular emptying. In the initial stages of MR, the left ventricle compensates by more complete emptying due to reduced afterload, leading to reduced end-systolic volume and increased ejection fraction. As MR becomes chronic, the LV end-diastolic volume increases, mitral annular diameter increases, and end-systolic volume returns to normal. High LV end-diastolic volume leads to increased wall stress and, coupled with increased annular size, leads to further MR ('MR begets MR'). In most patients with chronic severe MR, the compensation is maintained for several years, but prolonged volume overload ultimately leads to myocardial decompensation. However, two studies have reported that patients with severe MR, even if asymptomatic, have a low likelihood of remaining asymptomatic and stable over 10 years of follow-up.[10,11]

Clinical features

Factors that influence symptoms in patients with chronic MR include severity and duration of MR, rate of progression, pressures in the left atrium and pulmonary artery, atrial arrhythmias, and associated valvular, myocardial, or coronary artery disease. Patients with chronic severe MR may be relatively asymptomatic during the initial course of the disease. Chronic weakness and fatigue due to low forward output are more common in MR than in MS. However, by the time symptoms of low output are apparent, serious and irreversible LV dysfunction may have developed. Unlike AS or regurgitation, angina pectoris is rare, unless coexisting coronary artery disease is present. Right-sided heart failure develops following development of pulmonary hypertension or severe acute MR. The rate of progression is higher in MR associated with Marfan syndrome or other connective tissue disorders.

Physical examination reveals sharp and rapid carotid upstroke, and hyperdynamic cardiac impulse which is displaced to the left. Cardiac auscultation demonstrates diminished first heart sound, and widely split second heart sound with accentuated pulmonary component. Third heart sound may be audible due to increased and rapid ventricular filling without concomitant ventricular dysfunction. A pansystolic murmur is the most prominent auscultatory finding. There is little correlation between murmur intensity and MR severity.

Laboratory evaluation

An ECG may reveal LA enlargement and atrial fibrillation; one-third of patients may have LV enlargement. A chest X-ray commonly reveals cardiomegaly with LA and LV enlargement in chronic severe MR. An echocardiogram reveals a dilated left atrium and left ventricle. Structural abnormality of the mitral apparatus, causing MR, and its suitability for repair is better delineated by transesophageal echocardiography. Cardiac catheterization with left ventriculography and coronary angiography is indicated in patients with discrepancy between clinical and echocardiographic findings and also to assess other valvular abnormalities or coexisting coronary artery disease.

Management

The role of pharmacologic therapy in chronic severe MR is debatable, since afterload is already reduced. Currently, there is no strong evidence for the use of angiotensin-converting enzyme (ACE) inhibitors or β-blockers in asymptomatic patients with normal blood pressure and normal ventricular function.[12] All patients with atrial fibrillation should receive anticoagulation and all patients with MR should receive endocarditis prophylaxis. Surgical therapy is indicated for symptomatic patients with severe MR or asymptomatic patients with evidence of progressive LV dilatation or onset of LV dysfunction. MV repair, if feasible, is preferable to replacement, as it has lower operative mortality, avoids the need for long-term anticoagulation, preserves LV geometry and function postoperatively, and eliminates the future risk of prosthetic valve dysfunction or endocarditis.

Acute MR

The predominant causes of acute MR include infective endocarditis, rupture of chordae tendinae, papillary muscle dysfunction, and prosthetic valve dysfunction. Acute severe MR causes a marked reduction in forward cardiac output, with abrupt elevation of LA pressure, leading to pulmonary edema. The murmur of an acute MR may be decrescendo, with an accentuated pulmonary component of second heart sound. An echocardiogram reveals hypercontractile LV with severe MR. Afterload reduction with nitroprusside with addition of dobutamine for positive inotropy is important in this setting and may be life saving. An intra-aortic balloon pump may further help in stabilization prior to surgery, which is the definitive therapy.

MITRAL VALVE PROLAPSE

MVP is the most common cause of isolated MR requiring surgery in the United States.[13] It is also the leading condition predisposing to infective endocarditis. Like MR, MVP could result from pathologic involvement of any component of the MV apparatus. It is twice as common in women and, by echocardiographic criteria, is believed to occur in 2.4% of the general population.[14] It is characterized by more than 2 mm displacement of mitral leaflet(s) above the annular plane. MR results when the leaflet edges do not coapt.

Etiology and pathology

The most common form of MVP is associated with connective tissue disorders such as Marfan syndrome, Ehlers–Danlos syndrome, and osteogenesis imperfecta. Pathologic findings include myxomatous proliferation of MV with increase in acid mucopolysaccharide.[15] The leaflets become redundant and prolapsed. The valve cusps, annulus, and chordae tendineae may all be affected by myxomatous proliferation. Associated collagen degeneration within chordae tendineae leads to loss of tensile strength with risk of chordal rupture.[16] Myxomatous changes may also involve other valves.

Clinical features

In some patients, MVP is transmitted as an autosomal dominant trait with variable penetrance. Most patients with MVP are asymptomatic. Many patients report non-specific symptoms; however, their relationship to MVP has not been demonstrated. Patients may complain of chest pain, shortness of breath, palpitations, presyncope, or syncope. Auscultation reveals non-ejection click followed by mid to late systolic murmur. The length of the murmur correlates with the severity of MR. Maneuvers which decrease LV volume lead to earlier occurrence of MVP, with prolongation of murmur and vice versa. Most patients remain asymptomatic for many years. The serious complications include atrial arrhythmias, infective endocarditis, embolic events, and congestive heart failure (CHF). Risk factors for progression to severe MR and endocarditis include the presence of systolic click with murmur, thickened (>5 mm) and redundant leaflets, men older than 50 years of age. Major risk factors for morbidity and mortality include moderate or severe MR and/or LV ejection fraction 0.50.[17]

Laboratory evaluation

The ECG is normal in the majority of patients, with a few demonstrating non-specific ST- and T-wave abnormalities. Premature atrial and

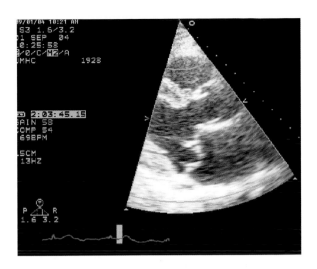

Figure 5.2 Transthoracic echocardiogram in a parasternal long-axis view showing mitral valve prolapse.

ventricular contractions, atrial and ventricular tachyarrhythmias, sinus and atrioventricular nodal dysfunction have been observed in MVP. It is also associated with Wolff–Parkinson–White syndrome. Echocardiography demonstrates myxomatous changes in valve leaflets, with prolapsing of leaflets into the left atrium above the mitral annular plane (Figure 5.2), location and severity of MR, cardiac chamber sizes, and LV function. Indications for angiography are similar to those for MR without MVP.

Treatment

Asymptomatic patients with no arrhythmias on ECG and without MR have an excellent prognosis and should be reassured and have follow-up examination, including an echocardiogram every 3–5 years. Patients with long systolic murmur should be evaluated annually. Endocarditis prophylaxis is recommended for patients with click and murmur or those with click associated with myxomatous changes of the mitral valve. Patients with history of palpitations, dizziness, and syncope should have Holter monitoring and exercise ECG. Electrophysiologic studies may be considered for further evaluation, as there is small risk of sudden death. Aspirin must be given to patients with embolic events not explained by any other coexisting disorder. The threshold for surgery when severe MR is present is lower in these patients than in patients having severe MR without MVP, since repair is usually feasible.

AORTIC STENOSIS

Aortic valve (AV) stenosis may be congenital, rheumatic, or degenerative. Isolated AS is more common in men and is rarely rheumatic in origin.[18,19] Congenital AS is most often due to a bicuspid aortic valve. A bicuspid AV is not usually stenotic at birth, but abnormal flow characteristics leads to fibrosis, rigidity, and calcification, leading to a stenotic valve in adulthood. Rheumatic AS results from commissural fusion, often associated with leaflet retraction, and leading to AS that is often combined with aortic regurgitation (AR). Degenerative AS is the most common cause of AS in adults.[20] It is secondary to leaflet calcification and leads to immobilization without commissural fusion. Increasing evidence suggests similar pathophysiologic features between degenerative AS and atherosclerosis, with experimental evidence suggesting that aggressive preventive measures may retard this process.[21]

Pathophysiology and clinical features

The normal AV area is 3–4 cm^2. Severe AS is defined as an AV area <1 cm^2. The natural history of AS has a long latent period during which there is gradually progressive obstruction to LV ejection, leading to increased afterload, which is compensated by left ventricular hypertrophy (LVH), which maintains cardiac output and reduces wall stress. The important clinical manifestations include angina, syncope, exertional shortness of breath, and CHF. Angina occurs in two-thirds of patients with critical AS, half of whom do not have significant epicardial coronary stenosis. In these patients, anginal symptoms are caused by impaired coronary vasodilator reserve[22] of the hypertrophied ventricle, resulting in an imbalance between oxygen supply and demand. Syncope is due to reflex-mediated bradycardia and vasodilation from activation of cardiac afferent nerves. The associated drop in blood pressure produces reduced cerebral perfusion and ultimately syncope in the most extreme cases.[23]

Symptoms and signs of CHF are usually late in the course of disease. Prognosis is poor in the absence of definitive treatment once symptoms develop. The average survival is 5 years after the onset of angina, 3 years after onset of syncope, and 2 years after onset of heart failure.[24]

The arterial pulse is slow rising, small, and sustained. A systolic blood pressure exceeding 200 mmHg is rare in severe AS. Carotid palpation reveals shudder due to coarse systolic vibrations. The cardiac apical impulse is sustained. A systolic thrill may be palpable in the aortic area and is specific for severe AS. Auscultation reveals a prominent ejection systolic murmur with audible fourth heart sounds, ejection click, and a diminished aortic component of second heart sound. When heart failure ensues, the systolic murmur becomes shorter and may disappear altogether.

Laboratory evaluation

LVH is the predominant finding on ECG; however, absence of LVH does not exclude severe AS. Other abnormalities include left atrium enlargement, pseudoinfarction pattern, atrial fibrillation, and atrioventricular conduction abnormalities. A chest X-ray reveals normal heart size in the absence of heart failure, and poststenotic dilatation of the ascending

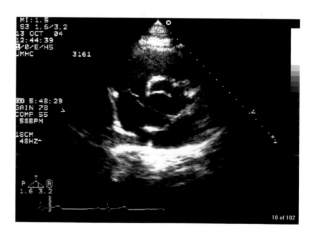

Figure 5.3 Transthoracic echocardiogram showing a bicuspid aortic valve in the parasternal short-axis view.

aorta. Echocardiography demonstrates valvular morphology (Figure 5.3), ventricular size, wall thickness and function, and coexisting valvular abnormalities. Doppler echocardiography allows the measurement of gradients across the aortic valve and calculation of the AV area. The principal indication for cardiac catheterization in patients with AS is to identify coexisting coronary artery disease if clinically indicated in patients being considered for surgery. Invasive hemodynamic assessment is indicated when there is a discrepancy between the clinical and echocardiographic assessments of severity.

Treatment

Asymptomatic patients have an excellent prognosis; however, they must be advised about endocarditis prophylaxis and to report any symptoms probably related to AS. Those with critical stenosis should be cautioned to avoid strenuous athletic and physical activity. Patients with mild AS should have a Doppler echocardiographic examination every 2 years and those with severe AS should have it every 6–12 months to assess decline in LV function. Exercise testing may help to unmask symptoms in patients with severe AS who may have modified their lifestyles to minimize symptoms.

Symptomatic patients with severe AS require aortic valve replacement (AVR). Surgery is also recommended if there is evidence of progression of LV dysfunction or abnormal hemodynamic response to exercise. Prophylactic AVR in asymptomatic patients with critical AS alone is not recommended.[25] The surgical risk is higher in patients with LV dysfunction; however, many patients in this group have significant improvement after surgery. Results with percutaneous balloon aortic valvuloplasty are disappointing due to high rates of restenosis at 6 months; however, it acts as a 'bridge' to valve replacement surgery in critically ill patients. Newer percutaneous methods for AVR in seriously ill patients are under development.

AORTIC REGURGITATION

AR may be caused by primary disease involving the leaflets or the wall of the aortic root. The leading causes of AR secondary to leaflet involvement include rheumatic heart disease, infective endocarditis, bicuspid aortic valve, myxomatous disease, and trauma. Aortic root dilatation is now more common than primary valve disease in patients undergoing AVR for pure AR.[26] The predominant conditions causing root dilatation include degenerative cystic medial necrosis, as seen in Marfan syndrome, root dilatation associated with a bicuspid AV, aortic dissection, and connective tissue disorders. An unexplained association exists between pregnancy and aortic dissection. The increase in blood volume, cardiac output, and blood pressure seen during pregnancy may contribute to it. Like MR, 'AR begets AR'.

Pathophysiology

In AR, the entire LV stroke volume is ejected into the aorta, which is a high-pressure chamber; however, the early systole is facilitated, as the diastolic aortic pressure is reduced. Volume overload of the left ventricle leads to eccentric hypertrophy of the dilated ventricle, which helps to keep the wall stress within the normal levels. As AR progresses, the wall thickening fails to keep up with the cavitary dilatation, leading to increase in wall stress and heart failure, with decline in ejection fraction.[27] In chronic severe AR, the myocardial oxygen demand is increased due to increased LV mass. The coronary perfusion pressure is reduced due to lower aortic diastolic pressure, which is the driving force for coronary flow and myocardial perfusion during diastole. These two factors together lead to myocardial ischemia.

Clinical features

Patients with AR have an asymptomatic course for several years.[28,29] Forty-five percent of patients with severe AR and normal LV function may remain asymptomatic for 10 years with development of symptoms or LV dysfunction at the average rate of less than 6% per year. Like AS, once the patient becomes symptomatic the downhill course is rapid. Four-year survival without surgery in patients with Class III or IV heart failure is 30%.[30] Symptoms due to reduced cardiac reserve and myocardial ischemia develop only after considerable cardiomegaly and myocardial dysfunction have developed. Predominant symptoms at this stage include angina, palpitations, fatigue, exertional dyspnea, orthopnea, and paroxysmal nocturnal dyspnea. Deterioration in LV function may occur even during the asymptomatic period. Depressed LV function is the most important determinant of mortality after AVR.

Physical examination reveals several peripheral signs secondary to increased stroke volume and wide pulse pressure. The apical cardiac impulse is displaced laterally and inferiorly. A carotid shudder, as seen in AS, may be palpable due to augmented stroke volume across the non-stenotic AV.[31] On auscultation, a high-frequency diastolic AR murmur is audible along the left sternal border. The length of the murmur and not its intensity usually correlate with AR severity. In patients with AR secondary to the aortic root disorders, the murmur may be better heard along the right sternal border. A harsh systolic ejection murmur due to increased LV stroke volume and ejection rate may be audible and conducted to carotids. However, it is less harsh and early peaking compared with the murmur of true AS.

Laboratory evaluation

An ECG reveals LVH and strain pattern with prominent Q waves in lateral leads. Intraventricular conduction disturbance may be noted late in the course of the disease and is usually associated with LV dysfunction. Marked cardiomegaly is noted on chest X-ray in chronic severe AR. Dilatation of ascending aorta is more marked than in AS. Severe aneurysmal dilatation of the ascending aorta suggests aortic root disease as the cause of AR. A two-dimensional echocardiogram demonstrates the valvular and aortic root morphology, cardiac chamber sizes, and function. Doppler echocardiography helps in assessment of AR severity (Figure 5.4). Serial echocardiographic studies help in assessment of progression of AR, its impact on LV remodeling, and timing of surgery in asymptomatic patients. Radionuclide imaging is helpful when echocardiographic

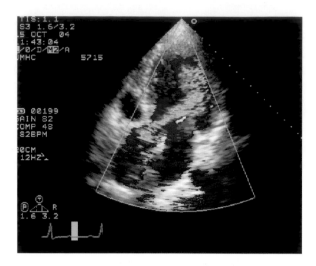

Figure 5.4 Color flow Doppler in apical 5-chamber view showing jet of aortic regurgitation.

images are suboptimal. It helps in assessment of regurgitant fraction and LV function at rest and with exercise. Cardiac magnetic resonance imaging (MRI) or computed tomography (CT) is the most accurate method for assessment of LV volumes, mass, regurgitant volumes, and regurgitant orifice area.

Management

All patients with AR should receive infective endocarditis prophylaxis. Symptomatic patients with severe AR need AVR. Asymptomatic patients with mild to moderate AR should have clinical and echocardiographic follow-up evaluations at 12–24-month intervals, whereas those with severe asymptomatic AR should be followed at intervals of 6 months. Cardiac catheterization and aortography may be indicated when there is discordance between clinical and non-invasive testing or if coronary angiography is needed. Patients with limited cardiac reserve or declining LV function should not engage in heavy exertion. Systolic hypertension, if present, should be treated, as untreated hypertension increases regurgitation volume. Vasodilator therapy has been shown to be beneficial and delay the need for surgery in asymptomatic patients.[32] It is indicated in patients with chronic severe AR with normal LV function; however, it is not a substitute for surgery if indicated. Surgery is not indicated in asymptomatic patients with severe AR and normal LV function.

Acute AR

Acute AR is most commonly caused by infective endocarditis, aortic dissection, or trauma. The normal-sized left ventricle cannot accommodate combined large-volume influx from the left atrium and aorta, leading to rapid increase in LV diastolic pressure and causing premature closure of the mitral valve.[33] Premature mitral closure protects the pulmonary venous bed from high LV diastolic pressures. The accompanying tachycardia shortens the diastole and reduces time for forward flow across the mitral valve, but compensates for reduced forward stroke volume. Patients with acute severe AR develop manifestations of cardiovascular collapse, with weakness, dyspnea, and hypotension. The peripheral signs of chronic AR are absent, and diastolic murmur is low-pitched and short. Prompt surgical treatment is indicated. While the patient is awaiting surgery, treatment with a positive inotropic agent and vasodilator is often necessary. The use of β-blockers and intra-aortic balloon pump is contraindicated.

TRICUSPID VALVE DISEASE

The two most common congenital abnormalities of the tricuspid valve (TV) are prolapse due to a floppy valve and Ebstein's anomaly. The most common acquired abnormality of the TV results from right ventricular dilatation, leading to annular dilatation, and regurgitation due to incomplete leaflet coaptation. Rheumatic involvement of TV leads to tricuspid stenosis (TS), which is usually associated with mitral and aortic valve disease. Like MS, TS is also more common in women. TS and regurgitation manifest with signs and symptoms of low cardiac output and right heart failure and mask the symptoms of MS. Other conditions causing TV disease include carcinoid syndrome, infective endocarditis in narcotic addicts, repeated

endomyocardial biopsy in transplant recipients, and exposure to methysergide and fenfluramine–phenteramine.

PULMONIC VALVE DISEASE

Pulmonary valve stenosis is most often congenital in origin. Rheumatic involvement of the pulmonary valve is uncommon. The pulmonic valve's involvement in carcinoid disease manifests in the form of pulmonary valve stenosis or a combination of pulmonary valve stenosis with regurgitation. The common causes of pulmonary regurgitation include dilatation of the pulmonary annulus secondary to pulmonary hypertension or infective endocarditis.

PROSTHETIC HEART VALVES

The prosthetic heart valve can be classified into two broad categories: mechanical and bioprosthetic. The mechanical valves are made of synthetic materials, which may include metal. These valves are more durable but generally require long-term (chronic) oral anticoagulation. Bioprosthetic valves are largely made of biologic materials, which may be a heterograft, such as from a pig (porcine), or an allograft, fashioned from human cadaveric tissue. These valves do not need chronic anticoagulation but generally are less durable. The design of prosthetic valves is under constant evolution, and newer valves have better hemodynamic characteristics and lower profiles and lower incidence of thrombosis. The most common mechanical valve in current use is the bileaflet St. Jude Medical valve.

Choice of a prosthetic valve in women of child-bearing age

Bioprosthetic valves have the advantage of not needing long-term anticoagulation but have the very significant disadvantage of accelerated degeneration in younger individuals, thus increasing the possibility of reoperation and replacement of the valve due to prosthetic valve failure. Use of mechanical prosthesis in this population is associated with the challenge of anticoagulation during pregnancy. Warfarin is teratogenic during the first trimester and can cause bleeding complications during the third trimester; therefore, it is best avoided during pregnancy. Warfarin should be discontinued as soon as pregnancy is detected, or even preferably, before conception.

Women tend to get smaller size valves due to smaller body size. All prosthetic valves are inherently stenotic and smaller-sized valves typically generate higher gradients across the valve. An increased hemodynamic burden, such as that seen during pregnancy, leads to an increased flow across the valve, thereby increasing the gradients even further and placing extra demand on the heart.

Aortic position of prosthetic valves is associated with a lower risk of thromboembolism compared with mitral position. A newer generation of mechanical valves such as the St. Jude Medical valve have a lower incidence of thromboembolism risk and therefore require a slightly less intense degree of anticoagulation.

PREGNANCY AND VALVULAR HEART DISEASE

Stenotic lesions are especially likely to cause symptoms during pregnancy. Patients with associated pulmonary hypertension and ventricular dysfunction are also at higher risk of complications. Patients at high risk of mortality during pregnancy are those with MS and atrial fibrillation, MS with NYHA Class III or IV symptoms, mechanical prosthetic valves, AS, and patients with pulmonary hypertension. Lower risk is encountered in patients with pulmonary valvular disease, patients with bioprosthetic valves, and patients with MS and NYHA Class I and II. There is also high risk of fetal and neonatal complication, including prematurity, low birth weight, spontaneous abortion, and neonatal mortality in patients with mechanical prosthetic valves.

Surgery during or immediately following pregnancy is associated with high maternal mortality. Surgery during pregnancy is associated with high fetal mortality. Therefore, surgery is reserved for emergencies and for patients failing to respond to medical therapy. For MS, percutaneous balloon valvuloplasty is associated with favorable outcomes and is the procedure of choice if feasible and necessary.

Drugs for valvular heart disease in pregnancy

No drug is absolutely safe in pregnancy and therefore the risk–benefit ratio should be assessed before commencing any drug therapy. However, β-blockers and digoxin are relatively safe. Heparin and furosemide can be used in pregnancy. Drugs that should be avoided during pregnancy are ACE inhibitors and warfarin.

VALVULAR HEART DISEASE ASSOCIATED WITH 'COLLAGEN' OR RHEUMATIC DISORDERS

Several rheumatic and other systemic disorders are associated with cardiac involvement. Many of these disorders, particularly SLE and scleroderma, are more common in women. Valvular involvement is found to a variable degree in these diseases. Table 5.1 summarizes valvular involvement in some of the more common rheumatic diseases.

Other conditions

The carcinoid syndrome is usually associated with right-sided valvular abnormalities such as leaflet thickening with resultant regurgitation. Sometimes, stenosis of the tricuspid and pulmonic valves may occur.

ENDOCARDITIS

Endocarditis is characterized by proliferation of microorganisms in the endothelium of the heart and is a serious, often devastating complication of valvular heart disease. It may be classified by the temporal course of disease, site of infection, cause of infection, and predisposing conditions such as intravenous drug abuse.

The majority of infections are caused by streptococci, staphylococci, and enterococci: 5–15% of patients with endocarditis have negative blood cultures, half of which are due to prior antibiotic administration. The risk of endocarditis is high in patients with a previous

Table 5.1 Valvular involvement of some common rheumatic diseases

Condition	Gender preponderance	Salient non-cardiac features	Cardiac involvement	Frequency of valvular involvement	Description of valvular involvement
Rheumatoid arthritis	Female	Joint pains with symmetrical polyarthritis	Predominantly pericardial. Conduction defects may occur	Uncommon	Aortic insufficiency
Ankylosing spondylitis	Male	Asymmetrical arthritis, including spine involvement	Aortic valve involvement common	Very common	Aortic insufficiency
Systemic lupus erythmatosus	Female	Antinuclear antibody, serositis, arthritis, glomerulonephritis, CNS dysfunction, anemia	Pericarditis, coronary arteritis, myocardial infarction, valvular involvement	Common (more than 50% of patients)	Non-bacterial (Libman–Sacks) endocarditis, thickened leaflets, regurgitation, stenosis
Antiphospho-lipid syndrome	Female	Positive APLA test and history of thrombosis	Valve thrombosis, non-bacterial endocarditis	Common (up to 30%)	Mitral regurgitation
Scleroderma (progressive systemic sclerosis, CREST syndrome)	Female	Skin 'hardening', arthralgia, proximal muscle weakness, esophageal dysmotility, telangectasia	Pericardial, endomyo-cardial fibrosis, PVCs, conduction abnor-malities, syncope, sudden death, pulmonary hypertension	Uncommon	Primary valvular involvement is rare
Polymyositis and dermato-myositis	Female	Skin lesions, proximal muscle weakness	Cardiomyopathy, conduction abnormality. Pericardial and coronary involvement rare. Pulmonary hypertension usually secondary	Uncommon	Primary valvular involvement is rare
Sarcoidosis	Female	Lung involvement, lymphadenopathy, arthropathy, skin, eye	Common: pericarditis. Uncommon: arrhythmias, conduction disorders, cardiomyopathy	Uncommon	Primary valvular involvement is rare

CNS, central nervous system; APLA, antiphospholipid antibody; PVCs, premature ventricular contractions.

history of endocarditis, patients with prosthetic valves, and in those with AR and MR, but it is lower in patients with stenotic lesions. Organisms enter the bloodstream from mucosal surfaces, skin, or other sites of infection.

The clinical manifestations result from cytokine production, damage to intracardiac structures, and embolization of vegetation fragments with infection and infarction of distant organs, and tissue injury due to an immunologic phenomenon. The diagnosis of endocarditis is established with certainty only when vegetations obtained at surgery or autopsy are examined histologically and micro-biologically. Duke criteria have been developed to assist in clinical diagnosis based on clinical, laboratory, and echocardiographic findings[34] (Figure 5.5). Transesophageal echocardiography is more sensitive than a transthoracic study in detecting vegetations.

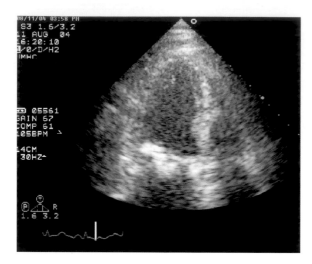

Figure 5.5 Apical three-chamber view showing a vegetation on the mitral valve.

Since all bacteria which are metabolically dormant and non-proliferating within the vegetation must be killed, therapy for endocarditis must be bactericidal and administered for prolonged periods. If fever persists for 7 days after appropriate antibiotic therapy, patients should be evaluated for paravalvular or metastatic abscesses. Surgical treatment may be indicated for certain intracardiac or peripheral complications of endocarditis. The American Heart Association has identified procedures that may precipitate bacteremia with organisms that cause endocarditis, cardiac lesions for which prophylaxis is advised, and regimens that may be used for this purpose.[7] Vulnerable patients should maintain good dental hygiene and aggressively treat local infections to reduce the risk for this serious complication.

REFERENCES

1. Bonow RO, Carabello B, Deleon AC, et al. ACC/AHA guidelines for management of patients with valvular heart disease: A report of the American College of Cardiology/American Heart Association Task Force on Practice Guidelines (Committee on Management of Patients with Valvular Heart Disease). J Am Coll Cardiol 1998; 32:1486.
2. Fligner CL, Reichenbach DD, Otto CM. Pathology and etiology of valvular heart disease. In: Otto CM, ed. Valvular Heart Disease, 2nd edn. Philadelphia: WB Saunders; 2004: 30.
3. Rahimtoola SH, Durairaj A, Mehra A, Nuno I. Current evaluation and management of patients with mitral stenosis. Circulation 2002; 106:1183.
4. Moreyra AE, Wilzon AC, Deac R, et al. Factors associated with atrial fibrillation in patients with mitral stenosis: a cardiac catheterization study. Am Heart J 1998; 135:138.
5. Popovic AD, Thomas JD, Neskovic AN, et al. Time related trends in the preoperative evaluation of patients with valvular stenosis. Am J Cardiol 1997; 80:1464.
6. Dajani AS, Taubert K, Ferrieri P, Peter G, Shulman, S. Treatment of streptococcal pharyngitis and prevention of rheumatic fever. Pediatrics 1995; 96:758.
7. Dajani AS, Taubert KA, Wilson W, et al. Prevention of bacterial endocarditis. Recommendations by the American Heart Association from the Committee on Rheumatic Fever, Endocarditis, and Kawasaki Disease, Council on Cardiovascular disease in the Young. JAMA 1997; 277:1794.
8. de Souza JAM, Martinez EE, Ambrose JA, et al. Percutaneous balloon mitral valvuloplasty in comparison with open mitral commisurotomy for mitral stenosis during pregnancy. J Am Coll Cardiol 2001; 37:900.
9. Carabello BA. Progress in mitral and aortic regurgitation. Curr Probl Cardiol 2003; 28:553.
10. Ling LH, Enriquez-Sarano M, Seward JB, et al. Clinical outcome of mitral regurgitation due to flail leaflet. N Engl J Med 1996; 335:1417.
11. Rosen SF, Borer JS, Hochreiter C, et al. Natural history of the asymptomatic patients with severe mitral regurgitation secondary to mitral valve prolapse and normal right ventricular performance. Am J Cardiol 1994; 74:374.
12. Host U, Kelbaek H, Hildebrant P, Skagen K, Aldershvile J. Effect of ramipril on mitral regurgitation secondary to mitral valve prolapse. Am J Cardiol 1997; 80:655.
13. Otto CM. Mitral valve prolapse. In: Otto CM, ed. Valvular Heart Disease, 2nd edn. Philadelphia: WB Saunders; 2004: 368.
14. Freed LA, Benjamin EJ, Levy D, et al. Mitral valve prolapse in the general population: the benign nature of the echocardiographic features in the Framingham study. J Am Coll Cardiol 2002; 40:1298.
15. Grande-Allen KJ, Griffin BP Calabro A, et al. Myxomatous mitral valve chordae. II: Selective elevation of glycosaminoglycan content. J Heart Valve Dis 2001; 10:325.
16. Barber JE, Ratliffe NB, Cosgrove DM 3rd, Griffin BP, Vesely I. Myxomatous mitral valve chordae. I: Mechanical properties. J Heart Valve Dis 2001; 10:320.

17. Avierinos JF, Gersh BJ, Melton LJ, et al. Natural history of asymptomatic mitral valve prolapse in the community. Circulation 2002; 106:1355.

18. Levinson GE, Alpert JS. Aortic stenosis. In: Alpert JS, Dalen JE, Rahimtoola SH, eds. Valvular Heart Disease, 3rd edn. Philadelphia: Lippincott, Williams and Wilkins; 2000: 183.

19. Carabello BA. Aortic stenosis. N Engl J Med 2002; 346:677.

20. Rajamannan NM, Gersh B, Bonow RO. Calcific aortic stenosis: from bench to bedside – emerging clinical and cellular concepts. Heart 2003; 89:801.

21. Chan C. Is aortic stenosis a preventable disease? J Am Coll Cardiol 2003; 42:593.

22. Marcus ML, Doty DB, Hiratzka LF, Wright CB, Eastham CL. Decreased coronary reserve: a mechanism for angina pectoris in patients with aortic stenosis and normal coronary arteries. N Engl J Med 1982; 307:1362.

23. Mark AL, Kioschos JM, Abboud FM, Heistad DD, Schmid PG. Abnormal vascular responses to exercise in patients with aortic stenosis. J Clin Invest 1973; 52:1138.

24. Ross J Jr, Brauwald E. Aortic stenosis. Circulation 1968; 38(Suppl V):61.

25. Bonow RO, Braunwald E. Valvular heart disease. In: Zipes D, Libby P, Bonow RO, Braunwald E, eds. Heart Disease, 7th edn. Philadelphia: WB Saunders; 2004: 1582.

26. Chan KL. Is aortic stenosis a preventable disease? J Am Coll Cardiol 2003; 42:593.

27. Bonow RO. Chronic aortic regurgitation: role of medical therapy and optimal timing of surgery. Cardiol Clin 1998; 16:449.

28. Bonow RO, Lakatos E, Maron BJ, Epstein SE. Serial long-term assessment of the natural history of asymptomatic patients with chronic aortic regurgitation and normal left ventricular systolic function. Circulation 1991; 84:1625.

29. Borer JS, Hochreiter C, Herrold EM, et al. Prediction of indications for valve replacement among asymptomatic and minimally symptomatic patients with chronic aortic regurgitation and normal left ventricular performance. Circulation 1998; 97:525.

30. Dujardin KS, Enriquez-Sarano M, Schaff HV, et al. Mortality and morbidity of aortic regurgitation in clinical practice. A long-term follow-up study. Circulation 1999; 99:1851.

31. Bonow RO. Chronic aortic regurgitation. In: Alpert JS, Dalen JE, Rahimtoola SH, eds. Valvular Heart Disease, 3rd edn. Philadelphia: Lippincott, Williams and Wilkins; 2000: 245.

32. Scognamiglio R, Rahimtoola SH, Fasoli G, Nistri S, Dalla Volta S. Nifedipine in asymptomatic patients with severe aortic regurgitation and normal left ventricular function. N Engl J Med 1994; 331:689.

33. Alpert JS. Acute aortic insufficiency. In: Alpert JS, Dalen JE, Rahimtoola SH, eds. Valvular Heart Disease, 3rd edn. Philadelphia: Lippincott, Williams and Wilkins; 2000: 269.

34. Durack DT, Lukes AS, Bright DK. New criteria for diagnosis of infective endocarditis: utilization of specific echocardiographic findings. Am J Med 1994; 96:200.

6

Cardiac arrhythmias

Saravanan Kuppuswamy and Greg Flaker

Heart rate differences between men and women • QT differences between men and women • Sudden cardiac death • Supraventricular tachycardia • Atrial fibrillation • Pregnancy and arrhythmia • Palpitations • Evaluation of palpitations/arrhythmia • Indications for electrophysiology testing • Treatment • Devices in pregnancy • Radiofrequency ablation • Conclusions

HEART RATE DIFFERENCES BETWEEN WOMEN AND MEN

Women have faster heart rates than men, and the differences are more pronounced at different ages. In the first year of life, the average heart rate for females is 132 bpm (beats/min) and 131 bpm for males. However, between ages 4 and 8 years the average heart rate for females is 93 bpm and for males is 89 bpm. Between ages 8 and 13 years the average heart rate for females is 87 bpm and for males is 80 bpm. Throughout the rest of life, the average heart rate for females is 2–7 bpm faster than for

males. By the sixth decade, the average heart rate for women is 73 bpm and for males is 70 bpm[1] (Table 6.1).

The reasons for the faster heart rates in women are uncertain. A variety of factors have been implicated, including direct or indirect influences of hormones on the sinus node. The fact that differences in heart rate become apparent in prepubertal females and persist into later life suggests that hormonal differences are not the only cause accounting for these differences.

Differences in heart rate variability have been described in men and women. Heart rate

Table 6.1 Mean (standard deviations) heart rates and QT intervals in various age groups

Age group	Male heart rate (bpm)	QT (ms)	Female heart rate (bpm)	QT (ms)
0–1	131 (17.9)	287 (28.2)	132 (17.5)	283 (25.5)
1–4	113 (12.4)	310 (18.9)	115 (14.1)	305 (21.3)
4–8	89 (14.5)	348 (25.6)	93 (13.9)	342 (24.0)
8–13	80 (13.1)	370 (26.6)	87 (14.9)	356 (27.7)
13–20	67 (11.2)	386 (27.0)	74 (11.1)	382 (27.0)
20–30	66 (10.8)	385 (28.9)	71 (10.5)	385 (27.3)
30–40	68 (11.6)	382 (29.8)	72 (11.0)	384 (28.6)
40–50	70 (11.7)	383 (30.0)	73 (11.3)	385 (30.1)
50–65	71 (12.4)	384 (31.4)	73 (11.4)	386 (31.0)
65–75	70 (13.1)	386 (33.7)	73 (10.9)	384 (30.7)

Adapted from Rautaharju et al.[1]

variability is the amount of heart rate fluctuation from the mean heart rate and is a measure of sympathetic and parasympathetic tone. Women younger than age 30 have lower heart rate variability than men, suggesting lower parasympathetic tone.[2]

With aging there is less heart rate variability, reflecting a decline in autonomic nervous system function. The decline of many parameters of autonomic function is more rapid in females.[3]

By age 50, differences in heart rate variability disappear, although some parameters of parasympathetic modulation differ between men and women even past age 60.[4–6] Collectively, these data are consistent with an effect on estrogen on the parasympathetic nervous system.

Differences in sympathetic nervous system function have been described in men and women. Young women have higher sympathetic nerve activity than young men. In contrast to parasympathetic activity, sympathetic activity increases with age.[7] Differences in sympathetic nerve function may also contribute to differences in heart rate between men and women. The decline of estrogens during menopause, which contributes to reduced parasympathetic activity, coupled with the increased sympathetic activity with age, help explain why sinus tachycardia is such a frequent complaint in women during menopause.[8]

Finally, there are data suggesting that intrinsic sinus node function is different between men and women. Administration of atropine and β-blocking agents result in a heart rate devoid of sympathetic and parasympathetic influences. Young women have a higher intrinsic heart rate than men, although the differences decrease with age,[9] suggesting that there are other factors accounting for the differences in heart rate. The differences in heart rate have also been related to differences in maximal exercise capacity between men and women.[10]

QT DIFFERENCES BETWEEN WOMEN AND MEN

The QT interval is also different between males and females, particularly in the first and second

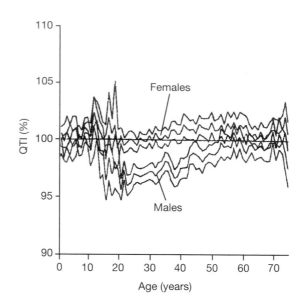

Figure 6.1
Mean values of the QT index (QTI = (QT/QT$_p$) × 100) with 95% confidence intervals calculated for each age subinterval of 1 year for males and females using the formula QT$_p$ = 656/(1 + 0.01 heart rate), showing a distinct decrease in rate-corrected QT values in males following puberty, followed by a linear increase through a major part of adult life. The slight non-significant age trend present in females at reproductive age disappears after inclusion of a correction term for QRS duration. Reproduced with permission from Rautaharju et al.[1]

decades of life. Rautaharju et al analyzed the QT interval on 14 379 children and adults aged from birth to 75 years and published the data on the variations in QT interval with age and gender[1] (Table 6.1, Figure 6.1).

Heart rate is an important variable affecting the QT interval and a variety of formulas have been proposed to correct for changes in heart rate – e.g. the QT index. Values for the QT index are different in men and women. During puberty, the QT index shortens in men, but remains constant in women. The QT index then gradually lengthens until 40–50 years of age in men and women[1] (see Figure 6.1). The shortening of the QT interval in men during puberty has correlated with the time when androgen levels are high. The QT$_c$ (QT interval corrected for heart rate) at rest does not differ among the three phases of the menstrual cycle, further arguing against a major hormonal contribution to the gender differences in the QT_c.[11]

Animal studies have supported the notion that androgens result in a relative shortening of the QT interval. When oophorectomized rabbits were randomized to receive placebo, dihydrotestosterone (DHT), or estradiol (E2), the QT interval increased in both DHT- and E2-treated rabbits. However, when quinidine was infused, the QT interval was increased significantly more with E2 than with DHT.[12] This differential effect of gonadal steroids on repolarization appears to be dependent on heart rate. At rapid heart rates, no differences were observed in the action potential duration; however, at slower heart rates, the action potential duration is longer in rabbits receiving E2 than in rabbits receiving DHT.[13]

Lengthening of the QT interval represents prolongation of the action potential in a group of cells in the ventricular myocardium. It implies that some groups of cells have prolonged action potential durations and some have shorter action potential durations. This heterogeneity of the ventricular tissue makes the heart vulnerable to life-threatening re-entrant ventricular arrhythmias. In addition, prolongation of the action potential can lead to deformities referred to as 'early after-depolarizations', which are important in the development of certain triggered ventricular arrhythmias. One of these types of ventricular arrhythmias is torsades de pointes, a polymorphic ventricular tachycardia characterized by polymorphic QRS complexes and a long–short initiation sequence. It is almost always seen in association with prolongation of the QT interval.

Lengthening of the QT interval may be acquired, due to a drug or electrolyte abnormality (Table 6.2), or it may be congenital. Genetic studies have identified at least six genes which regulate sodium and potassium flow into and out of the ventricular myocardium via ion channels. In the full expression of these syndromes, patients have prolongation of the QT interval, syncope, or sudden death due to ventricular arrhythmias. Presumably, partial expressions of these genes are present in some individuals, which result in repolarization abnormalities only when exposed to certain

Table 6.2 Common drugs that may prolong the QT interval.	
Drug	*Class*
Amantidine	Antiviral/parkinsonism
Amiodarone	Antiarrhythmic
Azithromycin	Antibiotic
Chloroquine	Antimalarial
Chlorpromazine	Antipsychotic
Clozapine	Antipsychotic
Clarithromycin	Antibiotic
Dofetilide	Antiarrhythmic
Erythromycin	Antibiotic
Fosphenytoin	Anticonvulsant
Haloperidol	Antipsychotic
Nicardipine	Antihypertensive
Ondansetron	Antiemetic
Quetiapine	Antipsychotic
Quinidine	Antiarrhythmic
Salmeterol	Bronchodilator
Sotalol	Antiarrhythmic
Tamoxifen	Selective estrogen receptor modifier (used in the treatment of breast cancer)
Vardenafil	Phosphodiesterase inhibitor/vasodilator
Venlafaxine	Antidepressant
Voriconazole	Antifungal

drugs, metabolic disorders, febrile states, or in heart failure.

Consequently, the relative prolongation of the QT interval in females during puberty may explain why female gender[14] is a predisposing factor in the development of the acquired form of torsades de pointes. Other factors which may contribute to the increased susceptibility of females to drug-induced cardiac arrhythmias include the observation that, when compared with males, female rabbits have lower densities of outward potassium channels, which affect action potential duration.[15] Estrogens also compete for metabolism by the cytochrome P450 enzyme system,[16] which is responsible for the metabolism of a variety of drugs that influence the QT interval.

Gender appears to play an important role in patients with the congenital form of long-QT syndrome. Gene mutations encode abnormal potassium channel proteins, which reduce the current of the rapidly activating, delayed inwardly rectifying potassium current. Females with this condition had a higher cardiac event rate, which suggests that gender plays a role in the expression of this ion channel.[17]

SUDDEN CARDIAC DEATH

Estimates of the incidence of sudden cardiac death vary widely. Based on multiple sources, recent studies have suggested that sudden cardiac death accounts for about 5.6% of the annual mortality in the United States.[18] Ventricular arrhythmias are the most common arrhythmia associated with this syndrome and epidemiologic data indicate that coronary artery disease is the cause of 80% of these arrhythmias.[19] Sudden death is more common in men than in women, at least in part due to the delayed onset of coronary artery disease in women. Women with cardiac arrest are more likely to have dilated cardiomyopathy or valvular heart disease than men who have cardiac arrest.[20]

Prior to the widespread use of implantable defibrillators, patients surviving a cardiac arrest often underwent electrophysiologic studies. Patients with inducible ventricular arrhythmias were thought to be more vulnerable to recurrent cardiac arrest and underwent sequential drug trials to prevent inducible ventricular arrhythmias. In general, patients with coronary artery disease and patients with sustained ventricular tachycardia were more likely to have inducible ventricular arrhythmias.[21] However, gender appeared to play an important role in the inducibility of arrhythmias. In one study, an induced arrhythmia was found in 87% of males with cardiac arrest but in only 39% of women.[22] Male gender was identified as an independent correlate of arrhythmia inducibility. These data suggest that the underlying substrate responsible for these life-threatening ventricular arrhythmias differs between males and females. Perhaps extracardiac factors are important in the genesis of cardiac arrhythmias in females. Alternatively, the differences in inducibility may simply reflect differences in the underlying heart disease in males and females. Subsequent studies have stratified for underlying disease. Although women are less likely to be inducible, when corrected for coronary artery disease there were no differences between genders.[20] Survival rates following implantation of defibrillators are better in females, although females who receive defibrillators tend to have better ventricular function and have less structural heart disease.[23]

SUPRAVENTRICULAR TACHYCARDIA

Most of the information available concerning supraventricular tachycardia (SVT) is from centers which perform catheter ablation. There are differences between males and females in the type of SVT reported from these centers. Atrioventricular (AV) nodal re-entry tachycardia is more common in females. Accessory pathways are more common in males.[24,25] Atrial tachycardia appear to be equally prevalent in males and females.[25]

Ovarian hormones may play a role in the frequency of SVT. In a study of 26 menstruating women with Holter-documented SVT, the duration and the number of episodes of SVT were related to plasma levels of progesterone and were negatively correlated with plasma levels of estradiol-17β.[26] In another study, 42 women who were referred for symptomatic SVT answered a specially designed questionnaire to determine if symptoms were related to the menstrual cycle. Seventeen (40%) were identified as having more cardiac arrhythmias during the perimenstrual phase of their cycles and/or after stopping estrogen replacement therapy. Six women had an initial negative electrophysiology study during mid-cycle or with estrogen replacement therapy. These 6 patients underwent repeat electrophysiology study when premenstrual or after estrogen therapy was withdrawn; all had inducible SVT.[27] These data suggest that estrogen protects against SVT, whereas progesterone may promote SVT. Estrogen inhibits the influx of extracellular calcium into vascular smooth muscle by an effect of cell membranes or L-type calcium channels,[28–30] but the effect appears only at high levels of estrogen. Since estrogens inhibit epinephrine release, and women who have low estrogen levels have increased epinephrine and norepinephrine levels compared with women with normal estrogen levels,[31] it is assumed that estrogen exerts its beneficial effect via alterations in sympathetic activity. The electrophysiologic effect of progesterone is not well studied.

ATRIAL FIBRILLATION

Atrial fibrillation is more prevalent in men than in women; however, approximately half of the patients with atrial fibrillation are women as a result of the higher proportion of women in older age groups.[32] Estimates on the prevalence of atrial fibrillation depend on symptoms during the arrhythmia; women with atrial fibrillation tend to have more symptoms than men.[33,34] Heart failure and hypertension are both risk factors for atrial fibrillation in men and women. Valvular heart disease is more commonly associated with atrial fibrillation in women than in men.[35] Even after correction for differences in risk factors, the relative risk of death is 1.5 in men and 1.9 in women.[36] The reasons for the differences in susceptibility to atrial fibrillation in men and the increased mortality associated with atrial fibrillation in women are uncertain.

Ischemic stroke is a dreaded complication of atrial fibrillation. Several small studies have suggested that women with atrial fibrillation have a higher risk of stroke than men.[37,38] In the Stroke Prevention in Atrial Fibrillation (SPAF) III trial[39] women >75 years were considered to be at high risk for stroke for reasons which have not been fully explained. It appears that women over 75 years have a high rate of cardioembolic stroke, and the benefits of anticoagulation in these women should be greater than for men.[40] At present, it is uncertain whether women are less likely to receive anticoagulation than men. At least one report has suggested that warfarin may be less efficacious in women.[41]

PREGNANCY AND ARRHYTHMIA

Pregnancy alters cardiac electrophysiology by multiple factors such as the hormonal changes, shifts in electrolytes, and alterations in adrenergic responsiveness. Estrogens have been postulated to increase the cardiac excitability and to sensitize the myocardium to catecholamines.[42]

Some arrhythmias occur more frequently in pregnant women. Although the essentials of treatment of the arrhythmias in pregnant women are similar to those for non-pregnant women, the treatment has to be individualized depending on the stage of the pregnancy and the risk–benefit ratio of exposing the fetus to the drugs. The principle is to avoid maternal hypotension and fetal hypoperfusion.

The most common cause of palpitations in pregnancy is sinus tachycardia.[43] Premature atrial contractions (PACs) and premature ventricular contractions (PVCs) are also common during pregnancy. In a study of 86 consecutive pregnant patients referred for palpitations, multiple PACs and PVCs or both were found in 18% of the patients.[44] These are more common during labor. PACs and PVCs are benign, frequently asymptomatic, and may not need any treatment. PVCs in asymptomatic patients with or without underlying heart disease do not need any treatment. If symptoms are severe, drug therapy may be considered after taking into consideration the potential side effects to the mother and the fetus. A thorough history of the relationship to caffeine, alcohol, or smoking should be obtained and any underlying electrolyte abnormalities or hypoxia should be corrected before initiating drug therapy.

SVT

The incidence of paroxysmal SVT has been shown to be increased in pregnancy.[45] Drugs used in the peripartum period, such as the oxytocics and tocolytic agents, are also responsible for the increased incidence of SVT during labor.

Atrial tachycardia

Atrial tachycardias are rare in pregnancy. In contrast to the non-pregnant women, these tend to occur in women with no structural heart disease. Although benign, prolonged tachycardia can lead to tachycardia-induced cardiomyopathy.

Atrial flutter and fibrillation

Atrial flutter and fibrillation are rare in pregnancy. Mendelsohn reported an incidence of <0.1% in women of childbearing age and an increased incidence of paroxysms of atrial fibrillation in pregnancy with underlying structural heart disease.[46] Thyrotoxicosis, valvular heart disease, hypertensive heart disease, pulmonary embolism, and cardiomyopathies should be excluded as the etiology of atrial fibrillation. Rheumatic heart disease has been the most reported underlying heart disease in atrial fibrillation in pregnancy.[47] As the incidence of mitral stenosis has decreased, congenital heart disease currently appears to be the common underlying heart disease in pregnant women with atrial fibrillation. The clinical manifestation depends on the ventricular response and the underlying heart disease. In mitral stenosis, atrial contraction and adequate diastolic filling time are essential to maintain cardiac output. In pregnancy, onset of atrial fibrillation is poorly tolerated with onset of dyspnea and pulmonary edema due to the loss of atrial contraction and shortened diastolic filling time.

Ventricular arrhythmia

Ventricular tachycardia is rare in pregnancy. Most of the case reports of ventricular tachycardia in pregnancy have been reported in patients with no structural heart disease or systemic disease.[48] In a series of 11 patients with ventricular tachycardia in pregnancy, all of the ventricular tachycardias had a monomorphic pattern and 73% of them originated from the right ventricular outflow tract. They disappeared completely during the postpartum period.[49] Right ventricular outflow tachycardia is characterized by the monomorphic pattern, left bundle branch block morphology, and inferior axis. Maternal and fetal outcomes are good. Other causes of ventricular tachycardia such as peripartum cardiomyopathy, ischemic heart disease, right ventricular dysplasia, obstructive and non-obstructive hypertrophic cardiomyopathy, and long QT syndrome must be considered in the etiology of ventricular tachycardia in pregnancy. Rashba reported that the postpartum interval is associated with a significant increase in risk for cardiac events among probands with the long QT syndrome, but not among first-degree relatives. They also

concluded that prophylactic treatment with β-blocker should be continued during the pregnancy and postpartum intervals in probands with the long QT syndrome.[50] Case reports of hyperthyroidism and hypomagnesemia associated with ventricular tachycardia have been reported.[51]

Bradyarrhythmias

The true incidence of bradyarrhythmias in pregnancy is unknown. Pregnancy does not seem to predispose to the development of bradyarrhythmias. Several cases of pregnancy with associated high-degree AV blocks have been reported, but the condition was usually present before the pregnancy and was first noted during pregnancy. The maternal and fetal mortality is related to the underlying heart disease and not the conduction defect.[46]

PALPITATIONS

Palpitations are a common complaint in women. They represent 15–25% of symptoms recorded by female cardiology patients.[8] Mitral valve prolapse syndrome is a common entity applied to a variety of pathogenic mechanisms involving the mitral valve, the mitral valve leaflets, the mitral valve annulus, or the chordae tendineae. The majority of patients with mitral valve prolapse remain asymptomatic throughout life, although life-threatening complications may occur, including progressive mitral regurgitation requiring mitral valve surgery, endocarditis, disabling chest pain, and cardiac arrhythmias. Mitral valve prolapse is a common condition that affects 2.5–5% of the population in general and is twice as frequent in women than men.[52]

There is an interesting body of literature concerning the evaluation of palpitations in young women that overlaps with the mitral valve prolapse literature.

A number of cardiac arrhythmias have been associated with mitral valve prolapse, including atrial arrhythmias,[53,54] ventricular arrhythmias,[55,56] and bradycardia.[57,58] The reason for these abnormalities is variable. Abnormalities of the mitral valve structure may be associated with congenital connections of a left-sided bypass pathway, which can result in supraventricular tachycardia.

Mitral valve prolapse patients may have high levels of catecholamines and respond in an exaggerated fashion to intravenous isoproterenol, which may account for certain atrial and ventricular arrhythmias.[59,60] These patients may also have abnormalities of autonomic function. Central modulation of baroreflexes has been described.[61] The excess sympathetic stimulation may result in a smaller than normal ventricle, which contributes to prolapse of the mitral leaflets into the left atrium during systole.

In addition, the associations of mitral valve prolapse with panic disorder[62] and generalized anxiety disorder[63] has been noted. This constellation of features – anatomic and metabolic abnormalities with an overlap of neuropsychiatric features – has made it imperative to establish an accurate diagnosis in order to initiate effective therapy when a young woman complains of palpitations.

EVALUATION OF PALPITATIONS/ARRHYTHMIA

Patients with rhythm disturbances can present with various symptoms, including palpitations, presyncope, and dyspnea. Although palpitations are mostly benign, they could represent life-threatening arrhythmias. The extensive differential diagnosis of palpitations and the fear of missing a diagnosis may lead to expensive investigations with minimal diagnostic value. The approach to a patient with palpitations and other symptoms of arrhythmia should begin with a thorough history, including a careful review of the medications and diet.

The patient's description of palpitations could give a clue to the etiology of the palpitations. The sensation of flip-flopping of the chest is generally caused by PACs or PVCs. A rapid fluttering sensation in the chest may be from sinus tachycardia, atrial or ventricular arrhythmias. The rhythm may indicate a probable mechanism. A rapid and regular pounding in the neck is typical of re-entrant supraventricular arrhythmias, particularly AV nodal tachycardia. This tachycardia is three times more common in women.[64]

The circumstances during which the palpitations occur are also important. Palpitations can be associated with anxiety or panic, but this diagnosis should not be accepted until other causes have been excluded. A study of 107 consecutive patients with SVT showed a tendency to ascribe palpitations to anxiety, especially in young women.[65]

Examples of palpitations that occur during periods of catecholamine excess include idiopathic ventricular tachycardias, mainly arising from the right ventricular outflow tract. Inappropriate sinus tachycardia is a rare disorder that causes palpitations after minimal exertion or minimal stress, is most frequently seen in young women, and may be from hypersensitivity to β-adrenergic stimulation.

AV nodal tachycardia often occurs while standing up straight after bending over and may end after lying down. A pounding sensation while lying in bed supine or left lateral position may be secondary to premature beats, as these tend to occur at slow heart rates. Associated symptoms of dizziness, syncope, or presyncope should raise the suspicion of ventricular tachycardia, but this can happen with supraventricular tachycardias with rapid heart rate.

The mode of onset and termination can also help in differentiating the etiology of the palpitations. Both supraventricular and ventricular tachycardia can have abrupt onset and termination, but termination with carotid sinus massage or the Valsalva maneuver is suggestive of supraventricular tachycardia. Asking the patient to tap out the rhythm with her own finger may help to differentiate regular and irregular rhythm.

A detailed drug and diet history should be obtained, including use of nasal decongestants, dietary supplements, and caffeine and alcohol intakes. Coexisting illness, such as chronic obstructive lung disease, thyrotoxicosis, and coronary artery disease, should be considered.

The initial investigations should begin with a 12-lead electrocardiogram. Particular attention should be paid to the PR interval and delta waves, the presence of which would suggest ventricular pre-excitation syndromes. Marked left ventricular hypertrophy may suggest hypertrophic cardiomyopathy. Evidence of left atrial enlargement suggests a substrate for atrial fibrillation. The presence of Q waves may raise the suspicion of a myocardial infarction with the substrate for the development of ventricular tachycardia.

Patients with underlying heart disease such as ischemic or non-ischemic, hypertrophic cardiomyopathy, clinically significant stenotic or regurgitant valvular lesions are at high risk for malignant arrhythmias and warrant further investigations. Patients with a family history of arrhythmia, syncope, and sudden cardiac death should also be included in the high-risk group.

Ambulatory electrocardiographic monitoring is useful in diagnosis. The Holter monitor is a continuous monitoring system that is worn for a day or two. Continuous event monitors record for a longer period of time and save the data only when the patient manually activates the monitor.

Echocardiography is indicated in patients with arrhythmias with clinical suspicion of heart disease, family history of genetically transmitted cardiac disease associated with arrhythmias such as tuberous sclerosis, rhabdomyoma or hypertrophic cardiomyopathy. It is not indicated for palpitations without corresponding arrhythmias or other cardiac signs or symptoms and for isolated PVCs without the clinical suspicion of heart disease.[66]

INDICATIONS FOR ELECTROPHYSIOLOGY TESTING

In patients with frequent or poorly tolerated episodes of tachycardia that do not respond to drug therapy and in whom electrophysiologic properties are essential for choosing appropriate therapy, an electrophysiologic study may be indicated. It may also be indicated in patients in whom there is concern about proarrhythmia or the effects of the drug on sinus node or AV node. It is not indicated for patients whose tachycardia is controlled by well-tolerated drug therapy.[67]

TREATMENT

The general treatment of SVT in the short term is terminating the tachycardia. This consists of vagal maneuvers or pharmacologic choices including adenosine, Class II and Class IV antiarrhythmic agents (Table 6.3). Non-pharmacologic approaches include atrial overdrive pacing or direct current cardioversion. Long-term therapy is aimed at preventing recurrences, and the choice of agents includes Class I through IV agents or radiofrequency (RF) ablation. RF ablation is equally successful in men and women.[68]

The treatment of atrial fibrillation revolves around rate control, conversion, and maintaining

---

Table 6.3 Vaughn–Williams classification of antiarrhythmic drugs

Class	Action	Drugs
I	Sodium channel blockers	
IA	Prolongs action potential	Quinidine, procainamide, disopyramide
IB	Shortens action potential	Lidocaine, mexiletine, tocainide, phenytoin
IC	Little effect on action potential, decreases conductivity	Encainide, flecainide, propafenone, moricizine
II	β-adrenergic blockade	Propranolol, esmolol, acebutolol, metoprolol, *l*-sotalol
III	Prolong action potential (potassium channel blockade)	Ibutilide, dofetilide, sotalol (*d*,*l*), amiodarone, bretylium
IV	Calcium channel blockade	Verapamil, diltiazem
Miscellaneous	Miscellaneous actions	Adenosine, digitalis, magnesium

sinus rhythm and prevention of thromboembolic complications. Recent studies have concluded that the management of atrial fibrillation with the rhythm-control strategy offers no survival advantage over the rate-control strategy, and there are potential advantages, such as a lower risk of adverse drug effects, with the rate-control strategy.[69]

In new-onset atrial fibrillation of less than 48 hours' duration, either pharmacologic or electrical cardioversion can be performed with minimal risk of thromboembolic complications. If the duration is more than 48 hours and if sinus rhythm has to be restored, an acceptable option is to first do a transesophageal echocardiogram. If no clots are visualized, proceed with cardioversion. To maintain sinus rhythm in the long term, propafenone of flecainide can be used if there is no underlying organic heart disease. In the presence of depressed left ventricular function, amiodarone is the drug of choice, and its use is limited by the side-effect profile. Dofetilide is a reasonable alternative. If the ventricular response is rapid in spite of maximal medical therapy, AV nodal ablation and a permanent pacemaker implantation is an alternative. In certain groups of patients, a pulmonary vein isolation procedure may be indicated. A recent study concluded that in a selected, risk-stratified population of patients with recurrent atrial fibrillation, a pill-in-the-pocket treatment strategy with either propafenone or flecainide is feasible and safe, with a high rate of compliance by patients, a low rate of adverse events, and a marked reduction in emergency room visits and hospital admissions.[70] Antiarrhythmics should be used cautiously as some of them have proarrhythmic effects, especially in women, in whom QT prolongation occurs more commonly.

Treatment of arrhythmias in pregnancy

In the treatment of symptomatic PVCs, β-blocker such as metoprolol and Class 1A agents such as quinidine and procainamide have been shown to be relatively safe in pregnancy.

Episodes of SVT should be treated initially with vagal maneuvers such as carotid sinus massage. If unsuccessful, the drug of choice would be adenosine. Adenosine has been shown to be safe in pregnancy, especially in the second and third trimester.[71] Fetal bradycardia has been noted, but no adverse fetal outcome was reported.[72] There is insufficient data for the use of adenosine in the first trimester.

Class IA: antiarrhythmic drugs

Quinidine has been used during pregnancy since 1930.[73] Quinidine is currently classified in the Food and Drug Administration (FDA) pregnancy risk category C (Table 6.4). A surveillance study involving 229 101 completed pregnancies reported one major birth defect among 17 newborns exposed to quinidine during the first trimester. However, no

Table 6.4 FDA pregnancy risk category

Category	Description
A	Adequate, well-controlled studies in pregnant women have not shown an increased risk of fetal abnormalities
B	Animal studies have revealed no evidence of harm to the fetus; however, there are no adequate and well-controlled studies in pregnant women. Or Animal studies have shown an adverse effect, but adequate and well-controlled studies in pregnant women have failed to demonstrate a risk to the fetus
C	Animal studies have shown an adverse effect and there are no adequate and well-controlled studies in pregnant women. Or No animal studies have been conducted and there are no adequate and well-controlled studies in pregnant women
D	Studies, adequate well-controlled or observational, in pregnant women have demonstrated a risk to the fetus. However, the benefits of therapy may outweigh the potential risk
X	Studies, adequate well-controlled, observational, in animals or pregnant women have demonstrated positive evidence of fetal abnormalities. The use of the product is contraindicated in women who are or may become pregnant

anomaly was observed in the six specified categories.[74] Quinidine appears to be relatively safe when antiarrhythmic therapy is considered necessary.

Procainamide is classified in FDA pregnancy risk category C. Although no teratogenic effects have been reported to date, because of the limited data available and the potential for unexpected side effects including drug-induced lupus, caution is recommended.

Disopyramide is also classified in FDA pregnancy risk category C and should be avoided, especially in the third trimester because of its effect on uterine contraction.[75]

Class IB

Lidocaine is in FDA pregnancy risk category C and appears to be safe during pregnancy. Fetal bradycardia and low Apgar scores have been reported with fetal acidosis and when the maternal drug levels are high. Mexiletine has also been used safely in pregnancy. Tocainide lacks significant human experience in pregnancy. Phenytoin should be avoided in pregnancy because of its teratogenic effects.

Class IC

Both flecainide and propafenone have been used safely in pregnancy for both maternal and fetal supraventricular arrhythmias and both are classified in FDA pregnancy risk category C.

Class II drugs: β-blockers

Both selective and non-selective β-blockers have been extensively used in pregnancy, and no teratogenicity has been reported. Intrauterine growth retardation has been reported with propranolol. β-Blockers can also increase the uterine contraction and result in premature delivery. In the newborn, bradycardia and hypoglycemia have been reported up to 72 hours after delivery.

Class III

Amiodarone is very effective, but potentially toxic for the fetus and the mother. Currently, the FDA pregnancy risk category for amiodarone is D and so this drug should only be used in extraordinary circumstances.

There are several case reports of the safety of sotalol in pregnancy. The current FDA risk category is B. In view of its potential maternal proarrhythmic effects, the use of this drug should be reserved for serious arrhythmias.

Class IV calcium channel blockers

Like most of the other antiarrhythmics, these drugs are currently in FDA pregnancy risk category C. Both oral and intravenous verapamil and diltiazem have been associated with prolonged hypotension.

Digoxin

Digoxin has been widely used in pregnancy. Adverse fetal outcomes have been associated with overdose. In therapeutic doses, digoxin appears to be safe in pregnancy.

In summary, antiarrhythmic drugs are better avoided in pregnancy. If indicated, drugs such as adenosine, β-blockers, digoxin, quinidine, and sotalol are preferred. It should also be taken into consideration that pregnancy may alter the pharmacodynamics of the drug. Decreased gastrointestinal motility may reduce the rate of absorption of certain drugs, and the slowed passage may increase the absorption of certain drugs. Increased volume of distribution, decreased protein binding, resulting in decreased total drug concentration, and increased renal clearance as a result of increase in renal blood flow and glomerular filtration rate should all be considered when drug therapy is considered in pregnancy.[76]

In any hemodynamically unstable arrhythmias, electrical cardioversion should be performed without much delay. This is even more important in pregnancy, as the fetus is also exposed to the risk of prolonged hypotension. Both synchronized cardioversion and defibrillation have been safely performed during all stages of pregnancy.[77]

In the event of cardiorespiratory arrest in late pregnancy, if the standard application of the

Advanced Cardiac Life Support (ACLS) algorithms has failed to restore effective circulation, a perimortem cesarean section should be performed within 4–5 minutes of the arrest. Most fetal survivors were delivered within 5 minutes of the maternal cardiac arrest.[68]

Anticoagulation for atrial fibrillation in pregnancy

As the majority of the atrial fibrillation in pregnancy is associated with underlying structural heart disease, anticoagulation is indicated except those with lone atrial fibrillation. The role of anticoagulation in preventing systemic arterial embolism has not been systematically studied in pregnant patients. Heparin, which does not cross the placenta, remains the drug of choice for anticoagulation in pregnancy. Warfarin should be avoided in the first trimester because of its association with teratogenic embryopathy and in the later stage of pregnancy because of the risk of fetal hemorrhage. The AHA/ACC guidelines recommend the following treatments.[78]

Class I (indicated)

Administer antithrombotic therapy (anticoagulant or aspirin) throughout pregnancy to all patients with atrial fibrillation, except those with lone atrial fibrillation. (Level of Evidence: C – expert opinion, case studies.)

Class IIb (may be considered)

Administer heparin to patients with risk factors for thromboembolism during the first trimester and last month of pregnancy. Unfractionated heparin may be administered either by continuous intravenous infusion in a dose sufficient to prolong the activated partial thromboplastin time (APTT) to 1.5–2 times the control value or by intermittent subcutaneous injection in a dose of 10 000 to 20 000 units every 12 hours, adjusted to prolong the mid-interval (6 hours after injection) APTT to 1.5 times control. (Level of Evidence: B – limited evidence from single randomized study or non-randomized studies.)

Limited data are available to support the subcutaneous administration of low-molecular-weight heparin for this indication. (Level of Evidence: C.) Administer an oral anticoagulant during the second trimester to patients at high thromboembolic risk. (Level of Evidence: C.)

DEVICES IN PREGNANCY

With the expanding indications for implantable defibrillators (ICDs), there are increasing numbers of pregnant patients with ICD. Although there are no reported cases of implantation of ICD in pregnancy, Natale et al reported a series of 44 pregnant patients with ICDs.[79] They concluded that the mere presence of an ICD should not deter women from becoming pregnant, and that pregnancy does not increase the risk of major ICD-related complications or result in a high number of ICD discharges. It is recommended that the ICD should remain activated during labor and should be switched off during cesarean section due to the interference with electrocautery.

RADIOFREQUENCY ABLATION

Electrophysiology studies expose the patient to a significant amount of radiation and are best avoided in pregnancy. Echocardiography-guided placement of EP catheters for the evaluation of syncope and ventricular tachycardia have been reported.[80] A few cases of ablation procedures performed during pregnancy with good fetal outcomes have been reported, but the long-term effects on the fetus are not known.[81,82]

CONCLUSIONS

Certain arrhythmias tend to occur more commonly in females than in males. The underlying mechanism of these arrhythmias may be different, as discussed earlier. Although there may be differences in the etiology of these arrhythmias, the basic principles of treatment of these arrhythmias remains the same, irrespective of the gender. Multiple factors have to be considered when treating arrhythmias in pregnant women.

The field of electrophysiology is rapidly advancing and the treatment modalities may be tailored to the individual patient. The results of recent trials have changed the way we manage patients with atrial fibrillation. The results of the ongoing clinical trials will give us more insight into managing the arrhythmias more effectively.

REFERENCES

1. Rautaharju PM, Zhou SH, Wong S, et al. Sex differences in the evolution of the electrocardiographic QT interval with age. Can J Cardiol 1992; 8(7):690.

2. Umetani K, Singer DH, McCraty R, Atkinson M. Twenty-four hour time domain heart rate variability and heart rate: relations to age and gender over nine decades. J Am Coll Cardiol 1998; 31:593.

3. Bonnemeier H, Wiegand WKH, Brandes A, et al. Circadian profile of cardiac autonomic nervous modulation in healthy subjects: differing effects of aging and gender on heart rate variability. J Cardiovasc Electrophysiol 2002; 14:791.

4. Liao D, Barnes RW, Chambless LE, et al for the ARIC investigators. Age, race, and sex differences in autonomic cardiac function measured by spectral analysis of heart rate variability – the ARIC study. Am J Cardiol 1995; 76:906.

5. Stein PK, Kleiger RE, Rottman JN. Differing effects of age on heart rate variability in men and women. Am J Cardiol 1997; 80:302.

6. Antelmi I, De Paula RS, Shinzato AR, et al. Influence of age, gender, body mass index, and functional capacity on heart rate variability in a cohort of subjects without heart disease. Am J Cardiol 2004; 93:381.

7. Ng A, Callister R, Johnson D, et al. Age and gender influence muscle sympathetic nerve activity at rest in healthy humans. Hypertension 1993; 21:498.

8. Rosano GC, Rillo M, Leonardo F, Pappone C, Chierchia SL. Palpitations: what is the mechanism, and when should we treat them? Int J Fertil 1997; 42(2):94.

9. Jose A, Collison D. The normal range and determinants of the intrinsic heart rate in man. Cardiovasc Res 1970; 4:160.

10. Burke JH, Goldberger JJ, Ehlert FA, et al. Gender differences in heart rate before and after autonomic blockade: evidence against an intrinsic gender effect. Am J Med 1996; 100:537.

11. Burke JH, Ehlert FA, Kruse JT, et al. Gender-specific differences in the QT interval and the effect of autonomic tone and menstrual cycle in healthy adults. Am J Cardiol 1997; 79:178.

12. Drici MD, Burklow TR, Haridasse V, Glazer RI, Woosley RL. Sex hormones prolong the QT interval and downregulate potassium channel expression in the rabbit heart. Circulation 1996; 94:1471.

13. Hara M, Danilo P Jr, Rosen MR. Effects of gonadal steroids on ventricular repolarization and on the response to E4031. J Pharmacol Exp Ther 1998; 285:1068.

14. Makkar RR, Fromm BS, Steinman RT, Meissner MD, Lehmann MH. Female gender as a risk factor for torsades de pointes associated with cardiovascular drugs. JAMA 1992; 270:2590.

15. Liu XK, Katchman, A, Drici MD, et al. Gender difference in the cycle length-dependent QT and potassium currents in rabbits. J Pharmacol Exp Ther 1998; 285:672.

16. Schubert W, Cullberg G, Edgar B, Hedner T. Inhibition of 17β-estradiol metabolism by grapefruit juice in ovariectomized women. Maturitas 1995; 20:155.

17. Priori SG, Schwartz PJ, Napolitano C, et al. Risk stratification in the long QT syndrome. N Engl J Med 2003; 348:1866.

18. Chugh SS, Jui J, Gunson K, et al. Current burden of sudden cardiac death: multiple source surveillance versus retrospective death certificate-based review in a large U.S. community. J Am Coll Cardiol 2004; 44:1268.

19. Zipes DP, Wllens HJJ. Sudden cardiac death. Circulation 1998; 98:2334.

20. Albert CM, McGovern BA, Newell JB, Ruskin JN. Sex differences in cardiac arrest survivors. Circulation 1996; 93:1170.

21. Schoenfield MH, McGovern B, Garan H, et al. Determinants of the outcome of electrophysiologic study in patients with ventricular tachyarrhythmias. J Am Coll Cardiol 1985; 6:298.

22. Freedman RA, Swerdlow CD, Soderholm-Difatte V, Mason JW. Clinical predictors of arrhythmia inducibility in survivors of cardiac arrest: importance of gender and prior myocardial infarction. J Am Coll Cardiol 1988; 12:973.

23. Kudenchuk P, Brady G, Poole JE, et al. Malignant sustained ventricular tachyarrhythmias in women: characteristics and outcomes of treatment with an implantable cardioverter defibrillator. J Cardiovasc Electrophysiol 1997; 8:2.

24. Calkins H, Yong P, Miller JM, et al for the Atakr Multicenter Investigators Group. Catheter ablation of accessory pathways, atrioventricular nodal reentrant tachycardia and the atrioventricular junction. Circulation 1999; 99:262.

25. Rodriguez LM, deChillou C, Schlapfer J, et al. Age at onset and gender of patients with different types of supraventricular tachycardias. Am J Cardiol 1992; 70:1213.

26. Rosano GMC, Leonardo F, Sarrel PM, et al. Cyclical variation in paroxysmal supraventricular tachycardia in women. Lancet 1996; 347(9004):786.

27. Myerburg RJ, Cox MM, Interian A, et al. Cycling of inducibility of paroxysmal supraventricular tachycardia in women and its implications for timing of electrophysiologic procedures. Am J Cardiol 1999; 83:1049.

28. Jiang C, Sarrel PM, Lindsay DC, Poole-Wilson PA, Collins P. Endothelium-independent relaxation of rabbit coronary artery by 17β-oestradiol in vitro. Br J Pharmacol 1991; 104:1033.

29. Kitazawa T, Hamada E, Kitazawa K, Gaznabi AKM. Non-genomic mechanism of 17β-oestradiol-induced inhibition of contraction in mammalian vascular smooth muscle. J Physiol (Lond) 1997; 499:497.

30. Freay AD, Curtis SW, Korach KS, Rubanyi GM. Mechanism of vascular smooth muscle relaxation by estrogen in depolarized rat and mouse aorta. Role of nuclear estrogen receptor and Ca^{2+} uptake. Circ Res 1997; 81:242.

31. Sarrel PM. Ovarian hormones and the circulation. Maturitas 1990; 12:287.

32. Go AS, Hylek EM, Phillips KA, et al. Prevalence of diagnosed atrial fibrillation in adults: national implications for rhythm management and stroke prevention: the AnTicoagulation and Risk Factors in Atrial Fibrillation (ATRIA) Study. JAMA 2001; 285(18):2370.

33. Flaker GC, Belew K, Beckman K, et al. AFFIRM Investigators. Asymptomatic atrial fibrillation: demographic features and prognostic information from the Atrial Fibrillation Follow-up Investigation of Rhythm Management (AFFIRM) study. Am Heart J 2005; 149(4):657.

34. Paquette M, Roy D, Talajic M, et al. Role of gender and personality on quality-of-life impairment in intermittent atrial fibrillation. Am J Cardiol 2000; 86:764.

35. Benjamin EJ, Levy D, Vaziri SM, et al. Independent risk factors for atrial fibrillation in a population-based cohort: the Framingham Study. JAMA 1994; 271(11):840.

36. Benjamin EJ, Wolf PA, D'Agostino RB, et al. Impact of atrial fibrillation on the risk of death. Circulation 1998; 98:946.

37. Friberg J, Scharling H, Gadsboll N, Truelsen T, Jensen GB. Comparison of the impact of atrial fibrillation on the risk of stroke and cardiovascular death in women versus men (The Copenhagen City Heart Study). Am J Cardiol 2004; 94:889.

38. Wang TJ, Massaro JM, Levy D, et al. A risk score for predicting stroke or death in individuals with new-onset atrial fibrillation in the community: the Framingham Heart Study. JAMA 2003: 290(8):1049.

39. Stroke Prevention in Atrial Fibrillation Investigators. Adjusted-dose warfarin versus low-intensity, fixed-dose warfarin plus aspirin for high-risk patients with atrial fibrillation: stroke prevention in atrial fibrillation III randomized clinical trial. Lancet 1996; 348:633.

40. Stroke Prevention in Atrial Fibrillation Investigators. Risk factors for Thromboembolism during aspirin therapy in patients with atrial fibrillation: The Stroke Prevention in Atrial Fibrillation Study. J Stroke Cerebrovasc Dis 1995; 5:147.

41. Hara K, Akiyama Y, Tajima T. Sex differences in the anticoagulant effects of warfarin. Jpn J Pharmacol 1994; 66(3):387.

42. Roberts JM, Insel PA, Goldfien A. Regulation of myometrial adrenoreceptors and adrenergic response by sex steroids. Mol Pharmacol 1981; 20:52.

43. Ostrezega E, Mehra A, Widerhorn J. Evidence of increased incidence of arrhythmias during pregnancy: a study of 104 pregnant women with symptoms of palpitations, dizziness or syncope. J Am Coll Cardiol 1992; 19:125

44. Shotan A, Ostrzega E, Mehra A, Johnson JV, Elkayum U. Incidence of arrhythmias in normal pregnancy and relation to palpitations, dizziness, and syncope. Am J Cardiol 1997; 79:1061.

45. Tawam M, Levine J, Mendelson M, et al. Effect of pregnancy on paroxysmal supraventricular tachycardia. Am J Cardiol 1993; 72:838.

46. Mendelsohn CL. Disorders of the heartbeat during pregnancy. Am J Obstet Gynecol 1956; 72:1268.

47. Szekely P, Snaith L. Atrial fibrillation and pregnancy. Br Med J 1961; 5237:1407.

48. Brodsky M, Doria R, Allen B, et al. New-onset ventricular tachycardia during pregnancy Am Heart J 1992; 123:933.

49. Nakagawa M, Katou S, Ichinose M, et al. Characteristics of new-onset ventricular arrhythmias in pregnancy. J Electrocardiol 2004; 37(1):47.

50. Rashba EJ, Zareba W, Moss AJ, et al., Influence of pregnancy on the risk for cardiac events in patients with hereditary long QT syndrome. Circulation 1998; 97:451.

51. Varon ME, Sherer DM, Abramowicz JS, Akiyama T. Maternal ventricular tachycardia associated with hypomagnesemia. Am J Obstet Gynecol 1992; 167:1352.

52. Levy D, Savage D. Prevalence and clinical features of mitral valve prolapse. Am Heart J 1987; 113(5):1281.

53. Josephson ME, Horowitz LN, Kastor JA. Paroxysmal and supraventricular tachycardia in patients with mitral valve prolapse. Circulation 1978; 57(1):111.

54. Winkle RA, Lopes MG, Fitzgerald JW, et al. Arrhythmias in patients with mitral valve prolapse. Circulation 1975; 52:73.

55. Gooch AS, Vicencio F, Maranhao V, Goldberg H. Arrhythmias and left ventricular asynergy in the

prolapsing mitral leaflet syndrome. Am J Cardiol 1972; 29:611.

56. Kligfield P, Hochreiter C, Niles N, Devereux RB, Borer JS. Relation of sudden death in pure mitral regurgitation, with and without mitral valve prolapse, to repetitive ventricular arrhythmias and right and left ventricular ejection fractions. Am J Cardiol 1987; 80:397.

57. Stein KM, Borer JS, Hochreiter, et al. Prognostic value and physiologic correlates of heart rate variability in chronic severe mitral regurgitation. Circulation 1993; 88:127.

58. Greenspon AJ, Schaal SF. AV node dysfunction in the mitral valve prolapse syndrome. Pacing Clin Electrophysiol 1980; 3:600.

59. Boudouglas H, Reynolds JC, Mazzaferri E, Wooley C. Metabolic studies in mitral valve prolapse syndrome. Circulation 1980; 61(6):1200.

60. Boudouglas H, Reynolds JC, Mazzaferri E, Wooley C. Mitral valve prolapse syndrome: The effect of adrenergic stimulation. J Am Coll Cardiol 1983; 2(4):638.

61. Coghlan HC, Phares P, Cowley M, Copley D, James TN. Dysautonomia in mitral valve prolapse. Am J Med 1979; 67:236.

62. Gorman JM, Shear MK, Devereux RB, King DL, Klein DF. Prevalence of mitral valve prolapse in panic disorder: effect of echocardiographic criteria. Psychosom Med 1986; 48(3/4):167.

63. Mazza DL, Martin D, Spacavento L, Jacobsen J, Gibbs H. Prevalence of anxiety disorders in patients with mitral valve prolapse. Am J Psychiatry 1986; 143(3):349.

64. Zimetbaum P, Josephson ME. Evaluation of patients with palpitations. N Engl J Med 1998; 338(19):1369.

65. Lessmeier TJ, Gamperling D, Johnson-Liddon V, et al. Unrecognized paroxysmal supraventricular tachycardia: potential for misdiagnosis as panic disorder. Arch Intern Med 1997; 157:537.

66. ACC/AHA/ASE 2003 Guideline update for the clinical application of echocardiography: summary article. A report of the American College of Cardiology/American Heart Association Task Force on Practice Guidelines (ACC/AHA/ASE Committee to Update the 1997 Guidelines for the Clinical Application of Echocardiography). Circulation 2003; 108:1146.

67. Zipes DP, DiMarco JP, Gillette PC, et al. Guidelines for clinical intracardiac electrophysiological and catheter ablation procedures: a report of the American College of Cardiology/American Heart Association Task Force on Practice Guidelines (Committee on Clinical Intracardiac Electrophysiologic and Catheter Ablation Procedures), developed in collaboration with the North American Society of Pacing and Electrophysiology. J Am Coll Cardiol 1995; 26:555.

68. Wilansky S, Willerson JT. Heart Disease in Women. Philadelphia: Churchill Livingstone; 2002: 578.

69. The Atrial Fibrillation Follow-up Investigation of Rhythm Management (AFFIRM) Investigators. A comparison of rate control and rhythm control in patients with atrial fibrillation. N Engl J Med 2002; 347:1825.

70. Alboni P, Botto GL, Baldi N, et al. Outpatient treatment of recent-onset atrial fibrillation with the 'pill-in-the-pocket' approach. N Engl J Med 2004; 351:2384.

71. Wolbrette D. Treatment of arrhythmias during pregnancy. Curr Women's Health Rep 2003; 3:135.

72. Elkayan U, Goodwin TM. Adenosine therapy for supraventricular tachycardia during pregnancy. Am J Cardiol 1995; 75:521.

73. Meyer J, Lackner JE, Schoechet SS. Paroxysmal tachycardia in pregnancy. JAMA 1930; 94:1901.

74. Rosa F. Personal communication, FDA; 1993. In: Briggs GG, Freeman RK, Yaffe SJ, eds. Drugs in Pregnancy and Lactation. A Reference Guide to Fetal and Neonatal Risk, 4th edn. Baltimore: Williams & Wilkins; 1994: 284, 693, 759.

75. Tadmor OP, Keren A, Rosenhak D, et al. The effect of disopyramide on uterine contractions during pregnancy. Am J Obstet Gynecol 1990; 162:482.

76. Rotmensch HH, Elkayam U, Frishman W. Antiarrhythmic drug therapy during pregnancy, Ann Intern Med 1983; 98:487.

77. Elkayam U, Gleicher N. Cardiac Problems in Pregnancy, 3rd edn. New York: Wiley-Liss; 1998: 167.

78. Fuster V, Ryden LE, Asinger RW, et al. ACC/AHA/ESC guidelines for the management of patients with atrial fibrillation. J Am Coll Cardiol 2001; 38:1231.

79. Natale A, Davidson T, Geiger MJ, Newby K. Implantable cardioverter-defibrillators and pregnancy: a safe combination? Circulation 1997; 96:2808.

80. Lee MS, Evans SJL, Blumberg S, Bodenheimer MM, Roth SL. Echocardiographically guided electrophysiologic testing in pregnancy. J Am Soc Echocardiogr 1994; 7:182.

81. Pagad SV, Barmade AB, Toal SC, Vora AM, Lokhandwala YY. 'Rescue' radiofrequency ablation for atrial tachycardia presenting as cardiomyopathy in pregnancy. Indian Heart J 2004; 56(3):245.

82. Gras D, Mabo P, Kermarrec A, et al. Radiofrequency ablation of atrioventricular conduction during the 5th month of pregnancy, Arch Mal Coeur Vaiss 1992; 85:1873.

7

Lipid abnormalities

David W Gardner

Introduction • Differences between men and women • Changes in lipids throughout life • Treatment of lipid abnormalities and the reduction in risk of cardiovascular disease • Pharmacotherapy for lipid abnormalities • Failure to address lipid problems • Summary

INTRODUCTION

With increasing awareness of the prevalence and risk of coronary heart disease (CHD) in women, there has been a great deal of interest in the role of lipids in the atherosclerotic process. A number of recent studies showed that treating lipid disorders, and even treating individuals with normal lipid levels, can have a dramatic effect on CHD risk. This chapter will focus primarily on the diagnosis and treatment of the lipid abnormalities for primary and secondary prevention of CHD. Other manifestations of hyperlipidemia such as acute pancreatitis, skin abnormalities, and tendinous xanthomas, also related to high levels of lipids, will not be covered in this chapter.

Many questions arise during diagnosis and treatment of lipid disorders in women. First and foremost, are there natural differences in lipid and lipoprotein levels between men and women? Secondly, do the many hormonal changes that women experience throughout life affect lipid levels and cardiovascular risk? CHD is the leading cause of death for Western women, just as it is for men, although there is a common misconception that women are at low risk for developing CHD.[1] For women, the increase in risk occurs about 10 years later in life than in men.[2] A major question has been whether abnormal lipid levels contribute to this risk. Additional questions deal with treatment of lipid disorders. Does modification of the lipid profile decrease CHD risk, and, if so, are women benefiting from lipid-lowering therapy? This chapter will attempt to answer these questions and make recommendations for treating women who have a lipid disorder.

DIFFERENCES BETWEEN MEN AND WOMEN

Men and women vary in terms of lipoprotein levels throughout life. These differences are seen as early as puberty and persist often until postmenopause. Because of these differences, assessing the role of lipids in CHD risk requires knowledge of what is 'normal' for women versus men.

Beginning in puberty and continuing beyond menopause, high-density lipoprotein (HDL) cholesterol levels are naturally about 10–14 mg/dl higher in women than in men.[1,3] It was originally believed that this difference was secondary to estrogen effects. However, the difference persists even when estrogen levels drop postmenopause. The difference may be related to male gender, leading to low HDL levels, a possible effect of testosterone,[4] rather than to women having high values.

Low-density lipoprotein (LDL) cholesterol levels rise throughout life in both genders. Prior to menopause, LDL values are significantly higher in men than women, but postmenopause this phenomenon is reversed.[3] Very low-density lipoprotein (VLDL) cholesterol levels also rise throughout life and are generally higher in men than in premenopausal women. Following menopause, VLDL cholesterol levels are more similar between men and women.

While lipid abnormalities carry significant risk for women, the risk is different than for men. Most prospective observational studies have found a strong relationship between increased total cholesterol and coronary artery disease (CAD) risk.[5] However, the Framingham Study[1,6] showed that the increase in risk is less in women than it is in men for the same increase in total cholesterol.

In women, low HDL cholesterol seems to be the strongest predictor of risk for CHD and plays a more important role than it does in men.[1,3,5,6] In the Lipid Research Clinics Prevalence Study, low HDL cholesterol was the lipid abnormality most predictive of early death in women.[1,6]

Finally, hypertriglyceridemia in women is an independent risk factor for CAD. In women, a strong association has been found between high triglyceride levels and CAD, while there is ongoing debate whether hypertriglyceridemia is even an independent risk factor for men.[1,3] In women, this association is independent of HDL cholesterol levels and total cholesterol levels.

These differences in lipid and lipoprotein levels between men and women should be taken into consideration when assessing risk and determining whether treatment is necessary. Differences must also be considered when trying to apply the results of lipid-lowering studies that enrolled only males to a female population.

CHANGES IN LIPIDS THROUGHOUT LIFE

Puberty

At puberty, there is a dramatic change in sex hormone levels and a significant increase in insulin resistance in both boys and girls. The level of testosterone and other androgens rise dramatically in males. Females experience a dramatic increase in estrogen and progesterone levels and a much smaller increase in androgen levels. In addition, there are extensive fluctuations in estrogen and progesterone levels that occur throughout the menstrual cycle. These

changes result in an average 14 mg/dl decrease in HDL cholesterol levels in males, whereas the lipid profile remains relatively unchanged in females.[1,3] The difference caused by this change persists throughout life; men continue to have lower average HDL than women. It is felt that this difference is related to the negative effect of testosterone on HDL cholesterol, rather than a positive effect of estrogen.[1,7]

The menstrual cycle

The menstrual cycle is associated with regular changes in circulating levels of both estrogen and progesterone. As estrogen levels climb during the follicular phase, LDL cholesterol levels decrease. Levels remain low during the progesterone-dominated luteal phase, only to rise again as progesterone drops and menses begin. HDL cholesterol levels remain constant in spite of rising estrogen levels. This finding is consistent with the finding that HDL cholesterol does not go up with puberty nor does it drop after menopause. Thus, it appears that, in the non-pregnant state, estrogen is not a major regulator of HDL cholesterol.[1]

Studies of triglyceride levels during the menstrual cycle have yielded varying results. Triglycerides have been reported to either remain unchanged or be increased by up to 34% during the follicular phase, when estrogen levels are rising.[1,7]

Pregnancy

Pregnancy results in very dramatic changes in circulating levels of sex steroids. These changes herald very important differences in both the quantity and quality of the circulating lipoproteins.[7] Estrogen levels increase throughout pregnancy, reaching a peak just before term. Triglycerides rise in a parallel fashion and at 36 weeks are two to three times higher than pre-pregnancy levels. This increase is for the most part due to an increase in the production of VLDL. There is also an increase in the triglyceride content of VLDL as well as the other lipoproteins. The increase in triglycerides is important to provide for the energy needs of the mother. This, and the increasing maternal insulin resistance seen in the second and third trimester, allow more glucose to be shunted through the placenta for use by the growing fetus.

LDL cholesterol and apolipoprotein (apo) B-100 levels also increase throughout pregnancy despite rising estrogen levels. The reason for this paradoxical rise in LDL cholesterol levels is not clear. It is possible that it results from the increase in VLDL, which is a precursor for LDL. In addition, the rising progesterone levels may contribute to the rise in LDL cholesterol concentrations. Although this has not been shown for natural progesterones, synthetic progesterones consistently increase cholesterol levels. There also appears to be an increase in the cholesterol content of the LDL particles, which results in an increase in particle size without an increase in particle number. An increase in particle size results in resistance to oxidation and thus potentially decreases the atherogenicity of the particles and helps to offset the potential risk from rising LDL cholesterol levels. The rising LDL cholesterol levels are probably adaptive. They provide the precursors for the dramatic increase in placental steroidogenesis which occurs during pregnancy. Pregnant women with defective LDL synthesis have low circulating levels of estrogen and progesterone.[7]

Although it might seem that the rising estrogen levels throughout pregnancy are associated with rising HDL cholesterol level, this is only true through mid-pregnancy when HDL levels peak twofold higher than at the pre-pregnancy level. A rise in HDL_2, the most cardiac protective of the HDL subfractions, is responsible for this increase. After mid-gestation, HDL_2 levels gradually fall until just before term. At that point, they are only 15% higher than baseline. The early rise in HDL cholesterol is due to the rising estrogen levels. The decrease that starts at midterm may be related to the increasing triglyceride levels and rising insulin levels that result from the increasing insulin resistance. It is likely that the rise in HDL cholesterol plays a role in protecting the mother from the atherogenic effects of the rise in triglycerides, LDL cholesterol, and apo B-100 levels.[3,6,7]

Many of the changes in lipoprotein levels during pregnancy should impart an increased risk for cardiovascular disease (CVD) during pregnancy. Despite this, there is no evidence that pregnant women experience higher rates of cardiovascular events than non-pregnant women. This is probably, in part, due to the increased HDL cholesterol level.[2] There has also been concern that the lipid changes during pregnancy may also predispose women with early or more frequent pregnancies to greater risk of cardiovascular events in the future. Although some studies have found this to be the case, most have not found any increase in risk.[7] These variable results suggest that if there is an increase in CHD risk from parity, it is a relatively small one.

In summary, the dramatic changes in lipoprotein levels that occur during pregnancy are adaptive and necessary to support the energy needs of the fetus and mother, as well as to allow the high rate of steroid hormone synthesis necessary to bring a pregnancy to a successful completion.

Menopause

Menopause brings about another dramatic change in sex steroid levels and, with it, a shift in lipids and lipoproteins (Figure 7.1). This is, in part, secondary to the drop in endogenous estrogen and progesterone that occurs with loss of functional follicles. In addition, the weight gain and increase in abdominal fat that is commonly seen at this period of time contributes to the change in lipids.[8–11]

During and after menopause, there is a significant increase in total cholesterol and LDL cholesterol.[8,10] Estrogen increases LDL receptors in the liver and is associated with an increase in LDL particle clearance. The drop in estrogen level at menopause is associated with a decrease in LDL receptor numbers. The decrease in receptors results in a decrease in the clearance of LDL by the liver and a rise in LDL concentration.[12] Although most studies have found no change in HDL cholesterol,[8,10,11] a few studies have reported a small decrease in HDL levels.[13]

One recent clinical trial studied lipids and lipoprotein values in pre-, transitional, and postmenopausal women.[8] This study also looked at the effects of body mass index (BMI)

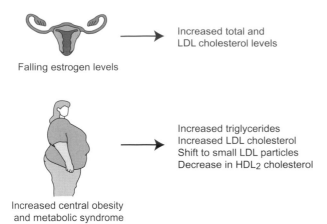

Falling estrogen levels → Increased total and LDL cholesterol levels

Increased central obesity and metabolic syndrome → Increased triglycerides Increased LDL cholesterol Shift to small LDL particles Decrease in HDL₂ cholesterol

Figure 7.1 Multiple etiologies for lipid changes after menopause. Menopause is associated with several changes in serum lipid levels. The loss of estrogen is associated with an increase in total cholesterol and low-density lipoprotein (LDL) cholesterol. There may also be an increase in abdominal fat. This may result in the development of the metabolic syndrome and its associated dyslipidemia: increased triglycerides, increased LDL cholesterol, a shift to small dense LDL particles, and a decrease in the concentration of the HDL₂ fraction of high-density lipoprotein (HDL) cholesterol.

and waist circumference. The transition to and through menopause was associated with an increase in LDL cholesterol, apo B, and triglycerides. There was also a gradual increase in BMI and waist circumference in many women. The rise in total cholesterol and LDL cholesterol levels was associated with the stage of menopause and estradiol levels. The increase in triglyceride levels was not associated with menopause stage, but with the increase in BMI and waist circumference. There was no change found in total HDL cholesterol levels but the HLD₂ subfraction decreased, thus changing the HDL₂/HDL₃ ratio. Thus, the change to an atherogenic lipid profile with increasing triglyceride level may be the result of increasing abdominal fat and the associated increase in insulin resistance and the metabolic syndrome.[8]

In general the rise in LDL cholesterol, apo B, and triglycerides is considered atherogenic and correlates with the significant rise in risk of cardiovascular disease that occurs after menopause. The well-documented increase in abdominal fat may be causing an increase in

metabolic syndrome and may contribute to these changes; additionally, the observed decrease in size of LDL particles is a finding which is associated with increased athero-genicity.[14]

Effects of treatment with sex steroids

Replacement of estrogen after menopause has been an attractive mechanism for reversing some of the adverse changes seen in lipid metabolism with the drop in estrogen production. In spite of the associated improvement in lipid profile with estrogen therapy, recent studies have failed to show any benefit in terms of reduction of CHD risk.

Treatment with estrogen generally has a positive effect on the lipid profile. It is well documented to decrease total cholesterol and LDL cholesterol concentrations as well as apo B levels. When given orally, estrogen also results in a significant increase in HDL cholesterol (HDL₂) and triglyceride levels.[1] These effects are primarily pharmacologic; at puberty, when endogenous estrogen levels are increasing, there is no change in HDL cholesterol level or triglyceride levels and at menopause there is no drop in HDL cholesterol or triglyceride levels.

Progestogens have an adverse effect on the lipid profile. They are associated with an increase in LDL cholesterol and apo B. They have also been associated with a decrease in HDL cholesterol, apo A-1, and HDL₂. These adverse effects are generally only seen with synthetic progestogens and are the result of their androgenic properties. When naturally occurring progestogens are administered, these adverse effects are minimized.[1]

Transdermal estrogen therapy yields somewhat different results. The effects on LDL cholesterol and HDL cholesterol are similar. However, triglyceride levels decrease rather than increase.[15,16] This difference is due to the lack of a first pass through the liver. Oral estrogens reach the liver in very high concentration and have pharmacologic effects on lipoprotein production. Transdermal estrogen is delivered to the periphery first and reaches the liver in much lower concentrations, having a much less dramatic effect on lipoprotein synthesis. These

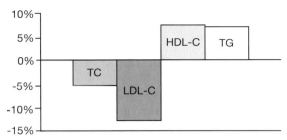

Figure 7.2 Effects on lipids of estrogen and progesterone therapy when compared with placebo. The beneficial effects of oral estrogen therapy on the total cholesterol (TC), low-density lipoprotein cholesterol (LDL-C), and high-density lipoprotein cholesterol (HDL-C), and the adverse effect on serum triglyceride (TG) levels. In spite of the beneficial changes in lipids, there was no improvement in cardiovascular outcomes from estrogen treatment.

expected results have therapeutic implications for women with hypertriglyceridemia. In general, if estrogen replacement is needed, the transdermal approach is preferable to oral delivery.

The lipoprotein changes associated with hormone replacement therapy (HRT) are complex, but appear to indicate protection from cardiovascular disease (Figure 7.2). Several epidemiologic studies have suggested HRT provides CVD protection. Results from two prospective trials are now available. The first trial looked at the effect of oral estrogen and progesterone in postmenopausal women with established coronary disease. At the end of 4.1 years there was no identifiable benefit.[17] An extension to 6.8 years also failed to show any benefit.[18] The second study, The Women's Health Initiative (WHI), looked at HRT in patients without a history of coronary disease. Despite mostly 'favorable' changes in the lipid profile (see Figure 7.2), neither estrogen combined with progesterone nor estrogen alone conferred any protection from cardiovascular events.[19,20] A great deal of debate about the reasons for these negative results has occurred. The results may be related to the increase in VLDL and triglycerides, a known cardiovascular risk factor in women and/or an increase in the risk for thrombosis.[21] A potential exists for transdermal therapy to have less of an adverse

effect on triglycerides and thrombosis,[22] but this has not yet been studied in prospective trials.

Polycystic ovarian syndrome

PCOS is not a stage of life, but instead is a very important condition that affects a large number of women during their reproductive years and is believed to be associated with a significant increased risk for cardiovascular disease.[23] It is currently estimated that between 4% and 10% of US women of reproductive age have PCOS.[24]

PCOS is defined as chronic anovulation (oligomenorrhea or amenorrhea), along with evidence of hyperandrogenism in the absence of hyperprolactinemia, virilizing adrenal or ovarian tumors, or congenital adrenal hyperplasia.[24]

The significance of PCOS for this discussion is its association with insulin resistance and the metabolic syndrome. Hyperinsulinism secondary to insulin resistance plays an important role in androgen excess and anovulation. Virtually all women with PCOS, whether obese or normal weight, have insulin resistance.[24] Metabolic syndrome is a group of cardiovascular risk factors that are closely linked to insulin resistance. These include, but are not limited to, impaired glucose tolerance or overt diabetes mellitus, hypertension, central obesity, and dyslipidemia.[25] PCOS is associated with a 31–35% incidence of impaired glucose tolerance and a 7–10% incidence of overt diabetes mellitus.[23,24,26] These numbers are almost three times higher than the rate of incidence found in women in the same age group without PCOS.[23]

The metabolic syndrome is associated with a distinct lipid and lipoprotein pattern, which is referred to as dyslipidemia. A similar pattern is seen in patients with type 2 diabetes. Dyslipidemia is characterized by high triglycerides and VLDL levels, low HDL cholesterol (particularly HDL$_2$), and low apo A-1 levels. In addition, there is strong evidence that the LDL particles in persons with metabolic syndrome are more dense and smaller (subpattern B) than in individuals without metabolic syndrome. These small LDL particles are more readily oxidized and therefore are considered more atherogenic than the larger particles.[14] In patients with PCOS, the triglycerides and VLDL levels are higher, and the HDL cholesterol and apo A-1 are lower than in women without the syndrome.[24] This is true for both obese and non-obese women with PCOS.[24,27] The difference persists when women, both with and without PCOS, are matched for BMI and other cardiovascular risk factors.[27] PCOS is also common in adolescent girls who have irregular menstrual cycles. Many adolescents diagnosed with PCOS have a lipid pattern typical of dyslipidemia, with reports showing that 50% have triglycerides >135 mg/dl and 28% have an HDL cholesterol <37 mg/dl.[24]

Hypertriglyceridemia and low HDL cholesterol are associated with a greater cardiovascular risk for women than for men. In addition, women seem to be more adversely affected by low HDL cholesterol levels than men.[1,3,5] It is very likely that much of the increased cardiovascular risk associated with PCOS is secondary to dyslipidemia.[24,27] Therefore, it is important that all patients who have been diagnosed with PCOS also be screened for dyslipidemia, along with screening for hypertension and glucose abnormalities. Lifestyle modifications can be instituted and, when clinically indicated (and when pregnancy is not an issue), medications can be started early in the disease process. Unfortunately, many lipid abnormalities are not identified until after vascular disease is clinically apparent. The diagnosis of PCOS offers an opportunity to make the diagnosis at a much earlier stage before permanent damage has occurred.

TREATMENT OF LIPID ABNORMALITIES AND THE REDUCTION IN RISK OF CARDIOVASCULAR DISEASE

One of the major concerns about lipid abnormalities is its association with an increased risk for cardiovascular disease. Hypercholesterolemia has long been recognized as a significant risk factor for early vascular disease.[6] This association is true for men and women, although for women a given total cholesterol concentration carries a somewhat lower risk.[3] This may be because women have higher HDL cholesterol levels, which contributes to the total cholesterol concentration.[28]

LDL cholesterol levels are a better predictor of cardiovascular events than total cholesterol. Total cholesterol reflects cholesterol in both atherogenic and antiatherogenic lipoproteins. Therefore, treatment of hypercholesterolemia is based on LDL cholesterol levels rather than on total cholesterol.[14] The average cholesterol level in patients with a myocardial infarction (MI) is not much higher than the general population. The majority of patients that experience an MI have 'normal' cholesterol and LDL cholesterol levels.[3] Many of these individuals have undesirable levels of HDL cholesterol, triglycerides, small dense LDL particles, or all three.[3,14]

The impact of dyslipidemia (high triglycerides and low HDL cholesterol) is of particular importance to women.[28] Whereas increased LDL cholesterol is a risk factor for CAD in women, low HDL cholesterol is the strongest predictor in women. An increase of 1% in HDL cholesterol is associated with a 3–5% decrease in risk for women but only a 2% decrease in risk for men.[2,29,30] The role of hypertriglyceridemia has also been well established and is much stronger for women than for men.[1,3]

Undesirable LDL cholesterol, low HDL cholesterol, and hypertriglyceridemia are all associated with significant cardiovascular disease in women. Unfortunately, women were often either excluded or underrepresented in the early intervention trials designed to demonstrate the benefit of lipid-lowering therapy in reducing risk for vascular events.[31] Recently, there have been a number of large studies published that did include women.

The AFCAPS/TexCAPS trial looked at the effects of lovastatin on acute coronary events in men and women without a history of coronary disease and average cholesterol levels. The participants were required to have low HDL cholesterol levels. There were 5608 men and 997 women who were randomized to either lovastatin or placebo. The study was ended after 5.2 years. Lovastatin reduced the incidence of a first acute major coronary event by 37%. The relative risk reduction in women was greater (46%) than in men (37%) but, because of the relatively lower number of events, there was no statistical difference in treatment effects between men and women.[32]

Table 7.1 Guidelines for treating lipids in women

Risk category	Features	Lipid goal
Highest risk	CAD or CAD equivalent with severe risk factors[a]	LDL <70 mg/dl
High risk	CAD or CAD equivalent	LDL <100 mg/dl
Moderate risk	Two or more risk factors, no CAD	LDL <130 mg/dl
Low risk	Less than two risk factors, no CAD	LDL <160 mg/dl
High triglycerides	LDL at goal and non-HDL cholesterol[b]	30 mg/dl higher than baseline
Low HDL cholesterol	LDL at goal and non-HDL cholesterol[b]	30 mg/dl higher than baseline

[a]Includes poorly controlled hypertension, diabetes, or metabolic syndrome.
[b]Non-HDL cholesterol = Total cholesterol − HDL cholesterol (does not have to be fasting).

The CARE trial was conducted in men and women with a past history of MI and average cholesterol levels.[33] Patients were randomized to treatment with either pravastatin or placebo. The primary end point was coronary death and non-fatal MI and secondary end points were combined coronary events (coronary death, non-fatal MI, percutaneous transluminal coronary angioplasty, or coronary artery bypass graft surgery) and stroke. There were 3583 men and 576 postmenopausal women in the study. The women had a 43% ($p = 0.035$) reduction in the primary end point, 46% ($p = 0.01$) reduction in combined coronary events, and a 56% ($p = 0.07$) reduction in stroke. Once again, the relative reduction was greater in women than in men.[33]

The Heart Protection Trial was conducted in patients with coronary heart disease, other vascular disease, or diabetes.[34] The trial studied 20 536 subjects: 15 454 men and 5082 women. Participants were randomized to either 40 mg of simvastatin or placebo, and the primary end point was mortality and fatal or non-fatal vascular events. There was a significant reduction in all-cause mortality and a 24% reduction in vascular events. Benefit from therapy was the same regardless of starting LDL cholesterol levels. Women had the same benefit as men, even though they had fewer events.[34]

In these three major trials with significant numbers of women enrolled, lipid-lowering therapy benefited women to the same or greater degree than men.[32–34] This is consistent with the observation that increased cholesterol and triglyceride level and low HDL cholesterol are risk factors in women. HMG CoA reductase inhibitors decrease total and LDL cholesterol and triglyceride levels and increase HDL cholesterol. There is not adequate data on the benefit of medications that target triglycerides and HDL cholesterol specifically (fibric acid derivatives and niacin) to draw any conclusions about their effects on CVD or mortality in women.

Cardiovascular disease is the leading killer of women in the Western world and mortality from it exceeds the next seven causes of mortality combined. This high risk, and the evidence of benefit from treating lipids in women, has led to the development of guidelines for preventing cardiovascular disease in women, which includes recommendations for lipid-lowering therapy.[35,36] These guidelines (Table 7.1) include the assessment of risk, and basing therapy on the overall risk, and do not differ significantly from the guidelines for prevention of cardiovascular disease in men. The recently published American Heart Association Guidelines[36] assigns the highest priority to individuals with a 10-year absolute risk of >20%. These are individuals with established CHD, cerebrovascular disease, peripheral arterial disease, abdominal aortic aneurysm, diabetes, and/or chronic kidney disease.[36] For these women, the goal is an LDL cholesterol of <100 mg/dl and a non-HDL cholesterol of

<130 mg/dl. This should be accomplished by simultaneously starting lifestyle modification and statin therapy. Because the Heart Protection Trial showed benefit regardless of the starting cholesterol levels, they recommend starting statin therapy even if the LDL cholesterol is less than 100 mg/dl.[34,36] In women at moderate risk (two or more risk factors and a 10-year absolute CHD risk of 10–20%), the recommendation is for lifestyle modification and to start statin therapy if the LDL cholesterol remains above 130 mg/dl. For women at low risk (a 10-year absolute risk of <10%), the goal is an LDL cholesterol of less than 160 mg/dl, along with the addition of statin therapy if the LDL cholesterol is greater than 190 mg/dl, combined with lifestyle changes. Because of the lack of data on the benefit of modifying triglyceride and HDL cholesterol levels in women, the guidelines recommend that if LDL cholesterol is at goal and either triglycerides or HDL cholesterol are not at goal, the non-HDL cholesterol be lowered to less than 130 mg/dl.[35] The NCEP also recommends that if triglycerides are very high (>500 mg/dl), the addition of a fibric acid derivative or niacin be considered as first-line therapy.[35]

PHARMACOTHERAPY FOR LIPID ABNORMALITIES

Pharmacotherapy of lipids is based on the concept that all patients have been instructed on lifestyle modification, which is referred to as therapeutic lifestyle changes (TLC).[35] The primary aim of pharmacotherapy is to decrease LDL cholesterol to the recommended levels. Thus, treatment with HMG CoA reductase inhibitors (statins) is the mainstay of therapy. These drugs are capable of reducing LDL cholesterol by more than 50% and have extensive safety data. They include lovastatin, simvastatin, pravastatin, atorvastatin, and rosuvastatin. It is important to recognize that statins are contraindicated during pregnancy (pregnancy risk category X) and should be used with caution in women with childbearing potential.

Other agents used to lower LDL cholesterol include bile acid binders and the relative new agent ezetimibe. These agents lower LDL by about 18–20%, and thus are reserved for second-line therapy when statins cannot be used or in combination with statin to obtain even greater reductions in LDL cholesterol. Ezetimibe can result in an additional 25% reduction in LDL cholesterol when added to a statin. Ezetimibe is classified as pregnancy risk category C.

Fibric acid derivatives (gemfibrozil and fenofibrate) and niacin are most often used to lower triglycerides and increase HDL cholesterol. They are only used as first-line therapy in patients with very high triglycerides (>400 mg/dl). They are also used in combination with statin when triglycerides are high (>200 mg/dl) or HDL cholesterol is low (>40 mg/dl) and the non-HDL cholesterol is above goal. Gemfibrozil interferes with the clearance of statin and may increase the risk of rhabdomyolysis. Fenofibrate has no effect on statin levels and thus is considered much safer to use in combination with statins. Both fibric acid derivatives are category C risk for pregnant patients.

FAILURE TO ADDRESS LIPID PROBLEMS

There is substantial evidence that lipid disorders in women at risk for cardiovascular disease are being underdiagnosed and undertreated in spite of the overwhelming evidence of benefit and nationally accepted guidelines for treatment.[37–40] In 1997, Schrott et al looked at postmenopausal women with heart disease in the HERS trial and reported on adherence to the 1988 and 1993 NCEP (National Cholesterol Education Program) adult treatment panel recommendations.[39] Their study found that although 47% of the women were taking lipid-lowering medications, 63% did not meet the 1988 goal of LDL cholesterol of <130 mg/dl and 91% did not meet the 1993 goal of LDL of <100 mg/dl. O'Meara et al looked at gender differences in treatment and control of lipids in hypertensive adults[38] and found that significantly more men than women with dyslipidemia were being treated with lipid-lowering drugs (25.5% vs 16.4%) and that significantly more men were at goal (8.6% vs 5.8%). In 2005,

Mosca et al looked at lipid management in 8353 high-risk women in a managed care setting[37] to evaluate whether they were achieving the American Heart Association recommended lipid levels for high-risk women.[36] At the time of the initial lipid evaluation, the women were drug naïve and only 7% had optimal levels for all lipids. Seventeen percent had an LDL cholesterol level of <100 mg/dl. After 36 months of follow-up, 32% had been placed on lipid-lowering therapy, with 12% achieving optimal lipid levels, and only 29% with LDL cholesterol of <100 mg/dl.[36]

Diabetes is well recognized as a coronary heart disease equivalent, and women who have diabetes experience the greatest increase in risk. Wexler et al recently looked at gender disparities in treating cardiac risk factors in diabetic patients.[40] Diabetic women without coronary heart disease were significantly less likely to be treated with lipid-lowering medications (adjusted odds ratio (AOR) = 0.82; $p = 0.01$), or to achieve an LDL cholesterol level of <100 mg/dl (AOR = 0.75; $p = 0.004$). There was no difference in treatment with lipid-lowering drugs between men and women with diabetes and coronary heart disease, but the women were still less likely to achieve the goal of an LDL of <100 mg/dl (AOR = 0.80; $p = 0.006$).

SUMMARY

There are significant differences in lipid and lipoprotein levels between men and women. These differences are the results of sex steroid hormone differences and the changes that take place in these hormones throughout a woman's life. In spite of these differences, lipids play an important role in the development of cardiovascular disease in women, and coronary artery disease is the leading cause of death in women. Recent interventional trials have demonstrated that lipid-lowering therapy is at least as beneficial in women as it is in men, and clear guidelines have been developed and published for the treatment of lipids in women. Several studies have shown that women are less likely than men to receive lipid-lowering therapy when indicated, and, when therapy is instituted, they are less likely to be treated to goal.

In order for women to benefit from the recent developments in the pharmacologic therapy of lipid abnormalities, there needs to be a greater awareness of the high risk for cardiovascular disease in this population and the role lipids play in this risk. In addition, women must be screened more frequently for lipid disorders, and healthcare providers must be more aggressive about starting and titrating medications to lower lipids to acceptable levels of risk.

REFERENCES

1. Miller VT. Dyslipoproteinemia in women. Special considerations. Endocrinol Metab Clin N Am 1990; 19(2):381.
2. O'Brien T, Nguyen TT. Lipids and lipoproteins in women. Mayo Clin Proc 1997; 72(3):235.
3. Kannel WB. Range of serum cholesterol values in the population developing coronary artery disease. Am J Cardiol 1995; 76(9):69C.
4. Li Z, et al. Effects of gender and menopausal status on plasma lipoprotein subspecies and particle sizes. J Lipid Res 1996; 37(9):1886.
5. Rich-Edwards JW, et al. The primary prevention of coronary heart disease in women. N Engl J Med 1995; 332(6):1758.
6. Kannel WB, et al. Serum cholesterol, lipoproteins, and the risk of coronary heart disease. The Framingham study. Ann Intern Med 1971; 74(1):1.
7. Salameh WA, Mastrogiannis DS. Maternal hyperlipidemia in pregnancy. Clin Obstet Gynecol 1994; 37(1):66.
8. Berg G, Mesch V, Boero L, et al. Lipid and lipoprotein profile in menopausal transition. Effects of hormones, age and fat distribution. Horm Metab Res 2004; 36(4):215.
9. Carr MC. The emergence of the metabolic syndrome with menopause. J Clin Endocrinol Metab 2003; 88(6):2404.
10. de Aloysio D, Gambacciani M, Meschia M, et al. The effect of menopause on blood lipid and lipoprotein levels. The Icarus Study Group. Atherosclerosis 1999; 147(1):147.
11. Hall G, Collins A, Csemiczky G, Landgren BM. Lipoproteins and BMI: a comparison between women during transition to menopause and regularly menstruating healthy women. Maturitas 2002; 41(3):177.
12. Abbey M, Owen A, Suzakawa M, Roach P, Westel PJ. Effects of menopause and hormone replacement therapy on plasma lipids, lipoproteins and LDL-receptor activity. Maturitas 1999; 33(3):259.

13. Tremollieres FA, et al. Coronary heart disease risk factors and menopause: a study in 1684 French women. Atherosclerosis 1999; 142(2):415.

14. Carmena R, Duriez P, Fruchart JC. Atherogenic lipoprotein particles in atherosclerosis. Circulation 2004; 109(23 Suppl 1):III2.

15. Erenus M, Karakoc B, Gurler A. Comparison of effects of continuous combined transdermal with oral estrogen and oral progestogen replacement therapies on serum lipoproteins and compliance. Climacteric 2001; 4(3):228.

16. Stevenson JC, Crook D, Godsland IF, Lees B, Whitehead MI. Oral versus transdermal hormone replacement therapy. Int J Fertil Menopausal Stud 1993; 38(Suppl 1):30.

17. Hulley S, Grady D, Bush T, et al. Randomized trial of estrogen plus progestin for secondary prevention of coronary heart disease in postmenopausal women. Heart and Estrogen/progestin Replacement Study (HERS) Research Group. JAMA 1998; 280(7):605.

18. Grady D, Herrington D, Bittner V, et al. Cardiovascular disease outcomes during 6.8 years of hormone therapy: Heart and Estrogen/progestin Replacement Study follow-up (HERS II). JAMA 2002; 288(1):49.

19. Anderson GL, Limacher M, Assaf AR, et al. Effects of conjugated equine estrogen in postmenopausal women with hysterectomy: the Women's Health Initiative randomized controlled trial. JAMA 2004; 291(14):1701.

20. Manson JE, Hsia J, Johnson KC, et al. Estrogen plus progestin and the risk of coronary heart disease. N Engl J Med 2003; 349(6):523.

21. Kuller LH; Women's Health Initiative. Hormone replacement therapy and risk of cardiovascular disease: implications of the results of the Women's Health Initiative. Arterioscler Thromb Vasc Biol 2003; 23(1):11.

22. Seed M, Knopp RH. Estrogens, lipoproteins, and cardiovascular risk factors: an update following the randomized placebo-controlled trials of hormone-replacement therapy. Curr Opin Lipidol 2004; 15(4):459.

23. Lobo RA, Carmina E. The importance of diagnosing the polycystic ovary syndrome. Ann Intern Med 2000; 132(12):989.

24. Bloomgarden ZT. American Association of Clinical Endocrinologists (AACE) consensus conference on the insulin resistance syndrome: 25–26 August 2002, Washington, DC. Diabetes Care 2003; 26(4):1297.

25. Guzick DS. Polycystic ovary syndrome. Obstet Gynecol 2004; 103(1):181.

26. Wild RA. Long-term health consequences of PCOS. Hum Reprod Update 2002; 8(3):231.

27. Wild RA. Polycystic ovary syndrome: a risk for coronary artery disease? Am J Obstet Gynecol 2002; 186(1):35.

28. Lewis SJ. Cholesterol and coronary heart disease in women. Cardiol Clin 1998; 16(1):9.

29. Gordon DJ, Probstfield JL, Garrison RJ, et al. High-density lipoprotein cholesterol and cardiovascular disease. Four prospective American studies. Circulation 1989; 79(1):8.

30. Legato MJ. Dyslipidemia, gender, and the role of high-density lipoprotein cholesterol: implications for therapy. Am J Cardiol 2000; 86(12A):15L.

31. Jacobs AK, Eckel RH. Evaluating and managing cardiovascular disease in women: understanding a woman's heart. Circulation 2005; 111(4):383.

32. Downs JR, Clearfield M, Weis S, et al. Primary prevention of acute coronary events with lovastatin in men and women with average cholesterol levels: results of AFCAPS/TexCAPS. Air Force/Texas Coronary Atherosclerosis Prevention Study. JAMA 1998; 279(20):1615.

33. Lewis SJ, et al. Effect of pravastatin on cardiovascular events in women after myocardial infarction: the cholesterol and recurrent events (CARE) trial. J Am Coll Cardiol 1998; 32(1):140.

34. Heart Protection Study Collaborative Group. MRC/BHF Heart Protection Study of cholesterol lowering with simvastatin in 20,536 high-risk individuals: a randomised placebo-controlled trial. Lancet 2002; 360(9326):7.

35. Expert Panel on Detection, Evaluation and Treatment of High Blood Cholesterol in Adults. Executive Summary of The Third Report of The National Cholesterol Education Program (NCEP) Expert Panel on Detection, Evaluation, and Treatment of High Blood Cholesterol In Adults (Adult Treatment Panel III). JAMA 2001; 285(19):2486.

36. Expert Panel/Writing Group. Evidence-based guidelines for cardiovascular disease prevention in women. Circulation 2004; 109(5):672.

37. Mosca L, Merz NB, Blumenthal RS, et al. Opportunity for intervention to achieve American Heart Association guidelines for optimal lipid levels in high-risk women in a managed care setting. Circulation 2005; 111(4):488.

38. O'Meara, JG, et al. Ethnic and sex differences in the prevalence, treatment, and control of dyslipidemia among hypertensive adults in the GENOA study. Arch Intern Med 2004; 164(12):1313.

39. Schrott HG, Bittner V, Vittinghoff E, Herrington DM, Hulley S. Adherence to National Cholesterol Education Program Treatment goals in postmenopausal women with heart disease. The Heart and Estrogen/Progestin Replacement Study (HERS). The HERS Research Group. JAMA 1997; 277(16):1281.

40. Wexler DJ, Grant RW, Meigs JB, Nathan DM, Cagliero E. Sex disparities in treatment of cardiac risk factors in patients with Type 2 diabetes. Diabetes Care 2005; 28:514.

8

Diabetes mellitus: focus on cardiovascular risk

Stephen A Brietzke

Introduction • Diagnosis and recognition of diabetes mellitus and related syndromes • Classification of diabetes mellitus • Cardiovascular morbidity and mortality in diabetes mellitus • Pathophysiology of diabetes mellitus-attributable coronary heart disease risk • Female-specific issues in diabetes mellitus: stages of life • Conclusions

INTRODUCTION

Diabetes mellitus (DM) is the end state of a group of dysglycemic disorders that include individuals at risk (based on hereditary and lifestyle characteristics), pre-diabetes (which includes impaired fasting glucose and impaired glucose tolerance), and overt diabetes (which is identified by fasting and postprandial hyperglycemia). These disorders are caused by impaired insulin secretion and/or action, and overlap among types that are common in mainstream clinical practice.

DM has been recognized as a major risk factor for cardiovascular disease for decades; indeed, cardiovascular events are the leading cause of death for patients with the most common form of diabetes, type 2 DM.[1] Patients with DM who suffer myocardial infarction (MI), stroke, and peripheral arterial disease of the lower extremities have historically suffered worse clinical outcomes than non-diabetic individuals with the same conditions.[2] In one major epidemiologic study, survival of DM patients who had never suffered MI was identical to that of non-DM patients who had had at least one MI.[3] In this same study, survival of diabetic patients who had MI was much worse than non-diabetic subjects post-MI. Symptoms

heralding the presence of serious coronary heart disease (CHD) are more likely to be absent in diabetic than in non-diabetic individuals, thus impeding a strategy of early diagnosis and intervention; declaration of CHD is thus more likely to be 'silent' MI or sudden cardiac death in patients with DM.[4] The frequency, severity, and lethality of atherosclerotic disease in diabetes is so compelling that the Adult Treatment Panel-III of the US National Cholesterol Education Project (NCEP) has assigned DM as a coronary heart disease equivalent. The tight weave between atherosclerotic disease and diabetes mellitus has led to a justifiable alternative definition of diabetes as 'a state of premature atherosclerosis associated with hyperglycemia.'[5]

Women are at least as susceptible to diabetes mellitus and its complications as are men. The early onset of DM in a woman obliterates the so-called 'estrogen advantage' that usually protects premenopausal women from atherosclerotic events prior to menopause. Diabetic women suffer early atherosclerotic events at the same rate as diabetic men, at a rate greater than non-diabetic men, and at a rate far in excess of non-diabetic age-matched women. Pregnancy and being at risk for unplanned pregnancy limits pharmacotherapy options in young women, as a result of known or potential deleterious effects of drugs on fetal development. In addition, young women present two distinct syndromes which are predictive of future diabetes: polycystic ovary syndrome and gestational diabetes mellitus (GDM). Each of these issues will be examined in ensuing sections of this chapter.

DIAGNOSIS AND RECOGNITION OF DIABETES MELLITUS AND RELATED SYNDROMES

The diagnosis of diabetes mellitus is based on identification of persistently abnormal fasting or random serum glucose concentration. The current classification scheme recognizes glucose concentrations between 'normal' and 'diabetic' as being 'pre-diabetic'; the latter group includes patients with impaired fasting glucose (IFG) and impaired glucose tolerance (IGT). Diabetes mellitus is diagnosed in the non-pregnant individual on the basis of two or more fasting plasma glucose values ≥126 mg/dl (≥7.0 mmol/l). Alternatively, diabetes mellitus may be diagnosed based on a non-fasting plasma glucose value ≥200 mg/dl (≥11.1 mmol/l) in the presence of symptoms of diabetes (polyuria, polydipsia, unexplained weight loss, blurred vision), or a 2-hour post-oral glucose challenge plasma glucose value ≥200 mg/dl during a 75 g anhydrous glucose (Glucola) oral glucose tolerance test (OGTT). Table 8.1 lists diagnostic criteria for normal glucose tolerance, impaired fasting glucose, impaired glucose tolerance, and

diabetes mellitus, based on the current classification scheme of the American Diabetes Association.[6,7]

CLASSIFICATION OF DIABETES MELLITUS

The syndrome of diabetes mellitus is suspected and confirmed based on the presence of classic symptoms of hyperglycemia (polyuria/nocturia, polydipsia, polyphagia, unexplained weight loss, and blurred vision), or on the basis of blood glucose screening tests obtained due to high risk of DM, based on a strong family history of diabetes, or personal risk characteristics known to confer high risk (sedentary lifestyle and obesity). The vast majority of patients encountered in clinical practice will have either type 1 or type 2 diabetes; an important additional type of DM, gestational diabetes, will be discussed in an ensuing section of this chapter.

Type 1 DM

In the United States, 5–10% of diabetic patients have type 1 diabetes.[8] This form of diabetes is defined by total or near-total absence of endogenous insulin secretion, usually on the basis of autoimmune destruction of β cells of the pancreatic islets. Most such patients can be identified at the time of diagnosis by clinical markers of islet cell autoimmunity, such as glutamic acid decarboxylase autoantibodies or anti-islet cell autoantibodies. Because the

Table 8.1 Diagnostic criteria for diabetes mellitus and other states of dysglycemia

Glucose tolerance classification	Fasting plasma glucose (FPG)	2-hour post-oral glucose challenge (2-hr OGTT) plasma glucose
Normal	<100 mg/dl (<5.6 mmol/l)	<140 mg/dl (<7.8 mmol/l)
Impaired fasting glucose	100–125 mg/dl (5.6–7.0 mmol/l)	<140 mg/dl (<7.8 mmol/l)
Impaired glucose tolerance	100–125 mg/dl (5.6–7.0 mmol/l)	140–199 mg/dl (7.8–11.1 mmol/l)
Diabetes mellitus	≥126 mg/dl (≥7.0 mmol/l)	≥200 mg/dl (≥11.1 mmol/l)

underlying pathophysiology responsible for diabetes in affected individuals is the absence of endogenous insulin secretion, insulin replacement therapy is obligatory in patients with 'classic' type 1 DM. In patients with severe insulin deficiency, oral antihyperglycemic therapy in the absence of insulin replacement therapy is ineffective and is therefore contraindicated.

Type 1 DM was once called 'juvenile-onset DM' because so many recognized patients were diagnosed during childhood or adolescence. It is now understood that type 1 DM can have onset at any age, including elderly persons. There is even an indolent-onset form of type 1 DM which can occur in middle-aged persons, and which has become known as 'latent autoimmune diabetes of adults' (LADA). Affected patients have serum markers of autoimmune-mediated islet cell disease (anti-GAD or anti-ICA autoantibodies), but demonstrate presence of endogenous insulin reserve. Individuals with LADA may respond to oral antihyperglycemic therapy for many years, but can develop progressive islet cell failure and thus may eventually require insulin replacement therapy. The natural history of patients recognized as having LADA is still being defined. Clinicians may suspect LADA in diabetic middle-aged adults with lean body habitus who exhibit low-grade, non-fasting ketonuria on office screening.[9]

Type 2 DM

Type 2 DM constitutes 90–95% of the total number of DM cases in the United States, and is thus by far the most common type of DM seen by practitioners.[10] The underlying metabolic defect in type 2 DM is a combination of inappropriately low insulin secretion in response to hyperglycemic stimulation, and insulin resistance, characterized by impaired cellular response to insulin signaling in target tissues such as muscle and adipose tissue. Patients with type 2 DM are heterogeneous with regard to the magnitude of these two defects, ranging from those with severely impaired insulin secretion and only slightly impaired insulin action, to those with marked

Table 8.2 Factors conferring increased risk for type 2 diabetes mellitus
Metabolic syndrome (three or more of the following components):   • Waist circumference (women) >35 inches (90 cm)   • Fasting serum triglycerides >150 mg/dl   • High-density lipoprotein (HDL) cholesterol <50 mg/dl   • Blood pressure ≥130/85 mmHg   • Impaired fasting glucose (IFG) or impaired glucose tolerance (IGT)   Sedentary lifestyle   Multiple first-degree relatives with diabetes   Ethnicity other than non-Hispanic white: • African-American/African-Caribbean   • Hispanic/Mexican-American   • Native American   • Pacific Islander   Polycystic ovary syndrome (PCOS)   History of gestational diabetes (GDM)

insulin hypersecretion and severely impaired target tissue response to insulin. Population-based studies, as in Pima Indians in the United States (Pima Indians have a 50% prevalence of type 2 DM), have demonstrated that insulin resistance presages the development of overt diabetes by many years.[11] In contrast to type 1 DM, patients with type 2 DM tend to have a strong family history of DM among first-degree relatives. A number of other components of the so-called metabolic syndrome also confer risk for type 2 DM. The more common of these individual risks are summarized in Table 8.2. Management of patients with type 2 DM includes dietary caloric restriction, exercise, oral antihyperglycemic drug therapy, and supplemental injected insulin.

CARDIOVASCULAR MORBIDITY AND MORTALITY IN DIABETES MELLITUS

Data from several large, well-designed population-based studies document a markedly increased risk for fatal and non-fatal cardiovascular events among women with DM. The

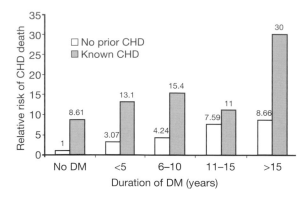

Figure 8.1 Relative risk of death from coronary heart (CHD) disease among participants in the Nurses' Health Study (1976–1996) as a function of duration of known diabetes mellitus (DM). Multivariate analysis adjusted for additional CHD risk factors, including smoking, age, hypertension, family history of CHD, and hypercholesterolemia. (Reproduced with permission from Hu et al.[12])

Nurses' Health Study, which ran from 1976 to 1996, accrued 2 341 338 person-years of data among an exclusively female study population. Compared with women who had neither DM nor CHD at the outset of the study, relative risk (RR) = 1.0, diabetic women exhibited an age-adjusted RR of coronary mortality of 8.7, whereas women with no history of DM but with a known history of coronary disease had an RR of coronary mortality of 10.6. For women known to have both DM and CHD at the time of study enrollment, the RR of fatal coronary disease was even higher, at 25.8.[12] In this same study, increasing duration of known DM correlated with increasing risk of CHD-related death (Figure 8.1). In the population-based Copenhagen City Heart Study, which assessed annual health status over a 20-year period in 7198 women, RR of new acute MI was 1.5–4.5 for those with known DM compared with those without DM, and RR for stroke was 2.0–6.5 for diabetic vs non-diabetic women.[13] The Rancho Bernardo population-based study in an older (mean age = 62 years) California community in the United States ran for 14 years and included a database of 2344 patients; among women with DM, the RR for CHD death was 3.3 (compared with non-diabetic women). For men with DM

in the Rancho Bernardo study, the relative risk of CHD death was only 1.8 compared with non-diabetic men; the authors of the study attribute the greater risk of CHD death in diabetic women to superior overall survival in the absence of DM.[14] The Women's Pooling Project identified a threefold increased risk of fatal stroke among women with DM and no prior history of stroke or known CHD, compared with non-diabetic women. This hazard ratio was exceeded only by women who had previously had a stroke.[15]

PATHOPHYSIOLOGY OF DIABETES MELLITUS-ATTRIBUTABLE CORONARY HEART DISEASE RISK

Explanations for the DM-attributable CHD risk are not definitive, but there are numerous observations to suggest the underlying pathophysiologic mechanisms: these include dyslipidemia, hypercoagulability, altered vascular reactivity, and endothelial dysfunction. A summary of these pathophysiologic contributors is provided in Table 8.3.

Table 8.3 Pathophysiology of diabetes mellitus-related cardiovascular disease

Dyslipidemia:
- Hypertriglyceridemia
- Low HDL-C
- Small dense LDL-C

Hypercoagulability:
↑ Fibrinogen
↑ Factor VIII activity
↑ von Willebrand factor activity
↑ Plasminogen activator inhibitor-1 (PAI-1) activity

Decreased large artery distensibility

Endothelial dysfunction:
↓ Nitric oxide activity/response
↑ Vasoconstrictor expression (ET-1, AII)
↑ Vascular smooth muscle growth factor production
↑↑ Inflammatory adhesion molecule expression

HDL-C, high-density lipoprotein cholesterol; LDL-C, low-density lipprotein cholesterol; ET-1, endothelin-1; AII, angiotensin.

Dyslipidemia

Decreased plasma high-density lipoprotein cholesterol (HDL-C) and hypertriglyceridemia very frequently coexist with DM (most especially, type 2 DM).[16] HDL-C <50 mg/dl and very low-density lipoprotein (VLDL) cholesterol (correlating with endogenous plasma triglyceride concentration) ≥20 mg/dl have been strongly associated with CHD mortality among women with DM.[17] Low-density lipoprotein cholesterol (LDL-C) plasma concentration is known to correlate with CHD risk, but LDL-C particle size modifies the atherogenic risk, based on the fact that larger, 'fluffier' LDL-C particles are more resistant to oxidation than are small, dense particles. When LDL-C particle size was directly measured, DM in women was strongly associated with smaller LDL-C compared with non-diabetic women.[18] This observation suggests that for any plasma concentration of LDL-C, the atherogenicity of the LDL-C is greater in the presence of DM.

Hypercoagulability

Abnormal platelet function has been recognized as a DM-associated abnormality for many years. Known abnormalities include reduced platelet survival, increased generation of vasoconstricting prostanoids, and decreased generation of vasodilating nitric oxide and prostacyclin.[19,20] In the aggregate, these abnormalities favor clot formation by predisposing to enhanced platelet aggregation and platelet-endothelial adhesion. The balance between systemic coagulability and fibrinolytic activity is also tipped towards hypercoagulability by DM-associated hyperfibrinogenemia, increased concentration of factor VIII, and reduced fibrinolysis due to increased levels of plasminogen activator inhibitor-1 (PAI-1).[19]

Altered vascular reactivity

As assessed by echocardiography, reduced abdominal aortic distensibility was found in women with type 1 DM as compared with diabetic men by Ahlgren and associates, and the degree of wall stiffness correlated with duration of DM.[21] Among premenopausal women with both type 1 and type 2 DM, Di Carli et al documented reduced coronary vasodilation and augmentation of myocardial blood flow in response to adenosine- and dipyridamole-induced hyperemia, as compared with non-diabetic women. Responses of the diabetic women to pharmacologic challenge resembled the response of non-diabetic, postmenopausal women to the same pharmacologic hyperemia challenge.[22] Although the relationship of these observations to cardiovascular risk is unclear, they, nonetheless, suggest fundamental difference in large-artery function in diabetic versus non-diabetic women.

Endothelial dysfunction

Vascular endothelium, the thin luminal-lining cell layer of blood vessels, is now known to produce numerous cytokines and substances responsible for vascular smooth muscle proliferation, maintenance of blood pressure, vascular inflammation, and coagulation. As a disease associated with microangiopathy and atherosclerosis, diabetes is known to be associated with numerous derangements of normal endothelial function; the significance of these derangements continues to be a ripe area of basic and clinical research. Production of the most potent locally derived vasodilatory substance, nitric oxide (NO), appears to be augmented in DM; however, the activity of NO appears to be paradoxically reduced.[23] In part, reduced NO activity is explained by increased endothelial generation of reactive oxygen species, resulting in a state of increased oxidative stress. Among other effects, oxidative modification of LDL-C results in enhanced atherogenicity of that particle. Other derangements of normal endothelial function in DM include increased generation and activity of locally derived vasoconstrictor substances, notably including endothelin-1 (ET-1) and angiotensin II (AII), increased generation and activity of promoters of vascular smooth muscle proliferation, including platelet-derived growth factor (PDGF) and fibroblast growth factor, and increased expression of proinflammatory adhesion molecules (ELAM, VCAM, and

ICAM).[24] In the aggregate, DM-associated alterations in endothelial function are associated with a milieu favoring hypertension, a proinflammatory vascular state, and vascular smooth muscle/atherosclerotic plaque proliferation.

FEMALE-SPECIFIC ISSUES IN DIABETES MELLITUS: STAGES OF LIFE

Women's issues which directly relate to diabetes risk include infertility and oligomenorrhea, pregnancy, the 'well woman' periodic health assessment, and aging.

The adolescent girl with oligomenorrhea

Adolescents with normal menarche and complaints of irregular menses, light 'spotting' sporadically, undesired facial hair growth affecting the chin and upper lip (requiring frequent depilatory treatments), a generally normal adolescent female appearance with a pattern of obesity that appears symmetrical, and no cutaneous striae, should raise the concern of polycystic ovary syndrome.

Syndrome recognition – polycystic ovary syndrome

After clinical evaluation and appropriate endocrinologic screening has excluded such conditions as Cushing's syndrome, thyroid dysfunction, hyperprolactinemia, and non-classic congenital adrenal hyperplasia, the most common explanation for this irregular pattern of menstruation (chronic anovulation) and mild hyperandrogenism (facial hirsutism) is the polycystic ovary syndrome (PCOS). An extremely common disorder of young women, it is now understood that PCOS is a substantial clinical risk factor for later type 2 DM and heightened cardiovascular risk. The pathophysiologic linkage between PCOS and dysglycemia appears to center around the nearly universal impaired insulin effect (insulin resistance) on ovarian steroidogenesis. Normal insulin action promotes efficient aromatization of androgenic precursors into estradiol; conversely, impaired insulin action inhibits aromatization and promotes the establishment and maintenance of an androgen-dominant ovarian microenvironment. At the ovarian level, mild hyperandrogenemia prevents or distorts luteinization, with clinical consequences resulting from the loss of the normal luteal phase of the menstrual cycle. These consequences include oligomenorrhea; acyclic bleeding (spotting); anovulation; and infertility. These problems are compounded by disordered gonadotropin secretion, which tends to perpetuate the hyperandrogenic milieu.

The importance of insulin's influence on ovarian function is reinforced by the higher-than-expected prevalence (18.8% vs 6.5% in age-matched, non-diabetic women) of PCOS among women with classic type 1 DM (who have absolute insulin deficiency, with generally normal insulin responsiveness). Since peripheral blood insulin levels in type 1 DM patients are much higher than in non-diabetic women as a consequence of chronic subcutaneous insulin injections, it is possible that the therapeutic hyperinsulinemia causes ovarian hyperandrogenism in this group of women.[25]

Risk of dysglycemia (impaired glucose tolerance and type 2 diabetes mellitus) in PCOS

Obesity is associated with individually determined insulin resistance, and is a major independent risk factor for both PCOS and type 2 DM. However, even non-obese women – body mass index (BMI) <30 kg/m^2 – with PCOS have approximately a fourfold relative risk of type 2 DM compared with eumenorrheic age-matched women.[26] In various population-based studies of women meeting the case definition of PCOS, when formal oral glucose tolerance has been performed, IGT has been identified in as many as 31% and diabetes in as many as 7.5% of the women studied.[27] Most of these women were in the 20–40-year-old age range; among similar-aged women with regular menstrual cycles, the prevalence of IGT averaged about 8% and diabetes about 1%. Based on these estimates and the estimated prevalence of PCOS, PCOS may contribute to 20% of the IGT and up to 40% of the type 2 DM seen in reproductive-aged women.[28]

PCOS-linked cardiovascular risk

The prevalence of the dyslipidemia phenotype (hypertriglyceridemia, low HDL-C, small dense LDL-C), hypertension, and visceral compartment obesity is much higher among women with PCOS when compared with eumenorrheic women. Fibrinogen and PAI-1 have measured significantly higher in PCOS vs non-PCOS women.[29] Despite these associations, increased CHD mortality has not been definitively established among women who underwent ovarian wedge resection as treatment for PCOS.[30] Notwithstanding, the high frequency of PCOS among reproductive-aged women and the strong association of PCOS with type 2 DM, the metabolic syndrome of insulin resistance, dyslipidemia, hypertension, and visceral compartment obesity, and serum markers of inflammation and hypercoagulability must be acknowledged, and a strategy of primary cardiovascular disease prevention is appropriate for young women who express PCOS.

Primary cardiovascular disease prevention in women with PCOS

At the time of recognition of the syndrome of PCOS, screening for abnormal glucose tolerance and dyslipidemia is an appropriate action. PCOS is considered by the American Diabetes Association to be one of the high-risk conditions for which a formal 2-hour oral glucose tolerance test is indicated. The recommended procedure is to obtain fasting serum (or plasma) glucose (serum triglycerides, HDL-C, and LDL-C can be obtained simultaneously), followed by the ingestion of a 75 g anhydrous glucose (Glucola) load, with subsequent measurement of serum (or plasma) glucose 2 hours after the test meal.

Cosmetic and reproductive aspects of PCOS can be managed by drug therapy (oral contraceptives and/or androgen receptor antagonists for hirsutism; oral contraceptives for oligomenorrhea; clomiphene for induction of ovulation), but it has been long appreciated that metabolic interventions also favorably modulate these aspects of PCOS. For patients with PCOS who are overweight, weight reduction (which ameliorates insulin resistance/hyperinsulin-

emia) frequently results in improved ovulatory function and fertility. In women at risk for future type 2 DM on the basis of IGT (but not PCOS specifically), a program of dietary caloric restriction (to promote and maintain weight loss) and regular aerobic physical exercise has been shown to prevent or delay the onset of diabetes.[31] Since these same interventions have also been shown to improve ovulatory function in PCOS, these therapeutic lifestyle modifications can be recommended enthusiastically to obese PCOS patients even without in-depth biomedical risk stratification (e.g. glucose tolerance testing, lipid profiles, etc.).

An important pharmacotherapeutic treatment option in patients with PCOS is metformin. As monotherapy, metformin has been shown to improve ovulatory menstrual cycles in over 50% of treated women; serum levels of insulin and androgens are concomitantly improved.[32] In clinical trials of metformin in PCOS, the usual dose is 500 mg three times daily; in clinical practice, many patients appear to benefit from doses as low as 500 mg twice daily. In addition to its effect on ovulation, there is evidence that metformin also favorably modifies future risk for type 2 DM. In the Diabetes Prevention Program (which did not specifically include women with PCOS, but rather those with IGT on OGTT), use of metformin was also shown to reduce the incidence of type 2 DM over a 6-year period by 31%, compared with an untreated control group.[31] Enthusiasm for the use of any oral medication in young women of reproductive potential is naturally tempered by the possibility of untoward effects of the drug on fetal development – particularly if the drug therapy increases the likelihood of pregnancy by improving ovulation and fertility. Although metformin is not approved by the US Food and Drug Administration (FDA) for use in pregnancy, available information about fetal development and pregnancy outcomes is reassuring. No adverse effects on fetal development have been identified, and the drug is classified as Class B in gestation. Further consideration of the risks and benefits of metformin use in pregnancy is provided in the ensuing section of this chapter.

The young woman with hyperglycemia in pregnancy

Young women with a positive family history of type 2 diabetes mellitus have higher risks of developing abnormal 100 g oral glucose (Glucola) challenge. With the abnormal glucose challenge, a diagnosis of gestational diabetes mellitus is entertained.

Case definition – gestational diabetes mellitus

The American Diabetes Association defines gestational DM as the onset or first recognition of hyperglycemia during pregnancy. Pointedly, this classification leaves open the possibility that diabetes mellitus may have pre-dated the pregnancy.[33] As with other forms of diabetes mellitus, diagnosis rests on the confirmation of fasting hyperglycemia, or hyperglycemia post-oral glucose challenge. The diagnostic cut-off points for GDM are summarized in Table 8.4. The rationale for screening at 28 weeks is the long-standing recognition that maternal glucose homeostasis is progressively challenged throughout the duration of pregnancy, peaking in the third trimester with rising placental production of somatomammotropin, which opposes the actions of insulin and promotes hyperglycemia.

Table 8.4 Diagnosis of gestational diabetes mellitus using 100 or 75 g oral anhydrous glucose challenge

Challenge	Plasma glucose	
	mg/dl	mmol/l
100 g oral glucose load:		
Fasting	95	5.3
1 h post-glucose challenge	180	10.0
2 h post-glucose challenge	155	8.6
3 h post-glucose challenge	140	7.8
75 g oral glucose load:		
Fasting	95	5.3
1 h post-glucose challenge	180	10.0
2 h post-glucose challenge	155	8.6

Future risk of type 2 DM and cardiovascular disease in GDM

A systematic review of studies tracking patients diagnosed with GDM and followed for postpartum glucose tolerance for periods of time ranging from 6 months to over 25 years reports that the incidence of type 2 DM peaks at 30–60% within 5 years of the index episode of GDM and peaks at about 70% over 25 years of follow-up. Importantly, 3–10% of women with GDM continue to have DM when studied 6 weeks to 6 months postpartum, implying that the DM was not, in fact, gestational (i.e. type 2 DM with recognition in pregnancy would be a more accurate nomenclature).[34]

Aside from the risk of persistent or future type 2 DM, patients with GDM have been shown to have several other metabolic and proinflammatory characteristics which are of themselves cardiovascular risks. Hyperhomocysteinemia has been recognized as an independent cardiovascular risk factor. Relative to women unaffected by GDM, GDM patients have been shown to have higher plasma homocysteine levels and lower folic acid levels.[35] In this study, the plasma homocysteine was proportional to 2-hour post-oral glucose challenge glucose. Using 8-isoprostane derived from placenta, skeletal muscle, and adipose tissue as a marker of oxidative stress, Lappas and colleagues were able to show substantially higher release of this substance from tissues derived from women with GDM compared with women with normal glucose tolerance.[36] Adiponectin is an anti-inflammatory, insulin-sensitizing cytokine product of healthy adipocytes. Serum adiponectin concentration has been shown to be lower in patients with type 2 DM and metabolic syndrome when compared with unaffected, age-matched patients. Adiponectin has recently been identified as lower in patients with current[37] and prior[38] GDM, when compared with pregnant or postpartum women with no history of GDM. Finally, endothelial dysfunction, as assessed by reduced hyperemic response to acetylcholine infusion, has been identified when women with prior GDM have been compared with age-matched women unaffected by GDM.[39,40]

Management of GDM

Management of GDM

Within the context of pregnancy, mainstays of treatment of GDM have been dietary caloric restriction and, when necessary to control hyperglycemia, injections of NPH insulin and regular insulin. Resistance (weight-training) exercise has been shown to improve insulin action and lower postprandial hyperglycemia.[41] A recent study randomizing women requiring more than dietary therapy for GDM to either glyburide or insulin treatment documented comparable glycemic control and no significant disparity in the incidence of fetal hypoglycemia, anomalies, or birthweight.[42] Thus, use of glyburide in pregnancy, while not currently approved by the FDA, may yet be a practical option in some patients.

With regard to primary prevention of cardiovascular disease, patients with GDM should be viewed as being at very high risk for type 2 DM; indeed, many will be found to actually have type 2 DM by virtue of abnormal fasting or random plasma glucose testing 6–8 weeks postpartum. Thus, screening for persistent diabetes within 2 months postpartum is important. Efforts to reduce the incidence of future diabetes would then be of paramount importance, and is the topic of the next section of this chapter.

The young woman with prior GDM, or otherwise at risk for type 2 DM

Young women may seek medical advice for preventing diabetes. Frequently, the woman has a prior history of gestational diabetes, treated with dietary therapy, during her pregnancy. Although currently asymptomatic, she is concerned about her strong family history of diabetes and her prior history of GDM. These women require specific monitoring and preventive strategies.

Risk factors for type 2 DM

Risk factors for type 2 DM

Risks for type 2 DM can be categorized in dichotomous fashion as either *heritable* (non-modifiable) or *acquired* (modifiable). Heritable risk factors include family history of type 2 DM (particularly in first-degree relatives) and ethnicity (greater risk for those with Native American, African-American/Afro-Caribbean, Mexican-American, and Pacific Islander ancestry). Acquired risk factors include obesity (acknowledging that obesity risk is in large part inherited) and sedentary lifestyle. Other potentially modifiable personal habits – including cigarette smoking and the use of alcoholic and caffeinated beverages – may positively or adversely affect the likelihood of developing type 2 DM. Multiple component features of the metabolic syndrome also represent risks for DM: in general, these components have both heritable and acquired aspects that can be considered in appraising individual risk.

Obesity

Obesity

The synergy between family history of DM and obesity as contributors to individual risk was well-documented by the TOPS (Take Off Pounds Sensibly) Club's US survey of over 32 000 female members. Body weight in excess of 75% above ideal body weight, in the absence of a known history of DM in first-degree relatives, was associated with an odds ratio (OR) for DM of 7.2, compared with women within 10% of ideal body weight who had no family history of DM. Lean women (i.e. weight within 10% of ideal body weight) with a positive family history of DM had an OR of 6.0, compared with lean women with no family history of DM. In contrast, women with positive family history of DM and who were >75% above ideal body weight had an OR for DM of 22.8 relative to lean women with a negative family history of DM.[43]

Beyond excess adiposity itself, the distribution of adiposity, as ascertained by waist-to-hip circumference measurement, or simply by waist circumference measurement, confers independent risk for DM and excessive cardiovascular risk. One of the criteria for the metabolic (insulin resistance) syndrome is waist circumference (women) >35 inches (90 cm). Risk for type 2 DM was well chronicled in the Nurses' Health Study, in which women in the top decile of waist circumference had an RR for DM of 5.1 compared with women in the lowest decile.

Likewise, women in the top decile of waist-to-hip ratio had an RR for type 2 DM of 3.1 compared with women in the lowest decile.[44] Data from the Nurses' Health Study also documented an association with the amount of weight gained after age 18 and future risk of DM: women who gained 8–11 kg had an RR of DM of 2.7, and those who gained 5–7.9 kg had an RR for DM of 1.9. Women who lost at least 5 kg after age 18 had a 50% risk reduction for DM.[45] In this same study, body mass index was found to correlate strongly with coronary heart disease as well as type 2 DM, with RR for CHD rising from 1.0 at BMI $<23\,kg/m^2$ and peaking at 3.21 for BMI $\geq35\,kg/m^2$.[46]

Lifestyle-related risk factors

Use of alcoholic beverages in light to moderate amounts ($<30\,g/day$) is associated with reduced risk of developing type 2 DM (RR = 0.42–0.78),[47] and among women with type 2 DM, regular ingestion of moderate amounts of alcohol are associated with reduced risk of coronary heart disease (RR for CHD compared with non-drinkers = 0.74 for $<5\,g$ daily and 0.48 for $\geq5\,g$ daily).[48] Based on this information, moderate use of alcoholic beverages need not be discouraged among young women who have or are at risk for type 2 DM. Likewise, caffeine (coffee) consumption need not be discouraged, and may arguably be protective against the development of type 2 DM (hazard ratio as low as 0.21 in a Finnish population-based study).[49] Cigarette smoking has not been shown to increase the risk of developing DM, but, as in non-diabetic individuals, smoking has been shown to substantially increase the risk of coronary heart disease (RR for diabetic women smoking ≥15 cigarettes daily = 7.67 vs non-smoking diabetic women).[50] Finally, sedentary patterns of behavior, including stationary activity at work and television viewing during leisure time, correlate with risk for obesity and type 2 DM in progressive fashion (risk for DM increases 7% per 2-hour increment of television viewing). Conversely, each 1 hour time period spent engaged in brisk walking has been found to be associated with a 34% reduction in DM risk.[51] Based on these observations, sedentary patterns of activity can be strongly discouraged among women otherwise at risk for DM.

Metabolic syndrome-related risk factors

Type 2 DM is often considered to be the end state of the metabolic (insulin-resistance) syndrome. Much of the cardiovascular morbidity and mortality in women with type 2 DM may in fact be attributable to non-DM components of the metabolic syndrome. In an Australian study which examined variables associated with the metabolic syndrome in diabetic women known to have CHD in comparison with diabetic women without overt CHD, indices of insulin resistance, plasma PAI-1, and serum triglycerides were greater in women with DM and CHD; mean LDL particle size was also significantly smaller, suggesting a preponderance of the pro-atherogenic 'small dense' LDL-C.[52] In a study of Pima Indian women (approximate lifetime risk for type 2 DM = 50%), higher HDL-C was found to be associated with decreased risk for DM over an observation period of nearly 10 years. Pima Indian women with HDL-C in the top decile had an RR of DM of 0.35 as compared with women with HDL-C in the lowest decile.[53]

Screening for and prevention of type 2 DM

For the young woman at risk for future development of type 2 DM, screening with fasting plasma glucose, HDL-C, and triglycerides is a prudent recommendation. Those women with normal fasting glucose, HDL-C $>50\,mg/dl$, and triglycerides $<100\,mg/dl$ probably constitute a low-risk group. Conversely, those with high-normal fasting glucose (approaching $100\,mg/dl$), HDL-C $<40\,mg/dl$, and triglycerides $>150\,mg/dl$ constitute the very high-risk group for developing DM over a period of 5 years. Targeting this latter group for lifestyle change recommendations and possibly drug therapy would appear to be a sound population-based strategy.

In the Nurses' Health Study, women with a BMI $<25\,kg/m^2$, a diet high in cereal fiber and polyunsaturated fat, and low in trans fat, abstinence from smoking, alcohol use averaging at least 5 g daily, and engaged in moderate physical exercise for at least one-half hour daily had an RR of diabetes of 0.09 compared with all other women. However, this low-risk group constituted only 3.4% of the study population.[54] The Diabetes Prevention Program enrolled patients (two-thirds were women) at high risk for DM based on an abnormal OGTT, and randomized to either a control (observation-only) group or a lifestyle modification group, which provided dietary counseling (to effect and maintain weight loss) and encouraged and monitored regular aerobic exercise (at least 150 minutes per week). After a mean follow-up of 2.8 years, the lifestyle intervention group enjoyed a 58% reduction in the incidence of DM, as compared with the control group.[31] Thus, a calorie-controlled diet, with the goal of decreasing excess adiposity, and regular aerobic exercise can be advised as low-risk, low-cost interventions of great potential pay-off in DM risk reduction. Exercise is also known to raise HDL-C, lower serum triglycerides, and improve insulin sensitivity – in other words, regular exercise can be expected to ameliorate non-DM aspects of the metabolic syndrome as well as to reduce the risk of DM itself.

Two available oral agents used in the treatment of DM, metformin and acarbose, have been shown to prevent or delay the onset of DM in randomized clinical trials. Enthusiasm for the use of oral agents in women at risk for becoming pregnant is naturally tempered by possible deleterious effects of these drugs on fetal development and pregnancy outcomes. In a study of 109 pregnancies in which mothers took metformin throughout the period of conception and throughout the entire pregnancy, no disproportionate incidence of birth defects, neonatal macrosomia, or infant psychomotor developmental abnormalities through 18 months of follow-up were identified (comparison with gender-specific Centers for Disease Control and Prevention expected incidence rates).[55] In the Diabetes Prevention Program, a second intervention group (unique from the lifestyle intervention group) was randomized to receive metformin, and this group enjoyed a 31% RR reduction in the incidence of DM, over a mean 2.8 years of

follow-up.[31] It might reasonably be inferred that combining metformin with lifestyle interventions would produce an additive risk reduction for DM, but such an inference remains to be validated by clinical trial. Acarbose, an α-glucosidase inhibitor which delays absorption of dietary carbohydrate, was likewise shown to be associated with a 32% RR reduction for DM in patients at risk (approximately 50% of the patients enrolled were women) on the basis of IGT on OGTT.[56] Like metformin, acarbose is scored as pregnancy risk Class B (no evidence of harm), and would thus be an attractive agent for use in a woman of reproductive potential. A third class of oral antihyperglycemic agent, the thiazolidinediones, is currently being evaluated for its effect on preventing onset of DM. However, the prototype member of this class, troglitazone, was removed from world markets based on cases of fatal hepatotoxicity; additionally, the currently available agents of this class, pioglitazone and rosiglitazone, are considered pregnancy risk Class C (effect on fetus cannot be ruled out).

The post-reproductive years and overt DM

Once overt DM has developed and pregnancy is no longer a consideration, the full spectrum of therapy for diabetes and its related conditions can be considered: antihyperglycemic therapy, which may include insulin secreto-gogues (sulfonylurea agents and metiglinides), inhibitors of gluconeogenesis (biguanides = metformin), insulin-sensitizing compounds (thiazolidinediones), inhibitors of dietary carbohydrate absorption (α-glucosidase inhibitors, such as acarbose). Any of these agents can be used as monotherapy, and agents from different classes can be combined, with general efficacy expectations of 1–2% decrease in HbA_{1c} for the first agent (monotherapy) and a subsequent 1% decrease in HbA_{1c} for each agent subsequently added. Consensus guidelines from the American Diabetes Association and the American Association of Clinical Endocrinologists advocate a target HbA_{1c} of <7% (ADA) or <6.5% (AACE).

Whereas the two largest clinical trials of intensive glycemic control of diabetes showed substantial reduction in risk for the major microvascular complications of DM (retinopathy, nephropathy, and neuropathy), the impact of this intervention as a stand-alone in the prevention of cardiovascular disease is not apparent. Most patients with overt type 2 DM have hypertension and dyslipidemia, as well as hyperglycemia. Several large studies afford an evidence foundation justifying aggressive management of these DM-associated (but independent) cardiovascular risks. The United Kingdom Prospective Diabetes Study (UKPDS) showed significant outcomes benefit with regard to both microvascular and atherosclerotic events with 'tight' blood pressure (BP) control (mean on-treatment BP = 144/82 mmHg in 'tight' control group vs mean on-treatment BP = 154/87 mmHg in control group) as the major intervention. In the UKPDS 'tight' blood pressure control study, 'tight' control was associated with a 32% reduction in risk for DM-related death, a 44% reduction in risk for stroke, and a 37% reduction in risk for any new microvascular complication.[57] The value of hypolipidemic therapy in type 2 DM was underscored by the Heart Protection Study, which demonstrated that in the subgroup of diabetic patients (including over 1800 women) treated with a statin drug (simvastatin) – regardless of pre-treatment baseline total or LDL-C – treatment with the statin was associated with a 22% RR reduction for CHD events.[58] As a final consideration, the Steno-2 trial employed a multiple risk factor intervention strategy for DM that included antihyperglycemic therapy (goal = HbA_{1c} <6.5%), antihypertensive therapy (goal = BP <130/80 mmHg), antihyperlipidemic therapy (goals = total cholesterol <175 mg/dl and fasting serum triglycerides <150 mg/dl), and use of daily aspirin therapy, versus a control group with less-stringent treatment goals. Treatment goals for glycemia were met in about 15%; for total cholesterol in about 72%; for triglycerides in about 58%; and for systolic blood pressure in about 50% of the subjects. Patients in the Steno-2 study were selected on the basis of microalbuminuria, which is an indicator of both early diabetic nephropathy and increased cardiovascular risk. Use of the multiple risk factor inter-vention strategy resulted in a 53% RR reduction for cardiovascular disease events and a more than a 50% risk reduction for any new-onset microvascular complication.[59]

CONCLUSIONS

Diabetes mellitus is the end state of dysglycemic conditions, also including impaired glucose tolerance and impaired fasting glucose, which are all associated with increased risk for cardiovascular disease. Two important conditions unique to women – the polycystic ovary syndrome and gestational diabetes mellitus – provide the opportunity to teach and employ lifestyle interventions (in the form of modest dietary calorie restriction and regular aerobic exercise) which are of low cost and low risk and therefore attractive in a population-based approach to health. Once DM has occurred, a comprehensive cardiovascular risk factor modification strategy, addressing not only glycemia but also blood pressure, serum lipids, and hypercoagulability, is the approach most likely to have a favorable effect on long-term health status.

REFERENCES

1. Geiss LS, Herman WH, Smith PJ. Mortality in non-insulin-dependent diabetes. In: Diabetes in America/National Diabetes Data Group, 2nd edn. Bethesda, MD: National Institutes of Health; 1995.
2. Beckman JA, Creager MA, Libby P. Diabetes and atherosclerosis: epidemiology, pathophysiology, and management. JAMA 2002; 287:2570.
3. Haffner SM, Lehto S, Ronnemaa T, et al. Mortality from coronary heart disease in subjects with type 2 diabetes and in nondiabetic subjects with and without prior myocardial infarction. N Engl J Med 1998; 339:229.
4. Valensi P, Sachs RN, Harfouche B, et al. Predictive value of cardiac autonomic neuropathy in diabetic patients with or without silent myocardial ischemia. Diabetes Care 2001; 24:339.
5. Fisher M. Diabetes: can we stop the time bomb? Heart 2003; 89(Suppl 2):ii28.
6. American Diabetes Association. Diagnosis and classification of diabetes mellitus. Diabetes Care 2005; 28(Suppl 1):S37.
7. Expert Committee on the Diagnosis and Classification of Diabetes Mellitus. Follow-up report on the diagnosis of diabetes mellitus. Diabetes Care 2003; 26:3160.

8. LaPorte RE, Matsushima M, Chang YE. Prevalence and incidence of insulin-dependent diabetes. In: Diabetes in America/National Diabetes Data Group, 2nd edn. Bethesda, MD: National Institutes of Health; 1995. NIH Publication No. 95-1468.

9. Pozzilli P, Di Mario U. Autoimmune diabetes not requiring insulin at diagnosis (latent autoimmune diabetes of the adult): definition, characterization, and potential prevention. Diabetes Care 2001; 24:1460.

10. Kenny SJ, Aubert RE, Geiss LS. Prevalence and incidence of non-insulin dependent diabetes. In: Diabetes in America/National Diabetes Data Group, 2nd edn. Bethesda, MD: National Institutes of Health; 1995. NIH Publication No. 95-1468.

11. Lillioja S, Mott DM, Spraul M, et al. Insulin resistance and insulin secretory dysfunction as precursors to non-insulin-dependent diabetes mellitus. Prospective studies of Pima Indians. N Engl J Med 1993; 329:1988.

12. Hu FB, Stampfer MJ, Solomon CG, et al. The impact of diabetes mellitus on mortality from all causes and coronary heart disease in women: 20 years of follow-up. Arch Intern Med 2001; 161:1717.

13. Almdal T, Scharling H, Jensen JS, Vestergaard II. The independent effect of type 2 diabetes mellitus on ischemic heart disease, stroke, and death: a population-based study of 13,000 men and women with 20 years of follow-up. Arch Intern Med 2004; 164:1422.

14. Barrett-Connor EL, Cohn BA, Wingard DL, Edelstein SL. Why is diabetes mellitus a stronger risk factor for fatal ischemic heart disease in women than in men? The Rancho Bernardo Study. JAMA 1991; 265:627.

15. Ho JE, Paultre F, Mosca L. Is diabetes mellitus a cardiovascular disease risk equivalent for fatal stroke in women? Data from the Women's Pooling Project. Stroke 2003; 34:2812.

16. Kannel WB. Lipids, diabetes, and coronary heart disease: insights from the Framingham study. Am Heart J 1985; 110:1100.

17. Goldschmid MG, Barrett-Connor E, Edelstein SL, et al. Dyslipidemia and ischemic heart disease mortality among men and women with diabetes. Circulation 1994; 89:991.

18. Haffner SM, Mykkanen L, Stern MP, Paidi M, Howard BJ. Greater effect of diabetes on LDL size in women than in men. Diabetes Care 1994; 17:1164.

19. Sowers JR. Diabetes mellitus and cardiovascular disease in women. Arch Intern Med 1998; 158:617.

20. Glassman AB. Platelet abnormalities in diabetes mellitus. Ann Clin Laboratory Sci 1993; 23:47.

21. Ahlgren AR, Sundkvist G, Wollmer P, Sonesson B, Lanne T. Increased aortic stiffness in women with type 1 diabetes mellitus is associated with diabetes duration and autonomic nerve function. Diabet Med 1999; 16:291.

22. Di Carli MF, Afonso L, Campisi R, et al. Coronary vascular dysfunction in premenopausal women with diabetes mellitus. Am Heart J 2002; 144:711.

23. Taylor AA. Pathophysiology of hypertension and endothelial dysfunction in patients with diabetes mellitus. Endocrinol Metab Clin North Am 2001; 30(4):983.

24. Calles-Escandon J, Cipolla M. Diabetes and endothelial dysfunction: a clinical perspective. Endocr Rev 2001; 22:36.

25. Escobar-Morreale HF, Roldan B, Barrio R, et al. High prevalence of the polycystic ovary syndrome and hirsutism in women with type 1 diabetes mellitus. J Clin Endocrinol Metab 2000; 85:4182.

26. Roumain J, Charles MA, De Courten MP, et al. The relationship of menstrual irregularity to type 2 diabetes in Pima Indian women. Diabetes Care 1998; 21:346.

27. Legro RS, Kunselman AR, Dodson WC, Dunaif A. Prevalence and predictors of risk for type 2 diabetes mellitus and impaired glucose tolerance in polycystic ovary syndrome: a prospective, controlled study in 254 affected women. J Clin Endocrinol Metab 1999; 84:165.

28. Legro RS. Diabetes prevalence and risk factors in polycystic ovary syndrome. Obstet Gynecol Clin North Am 2001; 28:99.

29. Talbott EO, Zborowski JV, Sutton Tyrrell K, McHugh-Pemu KP, Guzick DS. Cardiovascular risk in women with polycystic ovary syndrome. Obstet Gynecol Clin North Am 2001; 28:111.

30. Wild S, Pierpoint T, McKeigue P, et al. Cardiovascular disease in women with polycystic ovary syndrome at long-term follow-up: a retrospective cohort study. Clin Endocrinol (Oxf) 2000; 52:595.

31. Diabetes Prevention Program Research Group. Reduction in the incidence of type 2 diabetes with lifestyle intervention or metformin. N Engl J Med 2002; 346:393.

32. Moghetti P, Castello R, Negri C, et al. Metformin effects on clinical features, endocrine and metabolic profiles, and insulin sensitivity in polycystic ovary syndrome: a randomized, double-blind, placebo-controlled 6-month trial, followed by open, long-term clinical evaluation. J Clin Endocrinol Metab 2000; 85:139.

33. American Diabetes Association. Position statement: diagnosis and classification of diabetes mellitus. Diabetes Care 2005; 28(Suppl 1):S37.

34. Kim C, Newton KM, Knopp RH. Gestational diabetes and the incidence of type 2 diabetes. Diabetes Care 2002; 25:1862.

35. Seghieri G, Breschi MC, Anichini R, et al. Serum homocysteine levels are increased in women with gestational diabetes mellitus. Metabolism 2003; 52:720.

36. Lappas M, Permezel M, Rice GE. Release of pro-inflammatory cytokines and 8–isoprostane from placenta, adipose tissue, and skeletal muscle from normal pregnant women and women with gestational diabetes mellitus. J Clin Endocrinol Metab 2004; 89:5627.

37. Ranheim T, Haugen F, Staff AC, et al. Adiponectin is reduced in gestational diabetes mellitus in normal weight women. Acta Obstet Gynecol Scand 2004; 83:341.

38. Winzer C, Wagner O, Festa A, et al. Plasma adiponectin, insulin sensitivity, and subclinical inflammation in women with prior gestational diabetes mellitus. Diabetes Care 2004; 27:1721.

39. Hannemann MM, Liddell WG, Shore AC, Clark DM, Tooke JE. Vascular function in women with previous gestational diabetes mellitus. J Vasc Res 2002; 39:311.

40. Hu J, Norman M, Wallensteen M, Gennser G. Increased large arterial stiffness and impaired acetylcholine induced skin vasodilation in women with previous gestational diabetes mellitus. Br J Obstet Gynaecol 1998; 105:1279.

41. Brankston GN, Mitchell BF, Ryan EA, Okun NB. Resistance exercise decreases the need for insulin in overweight women with gestational diabetes mellitus. Am J Obstet Gynecol 2004; 190:188.

42. Langer O, Conway DL, Berkus MD, Xenakis EM, Gonzales O. A comparison of glyburide and insulin in women with gestational diabetes mellitus. N Engl J Med 2000; 343:1134.

43. Morris RD, Rimm DL, Hartz AJ, Kalkhoff RK, Rimm AA. Obesity and heredity in the etiology of non-insulin-dependent diabetes mellitus in 32,662 adult white women. Am J Epidemiol 1989; 130:112.

44. Carey VJ, Walters EE, Colditz GA, et al. Body fat distribution and risk of non-insulin-dependent diabetes mellitus in women: the Nurses' Health Study. Am J Epidemiol 1997; 145:614.

45. Colditz GA, Willett WC, Rotnitzky A, Manson JE. Weight gain as a risk factor for clinical diabetes mellitus in women. Ann Intern Med 1995; 122:481.

46. Cho E, Manson JE, Stampfer MJ, et al. A prospective study of obesity and risk of coronary heart disease among diabetic women. Diabetes Care 2002; 25:1142.

47. Wannamethee SG, Camargo CA, Manson JE, Willett WC, Rimm EB. Alcohol drinking patterns and risk of type 2 diabetes mellitus among younger women. Arch Intern Med 2003; 163:1329.

48. Solomon CG, Hu FB, Stampfer MJ, et al. Moderate alcohol consumption and risk of coronary heart disease among women with type 2 diabetes mellitus. Circulation 2000; 102:494.

49. Tuomilehto J, Hu G, Bidel S, Lindstrom J, Jousilahti P. Coffee consumption and risk of type 2 diabetes mellitus among middle-aged Finnish men and women. JAMA 2004; 291:1213.

50. Al-Delaimy WK, Manson JE, Solomon CG, et al. Smoking and risk of coronary heart disease among women with type 2 diabetes mellitus. Arch Intern Med 2002; 162:273.

51. Hu FB, Li TY, Colditz GA, Willett WC, Manson JE. Television watching and other sedentary behaviors in relation to risk of obesity and type 2 diabetes mellitus in women. JAMA 2003; 289:1785.

52. Stoney RM, O'Dea K, Herbert KE, et al. Insulin resistance as a major determinant of increased coronary heart disease risk in postmenopausal women with type 2 diabetes mellitus. Diabet Med 2001; 18:476.

53. Fagot-Campagna A, Naryan KM, Hanson RL, et al. Plasma lipoproteins and incidence of non-insulin-dependent diabetes mellitus in Pima Indians: protective effect of HDL cholesterol in women. Atherosclerosis 1997; 128:113.

54. Hu FB, Manson JE, Stampfer MJ, et al. Diet, lifestyle, and the risk of type 2 diabetes mellitus in women. N Engl J Med 2001; 345:790.

55. Glueck CJ, Goldenberg N, Pranikoff J, et al. Height, weight, and motor-social development during the first 18 months of life in 126 infants born to 109 mothers with polycystic ovary syndrome who conceived on and continued metformin through pregnancy. Hum Reprod 2004; 19:1323.

56. Chiasson JL, Josse RG, Hanefeld GR, Karasik A, Laakso M. Acarbose for prevention of type 2 diabetes mellitus: the STOP-NIDDM randomized trial. Lancet 2002; 359:2072.

57. United Kingdom Prospective Diabetes Study Group. Tight blood pressure control and risk of macrovascular and microvascular complications in type 2 diabetes: UKPDS 38. BMJ 1998; 317:703.

58. Heart Protection Study Collaborative Group. MRC/BHF Heart Protection Study of cholesterol-lowering with simvastatin in 5963 people with diabetes: a randomized placebo-controlled trial. Lancet 2003; 361:2005.

59. Gaede P, Vedel P, Larsen N, et al. Multifactorial intervention and cardiovascular disease in patients with type 2 diabetes. N Engl J Med 2003; 348:383.

9

Preoperative evaluation

Sanjeev Wasson and Kevin C Dellsperger

Introduction • Preoperative assessment • Preoperative cardiac risk evaluation • Perioperative interventions • Valvular heart disease • Postoperative care • Summary

INTRODUCTION

Preoperative management of female patients is an evolving dynamic process that is aimed at improving surgical outcome. Identifying women at risk, and recognizing potential complications associated with specific surgical procedures can allow risk factor modification and planning perioperative management in conjunction with an anesthesiologist, the woman's primary care provider, and medical specialists, as indicated. Therefore, preoperative management must be thorough, streamlined, and cost-effective.

However, under-representation of female patients in clinical trials has led to a lack of available evidence examining the impact of gender on preoperative cardiac risk.

PREOPERATIVE ASSESSMENT

Routine history and physical examination is generally sufficient in young, healthy, asymptomatic women with a benign cardiac history.[1] However, elderly patients over 60 years or with significant history or physical findings or those undergoing major surgery require more detailed cardiac evaluation. During preoperative evaluation, all patients should be asked about their exercise capacity and history about previous ischemia, congestive heart failure, aortic stenosis (AS), severe hypertension, and peripheral

vascular disease. The physical examination should include blood pressure measurements in both arms, presence of bruits in carotid artery and jugular venous distension, auscultation of the lungs, evidence of congestive heart failure or murmur of AS, abdominal palpation, and examination of the extremities for edema and vascular integrity. Consider postponing elective surgery in patients with blood pressures above 180/110 mmHg. Cardiac sequelae can be avoided by maintaining stable diastolic blood pressures of less than 110 mmHg.

Selective laboratory investigations[2] should be requested only if the clinical evaluation indicates a likelihood of disease. These may include a pregnancy test; hemoglobin for surgery with expected major blood loss; serum creatinine if major surgery, hypotension is expected, nephrotoxic drugs will be used, or the patient is above age 50; and chest X-ray for patients above 60 years or with suspected cardiac or pulmonary disease.[3] Routine preoperative electrocardiograms (ECGs) are recommended.[4] in women older than 55 years; in women with known cardiac disease or with clinical evaluation that suggests cardiac disease; in women with significant risk factors for cardiovascular disease such as diabetes mellitus or hypertension; in women at risk for electrolyte abnormalities such as diuretic use; or in women undergoing major surgical procedures. A rhythm other than sinus, premature

---

Table 9.1 American Society of Anesthesiology (ASA) classification of physical status

Class	Status
I	Healthy patient
II	Controlled medical condition, no systemic effects (e.g. anemia, morbid obesity)
III	Medical conditions with significant systemic effects intermittently associated with significant functional compromise (e.g. healed myocardial infarction, diabetes with vascular complications)
IV	Incapacitating and life-threatening systemic disease (e.g. advanced hepatic or renal insufficiency)
V	Critical medical condition with little chance of survival (e.g. major cerebral trauma, massive pulmonary embolus)

Adapted from Dorman et al.[7]

Table 9.2 Clinical predictors of increased perioperative cardiovascular risk

Major clinical predictors
Abnormal ECG
Symptomatic or significant arrhythmia
High-grade atrioventricular block
Coronary artery disease
Unstable or severe angina (Canadian class III or IV)
Acute (within 7 days) or recent myocardial infarction (within 7–30 days)
Decompensated CHF
Severe valvular disease

Intermediate clinical predictors
Abnormal ECG
History of previous myocardial infarction or pathologic Q waves
Chronic stable or mild angina pectoris
Compensated CHF or history of CHF
Diabetes mellitus
Renal insufficiency

Minor clinical predictors
Abnormal ECG (left ventricular hypertrophy, left bundle-branch block, ST-T abnormalities)
Non-sinus rhythm
Advanced age
Uncontrolled hypertension
History of stroke
Low functional capacity

CHF, congestive heart failure; ECG, electrocardiogram.
From Eagle et al.[11]

---

atrial contractions, or more than five premature ventricular beats on a preoperative ECG all increase the risk of perioperative cardiac events.[5] On the other hand, the presence of bundle branch block does not significantly influence the risk of cardiac complications following non-cardiac surgery.[6] High-risk patients with advanced age, smoking, obesity, and known pulmonary disease require pulmonary function tests (PFTs) and an arterial blood gas (ABG) determination. Consider postponing elective surgery in patients with PaO_2 <50 mmHg and/or $PaCO_2$ >50 mmHg on ABG, or forced expiratory volume (FEV_1) in 1 second less than 2 litres. Following a complete history, examination and laboratory evaluation, surgical risk has been identified using the American Society of Anesthesiology (ASA) classification of physical status (Table 9.1).[7]

PREOPERATIVE CARDIAC RISK EVALUATION

Perioperative myocardial infarction (MI) is a major morbidity among patients undergoing non-cardiac surgery.[8] About 27 million patients in the United States receive anesthesia every year and approximately 50 000 of these patients suffer a perioperative myocardial infarction.[9] Several physiologic factors associated with surgery predispose to myocardial hypoxia, including the stress of surgery leading to increased myocardial oxygen demand, volume shifts and blood loss, and increased platelet reactivity, or vulnerable plaque rupture.[10] The ideal approach is to identify women at high risk or with undiagnosed cardiac disease, so that appropriate testing and therapeutic measures can be undertaken.

The American College of Cardiology/American Heart Association (ACC/AHA) Task Force Practice guidelines[11] for perioperative cardiac risk stratification for non-cardiac surgery were derived from studies with gross under-representation of women.[12] These guidelines mainly involve three elements: clinical risk

Table 9.3 Mnemonics for cardiac risk of non-cardiac surgical procedures

High risk: EVA (risk >5%)	**E**mergency major operation, particularly in elderly patients **V**ascular procedures (major) **A**nticipated prolonged surgical procedures associated with large fluid shifts and/or blood loss
Intermediate risk: CHOPIN (risk <5%)	**C**arotid endarterectomy **H**ead procedures **O**rthopedic procedures **P**rostate procedures **I**ntraperitoneal and intrathoracic procedures **N**eck procedures
Low risk: ABCDE (risk <1%)	**A**mbulatory procedures **B**reast procedures **C**ataract procedures **D**ermatologic procedures **E**ndoscopic procedures

From Eagle et al.[11]

profile (Table 9.2) including functional capacity; surgical risk (Table 9.3);[11] and non-invasive testing.

Clinical risk profile

Various multivariate risk indices have been utilized for perioperative cardiac risk stratification. The Goldman cardiac risk index[6] utilizes nine independent correlates for estimating cardiac morbidity, categorized further into four risk classes according to the total points. Only lifesaving surgery should be entertained in patients with a risk index of 26 or more points. Routine preoperative cardiac evaluation should be done in patients with index scores of 13–25 points.[13] Under-representation of women is present, with the gender distribution of 57% male and 43% female,[6] in the study leading to Goldman's criteria. However, several limitations of the Goldman index, including its weakness of poor discriminative capability among intermediate-risk patients, institution-dependence, and its decreased usefulness for vascular surgery patients led to the development of the Eagle criteria. Eagle and colleagues[14] correlate five clinical and two nuclear test predictors to postoperative ischemic risk in patients undergoing major

Table 9.4 Detsky modified risk index

Variables	Total points
Coronary artery disease:	
Myocardial infarction in <6 months earlier	10
Myocardial infarction in >6 months earlier	5
Angina (Canadian Cardiovascular Society classification):	
Class III	10
Class IV	20
Pulmonary edema:	
Within 1 week	10
Ever	5
Critical aortic stenosis	20
Arrhythmias:	
Rhythm other than sinus or premature atrial contraction	5
>5 premature ventricular contractions on ECG	5
Poor general medical condition (pO_2 <60 mmHg, pCO_2 >50 mmHg, potassium level <3 mmol/l, elevated renal function, bedridden patient)	5
Age >70 years	5
Emergency surgery	5

From Detsky et al.[18]

vascular surgery. A revised Goldman cardiac risk index, using six simplified independent predictors, showed 0.4, 0.9, 7, and 11% of complication rates in the presence of 0, 1, 2, or 3 or more factors, respectively.[15] The American College of Physicians[16,17] recommendations for cardiac risk assessment involve the Detsky modified risk index (Table 9.4)[18] and stress test results (dipyridamole thallium imaging or dobutamine stress echocardiography).

Although both men and women share several cardiovascular risk factors, there are gender-specific differences in clinical risk factors and their relative significance among the sexes which alter perioperative cardiovascular risk of non-cardiac surgery.[19] For men, the presence of ECG Q waves and a history of heart failure have been shown to be independent predictors of both perioperative and late events, whereas diabetes and angina are predictive of late events only. In contrast, in females, prior angina confers an increased risk for perioperative events, whereas Q waves and diabetes were of no prognostic value and a history of heart failure is predictive of long-term events only.[20]

There is a less probability of coronary artery disease (CAD) at any level of the major cardiac risk factors in women than in men. Therefore, the clinical risk stratification for the perioperative cardiac risk into major, intermediate, or minor predictors for women should be different than for men (see Table 9.2). Clinical presentations of CAD are also dissimilar among sexes and have been described in detail in Chapter 3. Chest pain is not a reliable indicator of CAD in women, and non-atherosclerotic causes of chest pain such as mitral valve prolapse and coronary artery spasm are more prevalent in women than in men. Therefore, classification of unstable angina as a major clinical predictor and stable angina as an intermediate clinical predictor of cardiac risk in the ACC/AHA guidelines is not well justified in women.[21] History of chest pain per se, that has not been demonstrated to be from CAD or in the absence of multiple risk factors for CAD, should not be considered an intermediate clinical predictor in women. Coronary angiography is also less likely to show CAD in women with chest pain syndromes,[22–24] with a less than 7% chance in

the presence of less than two risk factors for CAD and a 55% chance with more than two risk factors.[24] Overall, 50% of women with angina in the Coronary Artery Surgery Study (CASS) registry were found to have minimal or no coronary stenosis compared with 17% of men[22] Thus, while following the ACC/AHA guidelines in women, cardiac testing should be considered only when multiple intermediate clinical predictors are present.

Women with CAD are at a greater risk for adverse outcomes than men. A retrospective analysis[25] of 206 women undergoing elective gynecologic surgery demonstrated that the Goldman cardiac risk index, the New York Heart Association (NYHA) functional classification, glucose intolerance, cardiac arrhythmia, and estrogen replacement therapy were not useful predictors of perioperative cardiac morbidity. However, hypertension and a history of CAD, proven by previously documented MI, a history of exertional angina lasting more than 15 minutes responsive to nitrate therapy, or more than 70% stenosis on coronary angiogram were useful predictors of cardiac morbidity in this population. This way, uncontrolled hypertension is a more significant predictor for perioperative cardiac risk in women as opposed to a minor clinical predictor such as the ACC/AHA guidelines.[11] The incidence rate of perioperative infarction is about 0.15–2%, which increases to 6.6% in patients with a history of previous MI. The reinfarction rate at 6 months is higher in women than in men (19% vs 12%).[26] Similarly, in-hospital mortality rates following MI are higher in women than in men (17.5% vs 12.3%),[27] especially for African-American women (48% mortality at 48 months).[26] Hence, the significance of an acute MI as a major clinical predictor of perioperative cardiac risk may be even greater in women than in men, and such women are at increased risk for reinfarction, if surgery is performed within 6 months of infarction. Hence it is strictly advisable to postpone elective surgery for at least 6 months in these women.

Thus, the modifications in risk stratification of women may be appropriate considering the prognostic values of these sex-specific clinical variables with regard to the perioperative cardiac morbidity and mortality.[20]

Functional capacity

Functional capacity is usually expressed in metabolic equivalents (1 MET is defined as 3.5 ml of O_2 uptake/kg/min, which is the resting oxygen uptake in a sitting position). Multiples of the baseline metabolic equivalents are used to express aerobic demands of specific activities. Energy expenditure[28] is 1 MET if a woman can take care of self, such as eat, dress, or use the toilet; 4 METS if she can walk up a flight of stairs; 4–10 METS if she can run a short distance or scrub floors; >10 METS if she can participate in strenuous sports. Perioperative cardiac risks are increased in patients unable to perform activities of greater than 4 METs.

Surgical risk profile

The ACC/AHA guidelines for perioperative cardiac risk assessment stratified surgical procedures into high, intermediate, and low risk (see Table 9.3)[16] according to perioperative cardiac events rates of >5%, <5%, and <1%, respectively. Women are more likely to have preoperative risk factors, advanced age, chronic obstructive pulmonary disease (COPD), and diabetes, and have 60% more perioperative cardiac complications despite having undergone the same preoperative cardiac evaluation protocol as men patients.[29] Women suffer more perioperative MI and have poorer long-term survival after vascular surgery.[30] This is true, despite higher detection rates of cardiac disease preoperatively with electrocardiography and stress testing in men.[31] Thus, women planned for vascular surgery require even more aggressive preoperative cardiac risk assessment than men.

Non-invasive stress testing

Exercise or pharmacologic stress testing with imaging may detect occult coronary disease and give an estimate of functional capacity. Non-invasive testing further stratifies patients at intermediate risk by clinical risk profile.[32–35] An AHA/ACC Practice Guidelines provides

---

Table 9.5 Recommendations for preoperative 12-lead rest electrocardiogram

Class I
- Recent chest pain or ischemic equivalent in clinically intermediate- or high-risk patients scheduled for an intermediate- or high-risk surgery

Class IIa
- Asymptomatic persons with diabetes mellitus

Class IIb
- Prior coronary revascularization
- Asymptomatic male more than 45 years old or female more than 55 years old with 2 or more atherosclerotic risk factors
- Prior hospital admission for cardiac causes

Class III
- Routine test in asymptomatic subjects undergoing low-risk operative procedures

From Eagle et al.[11]

Table 9.6 Recommendations for preoperative non-invasive evaluation of left ventricular function

Class I
Current or poorly controlled heart failure

Class IIa
Prior heart failure and those with dyspnea of unknown origin

Class III
Routine test of left ventricular function in patients without prior heart failure

From Eagle et al.[11]

---

specific indications for the ECG (Table 9.5), non-invasive assessment of left ventricular function (Table 9.6),[36] and exercise or pharmacologic stress testing for preoperative evaluation of patients with coronary artery disease (Table 9.7).[11]

Special consideration should be given to the merits and demerits of a specific modality for stress testing in women, as described in Chapter 3. The studies examining the usefulness of the exercise stress test as a preoperative

Table 9.7 Recommendations for exercise or pharmacological stress testing

Class I
- Intermediate pretest probability of CAD
- Prognostic assessment of CAD patients; evaluation of subjects with significant change in clinical status
- Demonstration of myocardial ischemia before coronary revascularization
- Evaluation of adequacy of medical therapy; prognostic assessment after an acute coronary syndrome

Class IIa
- Evaluation of exercise capacity when subjective assessment is unreliable

Class IIb
- Diagnosis of CAD patients with high or low pretest probability (resting ST depression <1 mm, digitalis therapy, or left ventricular hypertrophy)
- Detection of restenosis in high-risk asymptomatic subjects within the initial months after PCI

Class III
- For exercise stress testing – resting ECG abnormalities that preclude adequate assessment, e.g. pre-excitation syndrome, electronically paced ventricular rhythm, rest ST depression >1 mm, or left bundle-branch block
- Severe comorbidity that limits life expectancy or candidacy for revascularization
- Routine screening of asymptomatic men or women without evidence of CAD
- Investigation of isolated ectopic beats in young patients

CAD, coronary artery disease; ECG, electrocardiogram; PCI, percutaneous coronary intervention.
From Eagle et al.[11]

diagnostic tool included more than 70% of men and, hence, their results may not be extended reliably to women.[37,38] The diagnostic and prognostic power of an exercise stress test for perioperative death or MI is limited by its low sensitivity, specificity, and positive predictive value in women.[11,39] Exercise stress testing in women has a lower false-negative rate and a higher false-positive rate as a result of the lower pretest probability of disease.[40] High false positivity has been explained by the differences in prevalence of multivessel CAD and prior

MI,[41–43] higher prevalence of syndrome X (microvascular angina), and mitral valve prolapse,[44] more baseline ECG changes due to hyperventilation or position change, inability of many women to perform adequate exercise due to comorbid conditions or general deconditioning, and microvascular function.[45] High false-positive results in women younger than 50 years, incapable of maximal exercise, those with diabetes, and those with an abnormal baseline ECG mandates addition of imaging procedures to the stress test and, probably, exercise stress test alone as a preoperative screening test does not have a place in the evaluation of women.[12]

Both dobutamine stress echocardiography (DSE) and dipyridamole thallium imaging (DTI) have high negative predictive values of nearly 100%, but have low positive predictive values of less than 20%.[46] DTI is an effective non-invasive means, with proven prognostic value for perioperative risk assessment in women prior to major non-cardiac surgery.[20] However, most of the studies examining DTI in vascular surgery patients either do not report gender distribution or include more than 65% of men.[47,48] Moreover, intrinsic gender factors such as breast artifact, small left ventricular chamber size, and a high prevalence of single-vessel coronary artery disease[49,50] adversely affect the diagnostic accuracy of nuclear perfusion imaging in women.[51]

A study by Hendel and coworkers[20] showed that transient thallium defects were predictive of perioperative MI and cardiac death in both sexes with good sensitivity (men, 81%; women, 79%) and acceptable specificity (men, 68%; women, 66%). The relative risk of perioperative cardiac events with a transient thallium defect was 3.9-fold in men (CI = 1.5–10.2) and 5.5-fold in women (CI = 1.4–22). In contrast, fixed perfusion defect increases the risk of long-term cardiac events by almost threefold in women; the magnitude of this effect was less important in men. Dipyridamole stress-induced ST-segment changes were shown to have a lower predictive value for perioperative events in women than in men.[20]

Positron emission tomography (PET) may be superior to single-photon emission computed tomography (SPECT) in terms of sensitivity (better contrast resolution), specificity (improved inferoposterior imaging in obese patients), discrimination between ischemia and scar, and better positive and negative predictive value for perioperative events of 45 and 92%, respectively.[52]

DSE is somewhat less sensitive (68 vs 88%) but more specific (84 vs 72%) than DTI.[53,54] Most of the studies evaluating the role of DSE in preoperative risk assessment of vascular surgery patients included >60% men.[55–60] When test referral bias is considered, the positive predictive value and adjusted sensitivity of DSE are lower in women than in men.[61] The prognosis after a normal DSE is more favorable in women than in men; however, the outcome of patients with abnormal DSE is not related to gender.[62]

The likelihood ratio of a positive test [sensitivity/(1 − specificity)] tells us how much the odds of a cardiac event increase when the test is positive, whereas the likelihood ratio of a negative test [(1 − sensitivity)/specificity] tells us how much the odds of a cardiac event decrease when the test is negative. The likelihood ratio of a positive or negative test should be >10 or <0.2, respectively, for a test to be considered to be useful in risk stratification, pointing towards a significant change in risk from the pretest level. Although the likelihood ratios of negative DSE and DTI are often good, the likelihood ratios of positive tests are usually much <10, indicating that these tests might not yield any useful information for risk stratification.[46]

ACC/AHA task force algorithm

Most of the studies from which the following algorithm of ACC/AHA Task Force for perioperative cardiac risk assessment[11] has been derived either do not include females or include only a minority of females. We propose a modified algorithm using the best available information for perioperative risk assessment in women (Figure 9.1).

Algorithms and flow diagrams have been used by the Task Force to guide practitioners in rational approaches to patients for a perioperative risk assessment.

First, the initial decision is the urgency of surgery. If the surgery is emergent, directly proceed to surgery. Alternatively, you may proceed direct to surgery:

- if the patient had coronary revascularization within 5 years and has no recurrent signs or symptoms
- if the patient had a coronary angiogram or stress test within 2 years and the results were favorable, and the patient had no change in symptoms
- in low-risk surgery (endoscopic procedure, superficial procedure, cataract surgery, breast surgery) in patients with no major clinical risk predictors.

Secondly, postpone non-cardiac surgery and perform coronary angiography or optimize medical management, if the patient has major clinical risk predictors:

- MI within past month
- unstable angina
- severe angina
- evidence of large ischemic burden by clinical symptoms or non-invasive testing
- decompensated heart failure
- high-grade atrioventricular block
- symptomatic arrhythmias in the presence of underlying heart disease
- supraventricular arrhythmias with uncontrolled ventricular rate
- severe valvular disease.

Thirdly, non-invasive cardiac testing to further define the patient's risk is indicated:

- if the patient has a major clinical predictor
- if the patient has an intermediate clinical predictor (mild angina, prior MI more than 1 month ago, compensated heart failure, creatinine concentration ≥2.0 mg/dl, or diabetes) and either has poor functional capacity of less than 4 METs (cannot climb a flight of stairs, walk on level ground at 4 mph, run a short distance, scrub a floor, or play a game of golf) or is undergoing high-risk surgery (vascular surgery, prolonged surgery with anticipated large fluid shifts and/or blood loss)

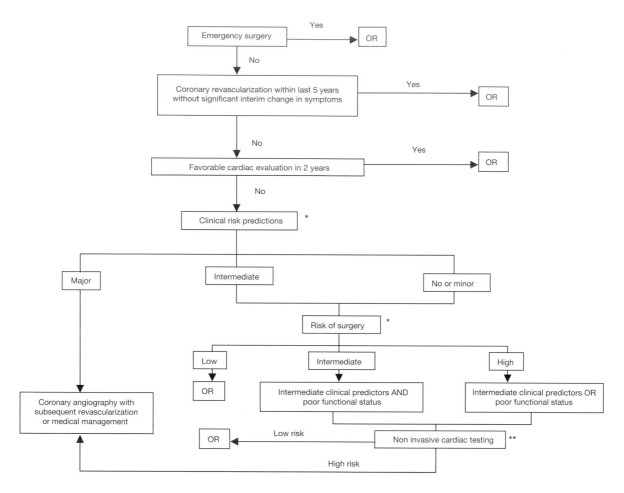

Figure 9.1 A modification to the ACC/AHA Task Force stepwise algorithm for preoperative evaluation. OR, operating room. * Women should be assigned different risk categories. ** Exercise stress testing alone without imaging has little role in women.

- if the patient has minor or no clinical risk predictors and poor functional capacity of less than 4 METs and is undergoing a high-risk surgery.

Fourthly, one can proceed with surgery in cases with low-risk non-invasive test results.

Fifthly, otherwise, consider coronary angiography in patients with high-risk non-invasive test results and determine therapy based on the results of the angiography. These options include subsequent revascularization or optimizing an anti-ischemic medical regimen with close intraoperative monitoring.

PERIOPERATIVE INTERVENTIONS

Various preoperative measures, including revascularization (Table 9.8), a medical regimen with β-blockers (Table 9.9),[11,63–67] antianginal medications and statins,[68–71] and aggressive hemodynamic monitoring, may further improve the postoperative cardiac outcome. β-Blockers (e.g. atenolol 25 mg orally each day) in the perioperative period may lower the cardiac risk sufficiently in patients with risk factors (e.g. age >65 years or known cardiovascular disease).

The issue of coronary revascularization prior to non-cardiac surgery in patients with significant

Table 9.8 Recommendations for coronary angiography in perioperative evaluation before (or after) non-cardiac surgery

Class I: patients with suspected or known CAD
- High-risk results of non-invasive test
- Medically uncontrolled angina
- Unstable angina in cases of intermediate-risk or high-risk non-cardiac surgery
- Equivocal non-invasive test results in high-risk clinical profile patients undergoing high-risk surgery

Class IIa
- Intermediate clinical risk patients planned for vascular surgery (non-invasive testing should be considered first)
- Moderate to large region of ischemia on non-invasive testing but without high-risk features and low ejection fraction
- Non-diagnostic non-invasive test results in intermediate clinical risk patients undergoing high-risk non-cardiac surgery
- Urgent non-cardiac surgery while convalescing from acute MI

Class IIb
- Perioperative MI
- Medically stabilized class III or IV angina and planned low-risk or minor surgery

Class III
- Low-risk non-cardiac surgery with known CAD and no high-risk results on non-invasive testing
- Asymptomatic after coronary revascularization with excellent exercise capacity (greater than or equal to 7 METs)
- Mild stable angina with good left ventricular function and no high-risk non-invasive test results
- Unsuitable candidate for coronary revascularization due to medical illness, severe left ventricular dysfunction (e.g. ejection fraction <0.20), or refusal to consider revascularization
- As part of evaluation for liver, lung, or renal transplantation in <40 years old patient, unless non-invasive testing reveals high-risk results

CAD, coronary artery disease; MI, myocardial infarction; METs, metabolic equivalents.
From Eagle et al.[11]

Table 9.9 Recommendations for perioperative medical therapy

Class I
- β-Blockers required in the recent past for angina or patients with symptomatic arrhythmias or hypertension
- β-Blockers: patients at high cardiac risk with evidence of ischemia on preoperative testing who are planned for vascular surgery

Class IIa
- β-Blockers: untreated hypertension, known coronary disease, or major risk factors for coronary disease on preoperative assessment

Class IIb
- α_2-Agonist: perioperative control of hypertension, or known CAD or major risk factors for CAD

Class III
- β-Blockers: contraindication to β-blockade
- α_2-2 Agonists: contraindication to α_2-agonists

CAD, coronary artery disease.
From Eagle et al.[11]

surgery vs the strategy of coronary revascularization followed by the non-cardiac surgery
- whether coronary revascularization significantly reduces the cardiac risk of subsequent non-cardiac surgery
- whether the recovery time from coronary revascularization would not unduly delay the non-cardiac surgery.

Moreover, several studies have shown worse outcomes of coronary artery bypass graft (CABG) surgery in women owing to their smaller caliber of coronary vessels.[72] The mortality rate for CABG is higher for women (3.9% vs 2.3% for men), and survivors of CABG with subsequent non-cardiac surgery have a mortality rate of 1.7%.[73]

Delaying surgery for at least 1 week after balloon angioplasty, for at least 6 weeks after placement of bare metal stents and for up to 6 months after implantation of drug-eluting stents is generally accepted.[74,75]

Retrospective analyses of the Coronary Artery Surgery Study (CASS) registry showed

coronary stenosis remains controversial. The decision of coronary revascularization before non-cardiac surgery should be based on:

- the relative risks and benefits of the strategy of proceeding directly to non-cardiac that[76] patients treated with CABG prior to non-cardiac surgery had a low risk for cardiac events during non-cardiac surgery (0.9 vs 2.4% in patients treated without revascularization). However, this benefit was partially offset by the 1.4% mortality associated with the CABG procedure itself. Subgroup analyses from the CASS registry have further suggested that the lower perioperative cardiac events and survival benefits with CABG were limited to patients with three-vessel CHD, low ejection fraction[77] and those who underwent high-risk surgery (abdominal, vascular, thoracic, and head and neck).[73] Thus, patients undergoing high-risk non-cardiac procedures with established indications for CABG, such as significant left main disease or three-vessel disease with impaired left ventricular function and in whom long-term outcome would likely be improved by CABG, should generally undergo revascularization before non-cardiac surgery.

On the other hand, the recently published Coronary Artery Revascularization Prophylaxis (CARP) trial, a randomized comparison of preoperative revascularization – with either percutaneous coronary intervention (PCI) or CABG – vs medical therapy in patients with stable coronary disease undergoing major vascular surgery[78] demonstrated no significant difference in the postoperative MI rate by cardiac enzymes, left ventricular ejection fraction at 3 months, and all-cause mortality among the revascularization and medical therapy groups. Although this trial had sufficient power to examine long-term mortality, it did not analyze perioperative events or evaluate the best screening approach or indications for angiography or revascularization in high-risk patients, such as those with large perfusion imaging defects or those with three-vessel disease plus left ventricular dysfunction. In addition, there was a mean delay of 36 days prior to major vascular surgery in the patients who underwent preoperative revascularization. Thus, the CARP trial suggested that the existing recommendations for all patients with CAD should be used when considering revascularization of patients undergoing non-cardiac surgery, with no further need for revising the threshold for revascularization due to subsequent planned surgery.

In conclusion, coronary revascularization is suitable for only a small subgroup of patients at high risk, especially in cases of women, who have a higher risk from CABG than men.

VALVULAR HEART DISEASE

An echocardiogram is indicated in women with murmurs on physical examination. Severe valvular disease is considered a significant risk factor for adverse cardiac outcomes with non-cardiac surgery according to the ACC/AHA guidelines, and should be evaluated with echocardiography, cardiac catheterization, and/or possible valve surgery and delay or cancellation of the proposed non-cardiac surgery. However, several reviews have suggested that patients with severe AS may undergo the indicated non-cardiac surgery safely without corrective valve surgery under intensive intraoperative and perioperative monitoring.[79,80] Similar literature is lacking for patients with severe mitral stenosis or severe valvular regurgitation planning for non-cardiac surgery without prior valve surgery.

POSTOPERATIVE CARE

Postoperative care in an intensive care unit should be considered in women with significant cardiovascular disease (e.g. history of left ventricular dysfunction), elderly women, and in women who have undergone surgical procedures with large blood loss and volume shifts. Certain postoperative conditions require special measures (Table 9.10).[81] Careful fluid management is required in an intensive care setting in women with malignant ascites, underlying renal or pulmonary disease, extensive gastrointestinal track manipulation, or resection. During the first 12 hours postoperatively, hourly assessment of intake and output is indicated. During the 48–72 hour period postoperatively, third space mobilization of extracellular fluid leads to late-onset pulmonary edema, manifested by tachypnea or hypoxia. Therefore, during the first 72 hours postoperatively, close cardiovascular monitoring is required.

Table 9.10 Guidelines for managing special perioperative conditions

Conditions	Indication or protocol
Cardiac medications	Aspirin or clopidogrel – discontinue 1 week prior to surgery and resume 48 hours after surgery β-blockers – continue to avoid postoperative adrenergic hyperactivity (may need to give intravenously)
Pulmonary artery catheter	Severe valvular disease, decompensated dilated or hypertrophic cardiomyopathy
Perioperative anticoagulation for prosthetic valves	Three options:[81] 1. Stop warfarin and start heparin preoperatively; stop heparin 2–4 hours preoperatively; proceed to surgery once INR is safe for operation; restart heparin postoperatively when safe; restart warfarin postoperatively when safe 2. Stop warfarin several days preoperatively and proceed to surgery once INR is at a safe level for operation; restart shortly after operation 3. Decrease dosing to keep INR low during procedure
Bacterial endocarditis prophylaxis	For procedures with high risk of bacteremia such as dental, respiratory, gastrointestinal, or genitourinary tract procedures
Pacemaker and implantable cardioverter-defibrillator	Due to electrocautery-induced electromagnetic interference, temporarily program pacemaker to fixed-rate mode to avoid temporary pacemaker inhibition; temporarily switch off ICD during surgery
Deep venous thrombosis prophylaxis	Prophylaxis for low-risk patients: encourage movement, elastic stockings Prophylaxis for moderate-risk patients: heparin 5000 U every 8 hours by subcutaneous injection or LMWH (dalteparin 2500 U qd or enoxaparin 40 mg qd) and/or sequential pneumatic compression stockings Prophylaxis for high-risk patients: heparin 5000 U subcutaneously every 8 hours or LMWH (dalteparin 5000 U qd or enoxaparin 40 mg qd and/or sequential pneumatic compression stockings

INR, international normalized ratio; ICD, implantable cardioverter-defibrillator; LMWH, low molecular weight heparin; U, units; qd, every day.

SUMMARY

Although optimal guidelines for preoperative cardiac evaluation in women are lacking, we have tried to provide the best-available information for safe perioperative evaluation and management in women. More prospective studies are required to evaluate clinical predictors of increased perioperative cardiac morbidity and mortality in women.

REFERENCES

1. Walton L. Preoperative management. In: Sciarra JJ, ed. Gynecology and Obstetrics, Vol 1. Philadelphia: Harper & Row; 1990: 1.

2. Owens WD, Felts JA, Spitznagel EL Jr. ASA physical status classifications: a study of consistency of ratings. Anesthesiology 1978; 49(4):239.

3. Kaplan EB, Sheiner LB, Boeckmann AJ, et al. The usefulness of preoperative laboratory screening. JAMA 1985; 253:3576.

4. Archer C, Levy AR, McGregor M. Value of routine preoperative chest x-rays: a meta-analysis. Can J Anaesth 1993; 40:1022.

5. Goldberger AL, O'Konski M. Utility of the routine electrocardiogram before surgery and on general hospital admission. Ann Intern Med 1986; 105:552.

6. Goldman L, Caldera DL, Nussbaum SR, et al. Multifactorial risk index of cardiac risk in noncardiac surgical procedures. N Engl J Med 1977; 297:845.

7. Dorman T, Breslow MJ, Pronovost PJ, et al. Bundle-branch block as a risk factor in noncardiac surgery. Arch Intern Med 2000; 160:1149.

8. Mangano DT. Perioperative cardiac morbidity. Anesthesiology 1990; 72:153.

9. Fleisher LA, Eagle KA. Lowering cardiac risk in noncardiac surgery. N Engl J Med 2001; 345:1677.

10. Dawood MM, Gupta DK, Southern J, et al. Pathology of fatal perioperative myocardial infarction: implications regarding pathophysiology and prevention. Int J Cardiol 1996; 57:37.

11. Eagle KA, Berger PB, Calkins H, et al. ACC/AHA guideline update for perioperative cardiovascular evaluation for noncardiac surgery – executive summary: a report of the American College of Cardiology/American Heart Association Task Force on Practice Guidelines (Committee to Update the 1996 Guidelines on Perioperative Cardiovascular Evaluation for Noncardiac Surgery). J Am Coll Cardiol 2002; 39:542.

12. Liu LL, Wiener-Kronish JP. Preoperative cardiac evaluation of women for noncardiac surgery. Cardiol Clin 1998; 16:59.

13. Bronson D, Halperin A, Marwick T. Evaluating cardiac risk in noncardiac surgery patients. Cleve Clin J Med 1995; 62:391.

14. Eagle KA, Coley CM, Newell JB, et al. Combining clinical and thallium data optimizes preoperative assessment of cardiac risk before major vascular surgery. Ann Intern Med 1989; 110:859.

15. Lee TH, Marcantonio ER, Mangione CM, et al. Derivation and prospective validation of a simple index for prediction of cardiac risk of major noncardiac surgery. Circulation 1999; 100:1043.

16. Guidelines for assessing and managing the perioperative risk from coronary artery disease associated with major noncardiac surgery. American College of Physicians. Ann Intern Med 1997; 127:309.

17. Palda VA, Detsky AS. Clinical guideline, part II. Perioperative assessment and management of risk from coronary artery disease. Ann Intern Med 1997; 127:313.

18. Detsky AS, Abrams HB, Forbath N, et al. Cardiac assessment for patients undergoing noncardiac surgery. Arch Intern Med 1986; 146:2131.

19. Lerner DJ, Kannel WB. Patterns of coronary heart disease morbidity and mortality in the sexes: a 26-year follow-up of the Framingham population. Am Heart J 1986; 111:383.

20. Hendel RC, Chen MH, L'Italien GJ, et al. Sex differences in perioperative and long-term cardiac event-free survival in vascular surgery patients. An analysis of clinical and scintigraphic variables. Circulation 1995; 91:1044.

21. Park KW. Preoperative cardiology consultation. Anesthesiology 2003; 98:754.

22. The National Heart, Lung, and Blood Institute Coronary Artery Surgery Study. A multicenter comparison of the effects of randomized medical and surgical treatment of mildly symptomatic patients with coronary artery disease, and a registry of consecutive patients undergoing coronary angiography. Circulation 1981; 63:I1.

23. Welch CC, Proudfit WL, Sheldon WC. Coronary arteriographic findings in 1,000 women under age 50. Am J Cardiol 1975; 35:211.

24. Waters DD, Halphen C, Theroux P, David PR, Mizgala HF. Coronary artery disease in young women: clinical and angiographic features and correlation with risk factors. Am J Cardiol 1978; 42:41.

25. Shackelford DP, Hoffman MK, Kramer PR Jr, Davies MF, Kaminski PF. Evaluation of preoperative cardiac risk index values in patients undergoing vaginal surgery. Am J Obstet Gynecol 1995; 173:80.

26. Tofler GH, Stone PH, Muller JE, et al. The MILIS Study Group. Effects of gender and race on prognosis after myocardial infarction: adverse prognosis for women, particularly black women. J Am Coll Cardiol 1987; 9:473.

27. Dietrich H, Gilpin E, NiCad P, et al. Acute myocardial infarction in women: influence of gender on mortality and prognostic variables. Am J Cardiol 1988; 62:1.

28. Hlatky MA, Boineau RE, Higginbotham MB, et al. A brief self-administered questionnaire to determine functional capacity (the Duke Activity Status Index). Am J Cardiol 1989; 64:651.

29. Roddy SP, Darling RC, Maharaj D. Gender-related differences in outcome: an analysis of 5880 infrainguinal arterial reconstructions. J Vasc Surg 2003; 37:399.

30. Mays BW, Towne JB, Fitzpatrick CM. Women have increased risk of perioperative myocardial infarction and higher long-term mortality rates after lower extremity arterial bypass grafting. J Vasc Surg 1999; 29:807.

31. Hendel RC, Chen MH, L'Italien GJ. Long-term outcome after early infrainguinal graft failure. J Vasc Surg 1997; 26:425.

32. Eagle KA, Singer DE, Brewster DC, et al. Dipyridamole-thallium scanning in patients undergoing vascular surgery. JAMA 1987; 257:2185.

33. Cutler BS, Leppo JA. Dipyridamole thallium 201 scintigraphy to detect coronary artery disease before abdominal aortic surgery. J Vasc Surg 1987; 5:91.

34. Boucher CA, Brewster DC, Darling RC, et al. Determination of cardiac risk by dipyridamole-thallium imaging before peripheral vascular surgery. N Engl J Med 1985; 312:389.

35. Sachs RN, Tellier P, Larmignat P, et al. Assessment by dipyridamole-thallium-210 myocardial scintigraphy of coronary risk before peripheral vascular surgery. Surgery 1988; 103:584.

36. Halm E, Browner W, Tubau J, et al. Echocardiography for assessing cardiac risk in patients having noncardiac surgery. Ann Intern Med 1996; 125:433.

37. Carliner NH, Fisher ML, Plotnick GD, et al. Routine preoperative exercise testing in patients undergoing major noncardiac surgery. Am J Cardiol 1985; 56:51.

38. Urbinati S, Di Pasquale G, Andreoli A, et al. Preoperative noninvasive coronary risk stratification in candidates for carotid endarterectomy. Stroke 1994; 25:2022.

39. Schlant RC, Blomqvist CG, Brandenburg RO, et al. Guidelines for exercise testing: a report of the Joint American College of Cardiology/American Heart Association Task Force on Assessment of Cardiovascular Procedures (Subcommittee on Exercise Testing). Circulation 1986; 74(3):653.

40. Weiner DA, Ryan TJ, Parsons L, et al. Long-term prognostic value of exercise testing in men and women from the Coronary Artery Surgery Study (CASS) registry. Am J Cardiol 1995; 75:865.

41. Okin PM, Kligfield P. Gender-specific criteria and performance of the exercise electrocardiogram. Circulation 1995; 92:1209.

42. Pratt CM, Francis MJ, Divine GW, Young JB. Exercise testing in women with chest pain: are there additional exercise characteristics that predict true positive test results? Chest 1989; 95:139.

43. Pryor DB, Shaw L, Harrell FE, et al. Estimating the likelihood of severe coronary artery disease. Am J Med 1991; 90:553.

44. Gibbons RJ, Balady GI, Beasley JW, et al. ACC/AHA guidelines for exercise testing: a report of the American College of Cardiology/American Heart Association task force on practice guidelines (Committee on Exercise Testing). J Am Coll Cardiol 1997; 30:260.

45. Barolsky SM, Gilbert CA, Faruqui A, Nutter DO, Schlant RC. Differences in electrocardiographic response to exercise of women and men: a non-Bayesian factor. Circulation 1979; 60:1021.

46. Grayburn PA, Hillis LD. Cardiac events in patients undergoing noncardiac surgery: shifting the paradigm from noninvasive risk stratification to therapy. Ann Intern Med 2003; 138:506.

47. Coley CM, Field TS, Abraham SA, et al. Usefulness of dipyridamole-thallium scanning for preoperative evaluation of cardiac risk for nonvascular surgery. Am J Cardiol 1992; 69:1280.

48. Stratmann H, Younis L, Wittry M, et al. Dipyridamole technetium-99m sestamibi myocardial tomography in patients evaluated for elective vascular surgery: prognostic value for perioperative and late cardiac events. Am Heart J 1996; 131:923.

49. Goodgold HM, Rehder JG, Samuels LD, Chaitman BR.

50. Hansen CL, Crabbe D, Rubin S. Lower diagnostic accuracy of thallium-201 SPECT myocardial perfusion imaging in women: an effect of smaller chamber. J Am Coll Cardiol 1996; 67:69.

51. Taillefer R, DePuey EG, Udelson JE, et al. Comparative diagnostic accuracy of Tl-201 and Tc-99m sestamibi SPECT imaging (perfusion and ECG-gated SPECT) in detecting coronary artery disease in women. J Am Coll Cardiol 1997; 29:69.

52. Marwick T, Shan K, Go R, et al. Use of positron emission tomography for prediction of perioperative and late cardiac events before vascular surgery. Am Heart J 1995; 130:1196.

53. Pasquet A, D'Hondt AM, Verhelst R, et al. Comparison of dipyridamole stress echocardiography and perfusion scintigraphy for cardiac risk stratification in vascular surgery patients. Am J Cardiol 1998; 82:1468.

54. Sicari R, Ripoli A, Picano E, et al. Perioperative prognostic value of dipyridamole echocardiography in vascular surgery: a large-scale multicenter study in 509 patients. Circulation 1999; 100:II269.

55. Poldermans D, Arnese M, Fioretti PM, et al. Improved cardiac risk stratification in major vascular surgery with dobutamine-atropine stress echocardiography. J Am Coll Cardiol 1995; 26:648.

56. Davila-Roman VG, Waggoner AD, Sicard GA, et al. Dobutamine stress echocardiography predicts surgical outcome in patients with an aortic aneurysm and peripheral vascular disease. J Am Coll Cardiol 1993; 21:957.

57. Eichelberger JP, Schwarz KQ, Black ER, et al. Predictive value of dobutamine echocardiography just before noncardiac vascular surgery. Am J Cardiol 1993; 72:602.

58. Lalka SG, Sawada SG, Dalsing MC, et al. Dobutamine stress echocardiography as a predictor of cardiac events associated with aortic surgery. J Vasc Surg 1992; 15:831.

59. Lane RT, Sawada SG, Segar DS, et al. Dobutamine stress echocardiography for assessment of cardiac risk before noncardiac surgery. Am J Cardiol 1991; 68:976.

60. Langan EM, Youkey JR, Franklin DP, et al. Dobutamine stress echocardiography for cardiac risk assessment before aortic surgery. J Vasc Surg 1993; 18:905.

61. Roger VL, Pellikka PA, Bell MR, et al. Sex and test verification bias: impact of exercise echocardiography. Circulation 1997; 95:405.

62. Biagini E, Elhendy A, Bax JJ, et al. Seven-year follow-up after dobutamine stress echocardiography: impact of gender on prognosis. J Am Coll Cardiol 2005; 45:93.

63. Mangano DT, Layug EL, Wallace A, et al for the Multicenter Study of Perioperative Ischemia Research Group. Effect of atenolol on mortality and cardiovascular morbidity after noncardiac surgery. N Engl J Med 1996; 335:1713.

64. Poldermans D, Boersma E, Bax JJ, et al. The effect of bisoprolol on perioperative mortality and myocardial infarction in high-risk patients undergoing vascular surgery. Dutch Echocardiographic Cardiac Risk Evaluation Applying Stress Echocardiography Study Group. N Engl J Med 1999; 341:1789.

65. Eagle KA, Froehlich JB. Reducing cardiovascular risk in patients undergoing noncardiac surgery (editorial). N Engl J Med 1996; 335:1761.

66. Poldermans D, Boersma E, Bax JJ, et al. Bisoprolol reduces cardiac death and myocardial infarction in high-risk patients as long as 2 years after successful major vascular surgery. Eur Heart J 2001; 22:1353.

67. Auerbach AD, Goldman L. Beta-blockers and reduction of cardiac events in noncardiac surgery: scientific review. JAMA 2002; 287:1435.

68. Lindenauer PK, Pekow P, Wang K, et al. Lipid-lowering therapy and in-hospital mortality following major noncardiac surgery. JAMA 2004; 291:2092.

69. Poldermans D, Bax JJ, Kertai MD, et al. Statins are associated with a reduced incidence of perioperative mortality in patients undergoing major noncardiac vascular surgery. Circulation 2003; 107:1848.

70. O'Neil-Callahan K, Katsimaglis G, Tepper MR, et al. Statins decrease perioperative cardiac complications in patients undergoing noncardiac vascular surgery. The Statins for Risk Reduction in Surgery (StaRRS) study. J Am Coll Cardiol 2005; 45:336.

71. Durazzo AE, Machado FS, Ikeoka DT, et al. Reduction in cardiovascular events after vascular surgery with atorvastatin: a randomized trial. J Vasc Surg 2004; 39:967.

72. Fisher LD, Kennedy JW, Davis KB, et al. Association of sex, physical size, and operative mortality after coronary artery bypass in the Coronary Artery Surgery Study (CASS): J Thorac Cardiovasc Surg 1982; 84:334.

73. Eagle KA, Rihal CS, Mickel MC, et al. Cardiac risk of noncardiac surgery: influence of coronary disease and type of surgery in 3368 operations. Circulation 1997; 96:1882.

74. Wilson SH, Fasseas P, Orford JL, et al. Clinical outcome of patients undergoing non-cardiac surgery in the two months following coronary stenting. J Am Coll Cardiol 2003; 42:234.

75. Auer J, Berent R, Weber T, Eber B. Risk of noncardiac surgery in the months following placement of a drug-eluting coronary stent. J Am Coll Cardiol 2004; 43:713.

76. Domanski M, Ellis S, Eagle KA. Does preoperative coronary revascularization before noncardiac surgery reduce the risk of coronary events in patients with known coronary artery disease? Am J Cardiol 1995; 75:829.

77. Rihal CS, Eagle KA, Mickel MC, et al. Surgical therapy for coronary artery disease among patients with combined coronary artery and peripheral vascular disease. Circulation 1995; 91:46.

78. McFalls EO, Ward HB, Moritz TE, et al. Coronary-artery revascularization before elective major vascular surgery. N Engl J Med 2004; 351:2795.

79. O'Keefe Jr JH, Shub C, Rettke SR. Risk of noncardiac surgical procedures in patients with aortic stenosis. Mayo Clin Proc 1989; 64:400.

80. Raymer K, Yang H. Patients with aortic stenosis: cardiac complications in noncardiac surgery. Can J Anaesth 1998; 45:855.

81. Stein PD, Alpert JS, Copeland J, et al. Antithrombotic therapy in patients with mechanical and biologic prosthetic heart valves. Chest 1995; 108(4 Suppl):371.

10

Oral contraceptives

James H Kerns

Introduction • Cardiovascular risks • Study types • Pathogenesis • Clinical entities • Cardiovascular accidents • Conclusions

INTRODUCTION

Oral contraceptives were introduced into US culture and society in August 1960 by GD Searle and Company. The Food and Drug Administration (FDA) approved Enovid-10, containing 9.85 mg of norethynodrel and 150 µg of mestranol,[1] for contraceptive use on June 23, 1960.[2] Many heralded this as a breakthrough in reproductive freedom for women.

Since that time, many companies have received FDA approval for manufacture and distribution of oral contraceptive pills. Table 10.1[3] is useful *in assessing the cardiovascular risks* of all women interested in using oral contraceptives.

Table 10.2[3] lists the biologic activity of the oral contraceptive products. This is useful, as the physician and the patient discuss the potential or current side effects prior to prescribing or changing the oral contraceptive pill.

CARDIOVASCULAR RISKS

The first combination oral contraceptive pill, containing 150 µg of estrogen, was associated with significant risk of thromboembolic complications. Since thromboembolic events were related to the estrogen dose, the dosage of estrogen has been gradually reduced from 50 µg to 30–35 µg dosing, and then to the current level of 20 µg.[4] While decreasing the estrogen dose to below 50 µg of estrogen reduced the incidence of thromboembolic events, concerns persisted about risks associated with vascular events with long-term combined oral contraceptive use.

In 1997, the WHO Scientific Group of Cardiovascular Disease and Steroid Hormone Contraception reviewed the current evidence of oral contraceptive use and risks for thromboembolic events, myocardial infarction, and stroke.[5]

During the last two decades clinicians and investigators have shared understanding that combination oral contraceptives have increased the risk of thrombosis, and the estrogen in the combination oral contraceptive pill caused this increased risk. Although not every study agreed, many epidemiologic studies, both case-controlled and cohort, showed a direct association between oral contraceptive pills and venous thrombosis. As the dose of estrogen increases, the risk of venous thrombosis increases. Similar associations were shown between combination oral contraceptives and stroke. Laboratory studies support that there is increase in the prothrombotic clotting factors in oral contraceptive pill users that is related to the estrogen dose and not the progestin used. This has provided biologic support for the epidemiologic data. The initial studies were carried out in the mid 1970s, and reflected the effects of the high-dose pills. More recent US studies indicate that the association between oral contraceptive pills and thrombosis is dose-related. Oral

Table 10.1 Oral contraceptives

Name	Progestin	Amount (mg)	Estrogen	Amount (µg)	Manufacturer
Monophasic					
Alesse	Levonorgestrel	0.1	Ethinyl estradiol	20	Wyeth
Brevicon	Norethindrone	0.5	Ethinyl estradiol	35	Watson
Demulen 1/35	Ethynodiol diacetate	1.0	Ethinyl estradiol	35	Searle
Demulen 1/50	Ethynodiol diacetate	1.0	Ethinyl estradiol	50	Searle
Desogen	Desogestrel	0.15	Ethinyl estradiol	30	Organon
Levlen	Levonorgestrel	0.15	Ethinyl estradiol	30	Berlex
Levlite	Levonorgestrel	0.1	Ethinyl estradiol	20	Berlex
Levora	Levonorgestrel	0.15	Ethinyl estradiol	30	Watson
Loestrin 1.5/30	Norethindrone acetate	1.5	Ethinyl estradiol	30	Parke-Davis
Loestrin 1/20	Norethindrone acetate	1.0	Ethinyl estradiol	20	Parke-Davis
Lo/Ovral	Norgestrel	0.3	Ethinyl estradiol	30	Wyeth
Low-Ogestrel	Norgestrel	0.3	Ethinyl estradiol	30	Watson
Mircette	Desogestrel	0.15	Ethinyl estradiol	20	Organon
Modicon	Norethindrone	0.5	Ethinyl estradiol	35	Ortho
Necon 0.5/35	Norethindrone	0.5	Ethinyl estradiol	35	Watson
Necon 1/35	Norethindrone	1.0	Ethinyl estradiol	35	Watson
Necon 1/50M	Norethindrone	1.0	Mestranol	50	Watson
Nelova 0.5/35	Norethindrone	0.5	Ethinyl estradiol	35	Warner-Chilcott
Nelova 1/35E	Norethindrone	1.0	Ethinyl estradiol	35	Warner-Chilcott
Nelova 1/50M	Norethindrone	1.0	Mestranol	50	Warner-Chilcott
Nordette	Levonorgestrel	0.15	Ethinyl estradiol	30	Wyeth
Norethin 1/35	Norethindrone	1.0	Ethinyl estradiol	35	Roberts
Norethin 1/50	Norethindrone	1.0	Mestranol	50	Roberts
Norinyl 1/35	Norethindrone	1.0	Ethinyl estradiol	35	Watson
Norinyl 1/50	Norethindrone	1.0	Mestranol	50	Watson
Norlestrin 1/50	Norethindrone acetate	1.0	Ethinyl estradiol	50	Parke-Davis
Ogestrel	Norgestrel	0.5	Ethinyl estradiol	50	Watson
Otho-Cept	Desogestrel	0.15	Ethinyl estradiol	30	Ortho
Ortho-Cyclen	Norgestimate	0.25	Ethinyl estradiol	35	Ortho
Ortho-Novum 1/35	Norethindrone	1.0	Ethinyl estradiol	35	Ortho
Ortho-Novum 1/50	Norethindrone	1.0	Mestranol	50	Ortho
Ovcon 35	Norethindrone	0.4	Ethinyl estradiol	35	Warner-Chilcott
Ovcon 50	Norethindrone	1.0	Ethinyl estradiol	50	Warner-Chilcott
Ovral	Norgestrel	0.5	Ethinyl estradiol	50	Wyeth
Zovia 1/35	Ethynodiol diacetate	1.0	Ethinyl estradiol	35	Watson
Zovia 1/50	Ethynodiol diacetate	1.0	Ethinyl estradiol	50	Watson
Multiphasic					
Estrostep	Norethindrone acetate	1.0(5d)	Ethinyl estradiol	20(5d)	Parke-Davis
	Norethindrone acetate	1.0(7d)	Ethinyl estradiol	30(7d)	Parke-Davis
	Norethindrone acetate	1.0(9d)	Ethinyl estradiol	35(9d)	Parke-Davis
Jenest	Norethindrone	0.5(7d)	Ethinyl estradiol	35(7d)	Organon
	Norethindrone	1.0(14d)	Ethinyl estradiol	35(14d)	Organon
Necon 10/11	Norethindrone	0.5(10d)	Ethinyl estradiol	35(10d)	Watson
	Norethindrone	1.0(11d)	Ethinyl estradiol	35(11d)	Watson
Nelova 10/11	Norethindrone	0.5(10d)	Ethinyl estradiol	35(10d)	Warner-Chilcott
	Norethindrone	1.0(11d)	Ethinyl estradiol	35(11d)	Warner-Chilcott
OrthoNovum 7/7/7	Norethindrone	0.5(7d)	Ethinyl estradiol	35(7d)	Ortho
	Norethindrone	0.75(7d)	Ethinyl estradiol	35(7d)	Ortho
	Norethindrone	1.0(7d)	Ethinyl estradiol	35(7d)	Ortho
OrthoNovum 10/11	Norethindrone	0.5(10d)	Ethinyl estradiol	35(10d)	Ortho
	Norethindrone	1.0(11d)	Ethinyl estradiol	35(11d)	Ortho

Table 10.1 Oral contraceptives – *continued*

Name	Progestin	Amount (mg)	Estrogen	Amount (µg)	Manufacturer
Ortho Tricyclen	Norgestimate	0.18(7d)	Fthinyl estradiol	35(7d)	Ortho
	Norgestimate	0.215(7d)	Ethinyl estradiol	35(7d)	Ortho
	Norgestimate	0.25(7d)	Ethinyl estradiol	35(7d)	Ortho
Tri-Levlen	Levonorgestrel	0.05(6d)	Ethinyl estradiol	30(6d)	Berlex
	Levonorgestrel	0.075(5d)	Ethinyl estradiol	40(5d)	Berlex
	Levonorgestrel	0.125(10d)	Ethinyl estradiol	30(10d)	Berlex
Tri-Norinyl	Norethindrone	0.5(7d)	Ethinyl estradiol	35(7d)	Watson
	Norethindrone	1.0(9d)	Ethinyl estradiol	35(9d)	Watson
	Norethindrone	0.5(5d)	Ethinyl estradiol	35(5d)	Watson
Triphasil	Levonorgestrel	0.05(6d)	Ethinyl estradiol	30(6d)	Wyeth
	Levonorgestrel	0.075(5d)	Ethinyl estradiol	40(5d)	Wyeth
	Levonorgestrel	0.125(10d)	Ethinyl estradiol	30(10d)	Wyeth
Trivora	Levonorgestrel	0.05(6d)	Ethinyl estradiol	30(6d)	Watson
	Levonorgestrel	0.075(5d)	Ethinyl estradiol	40(5d)	Watson
	Levonorgestrel	0.125(10d)	Ethinyl estradiol	30(10d)	Watson
Progestin only					
Micronor	Norothindrone	0.35	None	–	Ortho
Nor-QD	Norethindrone	0.35	None	–	Watson
Ovrette	Norgestrel	0.075	None	–	Wyeth

From Dickey.[3]

Table 10.2 Biologic activity of oral contraceptives

Class of compound	Progestational activity	Estrogenic activity	Androgenic activity	Fndometrial activity	Andro:Prog activity ratio
Progestins:					
19 nortestosterone					
Estrane progestins:					
Norethindrone	1.0	1.0	1.0	1.0	1.0
Norethindrone acetate	1.2	1.5	1.6	0.4	1.3
Ethynodiol diacetate	1.4	3.4	0.6	0.4	0.4
5(10) Estrane progestins:					
Norethynodrel	0.3	8.3	0	0	0
Gonane progestins:					
Levonorgestrel	5.3	0	8.3	5.1	1.6
dl-Norgestrel	2.6	0	4.2	2.6	1.6
Norgestimate	1.3	0	1.9	1.2	1.5
Desogestrel	9.0	0	3.4	8.7	0.4
Gestodene	12.6	0	8.6	12.6	0.7
Pregnane progestins:					
Chlormadinone acetate	1.0	0	0	NA	0
Megestrol acetate	0.4	0	0	NA	0
Medroxyprogesterone	0.3	0	0	NA	0
Estrogens:					
Ethinyl estradiol	0	100	0	0	0
Mestranol	0	67	0	0	0

From Dickey.[3]

contraceptive formulations have continued to change to lower both the estrogen and progestin doses; therefore, the older studies of the high-dose combination oral contraceptives are limited in their value. Earlier studies are limited in value because they had little information regarding other factors that could directly or indirectly influence thrombosis.[6]

STUDY TYPES

In the era of evidence-based medicine, clinicians and investigators evaluate and weigh the strength of clinical studies according to the following hierarchy, which reflects quality:

- randomized controlled trials
- non-randomized controlled trials
- cohort and case-controlled studies
- ecologic studies
- uncontrolled experiments
- descriptive cross-sectional studies
- expert opinion.

This hierarchy is useful for evaluating where new studies fit into the existing information. Within each group, individual studies vary with respect to quality and appropriateness of the data analysis and the interpretation of the results. Randomized controlled trials are the closest human equivalent to laboratory experimentation in which extraneous factors can be balanced and biases can be avoided. Up to this point, no studies regarding cardiovascular outcomes and combination oral contraceptives have used the randomized controlled trial design. Since cardiovascular events are rare in young women, it is not possible at a practical level to use the randomized controlled trial to answer the questions about cardiovascular events. For example, venous thrombosis occurs in about 1 per 10 000 women-years; a randomized controlled trial designed to compare the incidence of venous thrombosis in women who use different combination oral contraceptives would need to enroll several hundred thousand women. In addition, women or their doctors choose oral contraceptives for specific practical reasons, making it impractical to assign women to a particular formulation for a given length of time. Thus, the knowledge up to this point about oral contraceptives comes from observational studies.[6]

PATHOGENESIS

Risk factors for cardiovascular disease identified in the Framingham Heart Study[7] include elevated low-density lipoprotein (LDL) cholesterol (>130 mg/dl), elevated triglycerides (>150 mg/dl), high-density lipoprotein (HDL) cholesterol (<50 mg/dl). The ratio of total cholesterol to HDL cholesterol of >4 or the LDL to HDL cholesterol ratio of >3 is associated with increased cardiovascular risk. Use of these ratios is beneficial for identifying women at risk when their total cholesterol is between 150 and 200 mg/dl. Other characteristics of women at risk include central obesity, insulin resistance, hypertension, and smoking.

Atherogenic triglyceride-rich particles are small and dense, and more atherogenic than the larger LDL particles. Blood concentrations of these particles rise in persons whose diets are high in saturated fats and cholesterol and in whom central obesity develops.

An increase in plasminogen activator inhibitor-1 level is another component of this syndrome. As the fibrin reaches the endothelial cell, tissue plasminogen activator is released and single-chain urokinase activates plasmin to dissolve the fibrin. These affected women also have high levels of uric acid and microalbuminaria, which are associated with coronary heart disease. Platelet clumping and unclumping, like fibrin deposition and removal, are a continuous process. Activated protein C helps to slow platelet clumping and fibrin deposition by inhibiting the production of thrombin. In 5–6% of persons with European origin, clotting occurs at 8 times the rate as the rest of the population because of a mutation known as Factor V Leiden. This results in an activated protein C resistance and increased thrombin production. Women with this mutation are therefore at particularly high risk for development of thrombosis.[8]

Hypertension, part of the risk profile, is common in the US population. It is estimated that 50% of women are hypertensive by the time they reach their fifties. According to the recent Third National Health and Nutritional Examination Survey, one-third of those with hypertension are unaware of their condition. The latest Joint National Committee on the Detection, Evaluation, and Treatment of High Blood Pressure has reasserted the new parameters of 130/85 mmHg for defining hypertension. Many in this group believe this limit should be 120/80 mmHg.[9]

Mileikowsky et al[10] suggested that inhibition of prostacyclin may be an important mechanism for the increased thrombosis in women who smoke and use oral contraceptives. Usually, prostacyclin causes vasodilatation and inhibits platelet aggregation by its effects on endothelial cells and platelets. Urinary excretion of prostacyclin was noted to be decreased. Thromboxane A_2, a vasoconstrictor, causes platelet aggregation and adhesiveness. Rangemark et al[11] found that the urinary excretion of thromboxane A_2 metabolites were elevated in proportion to the number of cigarettes smoked per day. Thus, the lower prostacyclin and elevated thromboxane A_2 levels in the urine correspond to altered levels in the blood, respectively.

The levels of estrogen have decreased in the combination oral contraceptives from the initial doses of 150 µg to the current doses of <50 µg and the risk of thrombotic events have decreased. During this same time, the progestins in the combination oral contraceptives have changed. Norethindrone, norethindrone acetate, and ethynodiol diacetate are regarded as first-generation progestins. Levonorgestrel, a second-generation progestin, and norgestimate, norgestrel, and desogestrel, third-generation progestins, have largely replaced the first-generation progestins. These new progestins are at a 10-fold lower dose.

Attention has turned to evaluating the progestin component of the oral contraceptive and its role in the process of thrombosis. Studies conducted by Spellacy et al[12] showed that oral contraceptives containing ethinyl estradiol with either levonorgestrel or norgestrel had adverse effects on lipid and carbohydrate metabolism by increasing LDL, decreasing HDL, and increasing blood glucose

and insulin levels. Godsland et al[13] and Gaspard and Lefebvre[14] reported similar findings. Wahl et al[15] found that norethindrone and desogestrel have a beneficial effect by decreasing LDL cholesterol, increasing HDL cholesterol, and leaving glucose and insulin levels unaffected. A WHO study conducted in Europe, Asia, Africa, and Latin America caused alarm in 1995 when it determined that desogestrel and gestodene increased the risk of venous thromboembolism. The odds ratio (OR) for users of levonorgestrel is 3.5 and for desogestrel or gestodene is 9.1 when compared with non-users.[16] A study of British women by Jick et al[17] confirmed that the rate of venous thromboembolism events for levonorgestrel is 16.1 per 100 000 woman-years, for desogestrel 29.3 per 100 000 woman-years, and for gestodene 28.1 per 100 000 woman-years.

It was believed that when the doses of estrogen and progesterone were lowered to their current levels that the risk of cardiovascular events had been resolved. The latest studies have shown that women who smoke heavily (>14 cigarettes/day) and use low-dose combination oral contraceptive pills have >20 times the risk of a non-smoker of dying from a cardiovascular event and the light smoker (<15 cigarettes/day) 3 times the risk of the non-smoker. In 1997, the WHO study also concluded that acute myocardial infarction is rare among oral contraceptive users <35 years of age and who do not smoke, whereas the relative risk (RR) among smokers >35 is 40 events per 100 000 woman-years.[8]

CLINICAL ENTITIES

Venous thromboembolism

Venous thromboembolism (VTE) is rare in the age group 20–24 and rises with age. The estimated risk for all users is 1–3/10 000 woman-years aged 15–44, whereas pregnancy carries a risk of 5.91/10 000 woman-years. Rates have been noted to be similar in smokers and non-smokers.[4] Newer combination oral contraceptives with the gonane progestins (desogestrel, gestodene, norgestimate, and norgestrel) have been reviewed. Gestodene is not currently available in the United States. Four observational studies[16–19] reported an increase in RR for VTE comparing desogestrel or gestodene with levonorgestrel. Data are too sparse to compare norgestimate with levonorgestrel. In some studies,[16,17,19,20] 20 µg of ethinyl estradiol showed a higher RR when compared with 30 µg. Some investigators believe this may be due to selection bias on the part of the patient or physician.

Factor V Leiden mutation, 5–6% of those with European descent, carries with it an increased risk of VTE. Users of combination oral contraceptives without this mutation have a fourfold increase over non-users without the mutation for the formation of DVT, whereas users of combination oral contraceptives with the mutation have a 30-fold increase over non-users without the mutation for the formation of deep venous thrombosis (DVT).[21] The Leiden Thrombophilia Study noted that those women with the mutation had an eightfold increase for VTE events over those without the mutation in the group who did not use combination oral contraceptives and those women with the mutation had a 30-fold increase for VTE events over those without the mutation in the group who did use combination oral contraceptives.[22]

The WHO Collaborative Study,[23] a case-controlled study of premenopausal women of childbearing age, conducted from 1989 to 1993 in 17 countries, found a fourfold increase in Europe and a threefold increase in the developing countries for oral contraceptive users when compared with non-users for VTE events. They also noted a 2.6-fold increased risk when comparing desogestrel or gestodene with levonorgestrel. This same study noted a 7.6-fold (95% CI 3.9–14.7) increased risk for desogestrel or gestodene with 30 µg of ethinyl estradiol and a 38.2-fold (95% CI 4.5–325) increased risk for desogestrel or gestodene with 20 µg of ethinyl estradiol over non-users.

Separate analyses of second- and third-generation oral contraceptives were carried out. Compared with non-users, there was an RR of 3.1 for second-generation oral contraceptives (levonorgestrel) and a 6.8 RR for third-generation oral contraceptives containing desogestrel or norgestrel. Third-generation oral contraceptives compared with second-generation oral contraceptives give an RR of 2.2 (95% CI of 1.1–4.2)

In the Transnational Study,[24] funded by the manufacturer of gestodene, conducted in 1993–1995, it was noted that the RR was elevated 4.4-fold for the third-generation oral contraceptives containing desogestrel or gestodene and threefold for second-generation oral contraceptives containing levonorgestrel, when compared with non-users. Comparing third- with second-generation oral contraceptive, the RR is 1.5 (95% CI 1.0–2.2).

Eighty cases were noted from the General Practice Research Database from which VTE events were identified. Levonorgestrel was noted to have 1.61 events per 10 000 woman-years, whereas desogestrel had 2.93 events and gestodene had 2.81 events. This study noted a twofold increased RR of VTE comparing desogestrel and gestodene with levonorgestrel.[25]

Rosenberg et al[25] reviewed 116 cases from the Meditel Study. Those women who were never-users were noted to have 1.18 events per 10 000 woman-years, users of combination oral contraceptives containing 30–35 µg of ethinyl estradiol had 3.05 events, and users of progestin-only pills have 3.03 events, as compared with pregnancy (5.91 events). Use of desogestrel or levonorgestrel in the oral contraception showed 3.46 events per 10 000 woman-years. Eighty-three additional cases were later identified in which desogestrel with 20 µg of ethinyl estradiol was noted to have a relative risk of 3.49 (95% CI 1.21–10.12) when compared with levonorgestrel. Other third-generation formulations were noted to have an RR of 1.18 (95% CI 0.66–2.17) when compared with levonorgestrel.

Table 10.3 shows the RR of VTE for low-dose oral contraceptives.

Myocardial infarction

The WHO study[5] noted that acute myocardial infarction (AMI) is rare in non-smoking, non-diabetic women under the age of 35, and that after the age of 40 the incidence of AMI is 0.2/10 000 women-years. Death from AMI is rarer. This WHO study also noted that smoking

Table 10.3 Relative risk (RR) of venous thromboembolism for low-dose combination oral contraceptives studies

Study	Reference	Second generation		Third generation		Ratio of risks: 3rd vs 2nd generation RR (95% CI)
		Exposed cases/ controls	RR (95% CI)	Exposed cases/ controls	RR (95% CI)	
WHO: Europe	WHO (1995)	102/163	3.6 (2.5–5.1)	53/51	7.4 (4.2–13)	
WHO: other	WHO (1995)	103/137	2.8 (2.1–3.8)	18/7	12 (0.8–31)	
WHO:	WHO (1995)					2.6 (1.6–4.3)
UK GPRD	Jick (1995)	23	4.2 (1.6–42)	52	7.5 (3.0–24)	2.2 (1.3–3.6)
Leiden	Bloemenkamp (1995)	35/34	3.3 (1.9–5.7)	37/15	8.7 (3.9–19)	2.5 (1.2–5.2)
Transnational	Spitzer (1996)	132/402	3.2 (2.3–4.3)	127/249	4.8 (3.4–6.7)	1.5 (1.1–2.1)
Denmark	Lidegaard (1998)	30/56	1.8 (1.1–2.9)	117/118	3.2 (2.3–4.4)	1.8 (1.1–3.1)
UK GPRD	Vasilakis (1999)	2/11	1.7 (0.3–11)	6/14	4.4 (1.0–19)	1.8 (0.3–11)
Netherlands	Hering (1999)	6		27		4.2 (1.7–10)
UK MediPlus	Todd (1999)	33/141		53/160		1.3 (0.8–2.2)
Overall			3.0 (2.5–3.5)		4.8 (3.0–5.9)	1.9 (1.5–2.2)

From Farley et al.[26]

is a key factor, as it acts synergistically with oral contraceptive use in increasing the risk for AMI. Furthermore, in the European portion of the study, those women who used oral contraceptives and smoked (>10 cigarettes/day) were at a 20-fold risk for AMI, whereas the non-users were at an 11-fold risk for AMI.[27]

The Royal College of General Practitioners' Study[28] found no increased risk for myocardial infarction in non-smokers using oral contraceptives. There is a 20-fold increase in the RR in users of oral contraceptives who smoke >15 cigarettes/day.

Rosenberg et al[29] noted that those women who smoked (>25 cigarettes/day) and did not use oral contraceptives had a ninefold increase in RR for having an AMI over non-smoker, non-users of oral contraceptives. Those women who smoked (>25 cigarettes/day) and used oral contraceptives had a 30-fold increased risk over the non-smoker, non-user of oral contraceptives.

Rosenberg et al[29] noted that the Transnational study showed that the RR for AMI for users of oral contraceptives containing desogestrel or gestodene is 1.0, for oral contraceptives contain-

ing levonorgestrel is 3.1, and comparing third- to second-generation oral contraceptives the RR is 0.36 (95% CI 0.1–1.0). However, the General Practice Research Database showed that there was no difference in RR for oral contraceptives using desogestrel, gestodene, or levonorgestrel for AMI events. In a recent US case-controlled trial, comparing oral contraceptives with >50 μg of estrogen with oral contraceptives with <50 μg of estrogen, the RR for AMI events was 1.65 (not statistically significant).

Chasan-Taber and Stampfer[30] found little or no increased risk for AMI in oral contraceptive users aged <40 who were non-smokers. They also noted, in the United States, the baseline events for fatal ischemic heart disease are 0.1–0.2/10 000 woman-years for women aged <35, 0.41/10 000 woman-years aged 35–39, and 1.0–2.1/10 000 woman-years aged ≥40. They also noted past use of oral contraceptives had an RR of 1.01 (95% CI 0.91–1.12) for AMI events when compared with never-users of oral contraceptives.

Pitsavos et al[31] found that baseline mortality from AMI is <0.4/100 000 woman-years in

Table 10.4 Relative risk (RR) of myocardial infarction in users of low dose oral contraceptives (OCs) compared with non-users

Study and exposure	Reference	Exposed cases/ controls	RR (95% CI)
WHO: Europe	WHO (1997)	28/33	4.7 (2.0–11)
WHO: developing countries	WHO (1997)	13/22	2.9 (1.2–7.0)
Transnational	Lewis et al (1997)	35/120	2.1 (1.2–3.6)
Kaiser, CA	Sidney et al (1996)	10/29	1.7 (0.5–5.9)
Washington State	Sidney et al (1998)	4/61	0.7 (0.2–2.3)
UK MICA study	Dunn et al (1999)	40/180	1.4 (0.8–2.5)
Overall			2.0 (1.5–2.7)
Blood pressure check:			
WHO: Europe	WHO (1997)	17/21	3.2 (1.1–9.4)
WHO: developing countries	WHO (1997)	5/12	2.3 (0.7–8.3)
Transnational	Lewis et al (1997)	not stated	1.1 (0.7–1.7)
Overall			1.4 (0.9–2.1)
No blood pressure check:			
WHO: Europe	WHO (1997)	11/12	7.6 (2.0–25)
WHO: developing countries	WHO (1997)	8/10	3.5 (1.1–11)
Transnational	Lewis et al (1997)	not stated	2.8 (1.4–5.6)
Overall			3.6 (2.1–6.1)
Second-generation OCs:			
WHO	WHO (1997)	13/17	1.6 (0.5–5.5)
Transnational	Lewis et al (1997)	28/71	3.0 (1.5–5.7)
UK MICA study	Dunn et al (1999)	20/119	1.1 (0.5–2.3)
Overall			1.9 (1.2–3.0)
Third-generation OCs:			
WHO	WHO (1997)	3/5	1.0 (0.1–7.0)
Transnational	Lewis et al (1997)	7/49	0.8 (0.3–2.3)
UK MICA study	Dunn et al (1999)	20/61	2.0 (0.9–4.4)
Overall			1.4 (0.7–25)

From Farley et al.[26]

women aged 15–24 and increases to 2–7/100 000 woman-years in women aged 35–44. They noted increased risk with oral contraceptive use, smoking, and age >35.

Table 10.4 gives the RR for myocardial infarction and low-dose oral contraceptives.

CARDIOVASCULAR ACCIDENTS

General information

Chasan-Taber and Stampfer[30] noted that many studies that look at stroke often do not discriminate between ischemic or hemorrhagic stroke or do not adjust for the risk factors associated with stroke. They noted that early studies suggested an increased risk for those having past use of combination oral contraceptives, but that these findings have not been supported by recent studies. They noted that some studies have shown inconsistent results. For example, the total stroke risk in the European study was 1.41 (95% CI 0.9–2.2), in developing countries 1.86 (95% CI 1.49–2.33), and from the Group Health Cooperative Study was 0.6 (95% CI 0.1–2.9). They noted that several studies suggested a positive interaction between smoking and oral contraceptive use. The RR for fatal stroke in the oral contraceptive users who do not smoke compared with the general population is 0.3 (95% CI 0.0–3.00), whereas those women who smoke and use oral contraceptives have an RR of 7.1 (95% CI 1.5–33.0).

Table 10.5. Relative risk (RR) of ischemic stroke in users of low-dose oral contraceptives compared with non-users

Study and exposure	Reference	Exposed cases/ controls	RR (95% CI)
WHO: developing countries	WHO (1996)	63/89	3.3 (2.2–4.9)
Transnational	Heinemann et al (1998)	103/236	2.8 (2.0–3.8)
WHO: Europe	WHO (1996)	20/52	1.5 (0.7–3.3)
Denmark	Lidegaard et al (1998)	48/185	1.6 (1.1–2.4)
Washington State	Schwartz et al (1997)	6/46	1.4 (0.5–3.8)
Kaiser, CA	Petitti et al (1996)	17/43	1.2 (0.5–2.6)
Overall			2.2 (1.9–2.7)
Without blood pressure check:			
WHO: developing countries	WHO (1996)	34/34	5.2 (2.9–9.1)
Transnational	Heinemann et al (1998)	36/54	4.5 (2.6–8.0)
WHO: Europe	WHO (1996)	6/20	1.5 (0.5–4.6)
Overall			4.2 (2.9–6.2)
With blood pressure check:			
WHO: developing countries	WHO (1996)	21/45	2.1 (1.1–3.8)
Transnational	Heinemann et al (1998)	58/180	2.1 (1.4–3.1)
Who: Europe	WHO (1996)	9/24	1.3 (0.5–3.5)
Overall			2.0 (1.5–2.7)

From Farley et al.[26]

The WHO Collaborative Study[32] reviewed 1455 stroke cases (489 ischemic, 715 hemorrhagic, and 251 unspecified) and found the prevalence in women who use oral contraceptives was 18.1% and 12.4% in the control group. This study noted that the OR for total stroke for use of desogestrel or gestodene is the same as for levonorgestrel, the OR for ischemic stroke is greater with use of levonorgestrel unless the woman has hypertension, and the OR for hemorrhagic stroke is 6.84 (95% CI 1.73–27.1) when gestodene (6 cases and 4 controls) is compared with desogestrel (5 cases and 19 controls).

Pitsavos et al[31] noted that the stroke mortality rises with age and is 3- to 5-fold higher than mortality from myocardial infarction. This study confirmed that the risk of stroke increases in those who use oral contraceptives, are over age 35 and smoke, or have hypertension.

Ischemic strokes

The WHO study[5] noted that ischemic and hemorrhagic strokes are rare in non-smokers younger than age 35. This study noted that the risk of stroke increased with age. Two US studies[33,34] and an additional WHO study[35] found no significant increased risk for ischemic stroke in users of oral contraceptives containing less than 50 µg of estrogen. These studies also noted substantial increased risk for ischemic stroke in users of oral contraceptives who smoke, have hypertension (unrelated to pregnancy), or migraine headaches. An additional WHO Collaborative study reviewed 697 cases of ischemic stroke and found the overall RR of 3 comparing users of oral contraceptives with non-users. The RR was noted to be less in the younger age group or with lower doses of estrogen. This study found a fivefold increased RR in smokers and a 10-fold increased RR in those with hypertension and use oral contraceptives as compared with the non-users. Lidegaard[36] noted that women with migraine headaches who use oral contraceptives have a 2.7-fold increased RR using oral contraceptives containing 30–40 µg of estrogen and a 1.7-fold increased RR using oral contraceptives containing 20 µg of estrogen compared with those who do not use oral contraceptives.

Table 10.6 Relative risk (RR) of hemorrhagic stroke in users of low-dose oral contraceptives compared with non-users

Study and exposure	Reference	Exposed cases/ controls	RR (95% CI)
WHO: developing countries	WHO (1996)	60/128	1.7 (1.2–2.4)
WHO: Europe	WHO (1996)	27/72	1.3 (0.7–2.3)
Washington State	Schwartz et al (1997)	14/46	1.4 (0.7–3.0)
Kaiser, CA	Petitti et al (1996)	21/50	1.1 (0.6–2.2)
Overall			1.5 (1.1–1.9)
OC use, age <35 years:			
WHO: developing countries	WHO (1996)	24/68	1.1 (0.6–1.8)
WHO: Europe	WHO (1996)	18/56	0.9 (0.4–1.9)
Kaiser, CA	Petitti et al (1996)	14/34	1.0 (0.4–2.2)
Overall			1.0 (0.7–1.5)
OC use, age ≥35 years:			
WHO: developing countries	WHO (1996)	36/60	2.5 (1.5–4.1)
WHO: Europe	WHO (1996)	9/16	2.1 (0.9–5.3)
Kaiser, CA	Petitti et al (1996)	7/93	1.4 (0.5–3.8)
Overall			2.2 (1.5–3.3)

From Farley et al.[26]

Rosenberg et al[25] noted that the RR for ischemic stroke in healthy users of oral contraceptives when compared with non-users was 1.18, with a 3.5-fold increase for users who smoke.

Table 10.5 gives the RR for ischemic stroke and low-dose oral contraceptives.

Hemorrhagic strokes

The WHO study[5] noted an increased risk for hemorrhagic stroke in women using oral contraceptives >35 who smoke or have hypertension. In contrast, those women <35 years of age who do not smoke or have hypertension using oral contraceptives are not at increased risk. An additional WHO Collaborative study reviewed 1068 cases of hemorrhagic stroke, including 420 intracerebral and 608 subarachnoid cases. The overall RR comparing users of oral contraceptives with non-users is 1.38. The RR is >2 for those over age 35, threefold for smokers, and 10- to 15-fold for those with hypertension. The type of progestin did not affect the RR for hemorrhagic stroke.

Rosenberg et al[25] noted the RR for hemorrhagic stroke in healthy users of oral contra-

ceptives compared with non-users was 1.0, with a 3.5-fold increase for users who smoke.

Table 10.6 depicts the RR for hemorrhagic stroke and low-dose oral contraceptives.

CONCLUSIONS

In spite of the debate about the rarity of cardiovascular events for women on combination oral contraceptives, the overall health benefits of oral contraceptives outweigh the risks. Women who have a personal or family history of thrombosis, are diabetic, hypertensive, or obese need to have individualized assessment of their risks for cardiovascular disease. All women, especially prospective oral contraceptive users, should be assessed for cardiovascular disease. Specialized testing for clotting disorders should be carried out if the family or personal history is suggestive.[37]

The summary of cardiovascular risks are as follows:

1. Oral contraceptives increase the risk of ischemic stroke by 1.5–2.5 × baseline.
2. Oral contraceptives increase the risk of VTE 3–4 × baseline.

3. The risk of VTE may be slightly greater for users of third-generation oral contraceptives (desogestrel).
4. The risk of ischemic stroke may be less with third-generation oral contraceptives.
5. The risk of MI may be less with third-generation oral contraceptives.
6. The risks are significantly increased in women who are older, smoke, or have hypertension.
7. The WHO Scientific Group on Cardiovascular Disease and Steroid Hormone Contraception conclude that the incidence and mortality rates of all cardiovascular diseases (VTE, AMI, stroke) in women of reproductive age are very low. Any additional cardiovascular disease incidence or mortality attributable to oral contraceptives is very small if the users do not smoke or have other cardiovascular risk factors.

REFERENCES

1. Althus MD, Brogan DR, Coates DJ, et al. Hormonal content and potency of oral contraceptives and breast cancer among young women. Br J Cancer 2003; 88(Suppl 1):50.
2. Junod SW. The pill at 40. FDA Consumer Magazine 2000. www.fda.gov/fdac/departs/2000/400_word.html
3. Dickey RP. Managing Contraceptive Pill Patient, 10th edn. Dallas, Texas: Emis Medical Publishers; 2000: 86.
4. Burkman RT, Collins JA, Shuman LP, Williams JK. Current perspectives on oral contraceptive use. Am J Obstet Gynecol 2001; 185(Suppl 2):4.
5. WHO Scientific Group on Cardiovascular Disease and Steroid Hormone Contraception. Cardiovascular disease and steroid hormone contraceptives. WHO Technical Report Series No. 877. Geneva: WHO; 1998.
6. Westhoff CL. Oral contraceptives and thrombosis: an overview of study methods and recent results. Am J Obstet Gynecol 1998; 179(Suppl 3):38.
7. Castelli WP. Cardiovascular disease in women. Am J Obstet Gynecol 1988; 158:1553.
8. Castelli WP. Cardiovascular disease: pathogenesis, epidemiology, and risk among users of oral contraceptives who smoke. Am J Obstet Gynecol 1999; 180(Suppl 6):349.
9. The Fifth Report on the Joint National Committee on Detection, Evaluation, and Treatment of High Blood Pressure (JNCV). Ann Intern Med 1993; 153:154.
10. Mileikowsky GN, Nadler JL, Huey F, Frances R, Roy S. Evidence that smoking alters prostacyclin formation and platelet aggregation in women who use oral contraceptives. Obstet Gynecol 1988; 159:1547.
11. Rangemark C, Benthin G, Granstom ET, et al. Tobacco use and urinary excretion of thromboxane A_2 and prostacyclin metabolites in women stratified by age. Circulation 1992; 86:1495.
12. Spellacy WN, Buhi WC, Birk SA. The effects of norgestrel on carbohydrate and lipid metabolism over one year. Am J Obstet Gynecol 1976; 125:984.
13. Godsland IF, Crook D, Simpson R, et al. The effects of different formulations of oral contraceptive agents on lipid and carbohydrate metabolism. N Engl J Med 1990; 323:1375.
14. Gaspard UJ, Lefebvre PJ. Clinical aspects of the relationship between oral contraceptives, abnormalities in carbohydrate metabolism, and the development of cardiovascular disease. Am J Obstet Gynecol 1990; 163:33.
15. Wahl P, Walden C, Knopp R, et al. Effect of estrogen/progesterone potency on lipid/lipoprotein cholesterol. N Engl J Med 1983; 308:862.
16. Farley TM, Meirik O, Chang CL, Marmot MG, Poulter NR. Effects of different progestagens in low oestrogen oral contraceptives on venous thromboembolic disease. WHO Collaboration Study of Cardiovascular Disease and Steroid Contraception. Lancet 1995; 346:1582.
17. Jick H, Jick SS, Gunewich V, Myers MW, Vasilakis C. Risk of idiopathic cardiovascular death and non-fatal venous thromboembolism in women using oral contraceptives with differing progestagen components. Lancet 1995; 36.1589.
18. Spitzer WO, Lewis MA, Heinemann LAJ, Thorogood M, MacRae KD, on behalf of Transnational Research Group on Oral Contraceptives and the Health of Young Women. Third generation oral contraceptives and risk of venous thromboembolic disorders: an international case-control study. BMJ 1996; 312:83.
19. Farmer RDT, Laurenson RA, Thompson CR, Kennedy JG, Hambleton IR. Population based study of risk of venous thromboembolism associated with various oral contraceptives. Lancet 1997; 349:83.
20. Lewis MA, Heinemann LAJ, MacRae KD, Bruppacher R, Spitzer WO, on behalf of Transnational Research Group on Oral Contraceptives and the Health of Young Women. The increased risk of venous thromboembolism and the use of third generation progestagens: role of bias in observational research. Contraception 1996; 54:5.
21. Vandenbroucke JP, Kosler T, Briet E, et al. Increased risk of venous thrombosis on oral contraceptive users who are carriers of factor V Leiden mutation. Lancet 1994; 344:1453.
22. Bloemenkamp KWM, Rosendaal FR, Helmerhorst FM,

Buller HR, Vandenbroucke JP. Enhancement of factor V Leiden mutation of risk of deep vein thrombosis associated with oral contraceptives containing third-generation progestagens. Lancet 1995; 346:1593.

23. Poulter NR, Chang CL, Farley TMM, Meirik O, Marmot MG. Venous thromboembolic disease and combined oral contraceptives: results of international multicentre case-control study. WHO Collaborative Study of Cardiovascular Disease and Steroid Hormone Contraception. Lancet 1995; 346:1575.

24. Poulter NR, Meirik O. Haemorrhagic stroke, overall stroke risk, and combined oral contraceptives: results of an international, multicentre case-control study. WHO Collaborative Study of Cardiovascular Disease and Steroid Hormone Contraception. Lancet 1996; 348:505.

25. Rosenberg L, Palmer JR, Sands MI, et al. Modern oral contraceptives and cardiovascular disease. Am J Obstet Gynecol 1997; 177:707.

26. Farley TMM, Meirik O, Collins J. Cardiovascular disease and combined oral contraceptives: reviewing the evidence and balancing the risk. Hum Reprod Update 1999; 5:721.

27. Acute myocardial infarction and combined oral contraceptives: results of an international, multicentre, case-control study. WHO Collaborative Study of Cardiovascular Disease and Steroid Hormone Contraception. Lancet 1997; 349:1202.

28. Croft P, Hannaford PC. Risk factors for acute myocardial infarction in women: evidence from the Royal College of General Practitioners' oral contraceptive study. BMJ 1989; 298:165.

29. Rosenberg L, Palmer JR, Lesko SM, Shapiro S. Oral contraceptive use and the risk of myocardial infarction. Am J Epidemiol 1990; 131:1009.

30. Chasan-Taber L, Stampfer MJ. Epidemiology of oral contraceptives and cardiovascular disease. Ann Intern Med 1998; 128:467.

31. Pitsavos C, Stefanadis C, Toutouzas P. Contraception in women at high risk or with established cardiovascular disease. Ann NY Acad Sci 2000; 900:215.

32. Poulter NR, Chang CL, Farley TMM, Marmot MG, Meirik O. Effect on stroke of different progestagens in low oestrogen dose oral contraceptives. Lancet 1999; 354:301.

33. Schwartz SM, Petitti DB, Siscovick DS, et al. Stroke and use of low-dose oral contraceptives in young women: a pooled analysis of two US studies. Stroke 1998; 29:2277.

34. Petitti DB, Sidney S, Bernstein A, et al. Stroke in users of low dose oral contraceptives. N Engl J Med 1996; 335:8.

35. WHO Collaborative Study of Cardiovascular Disease and Steroid Hormone Contraception. Ischaemic stroke and combined oral contraceptives: results of an international, multicentre case-control study. Lancet 1996; 348:498.

36. Lidegaard O. Oral contraception and risk of cerebral thromboembolic attacks: results of a case-control study. BMJ 1993; 306:956.

37. Cohen J. Consensus conference on combination oral contraceptives and cardiovascular disease. Fertil Steril 1999; 71(Suppl 6):1.

11

Hormone replacement therapy

John W Cassels Jr

Introduction • Coronary heart disease • Women's Health Initiative • Venous thromboembolic disease • Stroke • Selective estrogen receptor modulators • Concurrent medication • Summary and recommendations

INTRODUCTION

During the second half of the 20th century, estrogen replacement therapy became a standard practice in the management of the perimenopausal transition and the menopause in women. Conjugated equine estrogens (CEE), in the form of Premarin, became available in Canada in 1941 and in the United States in 1942 after development in the laboratories of Ayerst. Popularized for the relief of vasomotor hot flushes and its ability to improve the overall sense of well-being of the aging woman, Premarin was one of the leading pharmaceuticals by prescriptions written and sales made by the mid 1980s.

Additional agents have been available, including estropipate (piperazine estrogen sulfate), estradiol valerate, ethinyl estradiol, esterified estrogens, and micronized estradiol. Routes of administration have been investigated to improve effectiveness and patient tolerance in the treatment of specific symptoms. Delivery by transdermal patch avoids first-pass hepatic effects, whereas use of vaginal estrogens in the form of cream, silicone ring, or tablet more directly treats the symptoms of urogenital atrophy without significant systemic effects.

By the mid 1970s another issue arose: the development of endometrial hyperplasia and endometrial cancers as a result of unopposed estrogen exposure. Work at Wilford Hall Air Force Medical Center by R Don Gambrell,[1] and by others, demonstrated that concurrent progestin administration reduced the risk of neoplasia experienced by patients on estrogen replacement. Over time, progestin therapy has evolved from cyclic therapy of 5 days per month to 14 days per month, to alternatives such as combining continuous lower-dose progestins with daily estrogen or administration of progestins only every 3 months. These progestin treatments provide similar endometrial protection. Various approaches have been utilized to improve metabolic responses to hormone exposure (i.e. improved lipid profiles, reduction of procoaguloant effects) and to gain greater patient acceptance from reduced breakthrough bleeding. In the United States, medroxyprogesterone acetate in doses of 2.5–10 mg has been the most commonly utilized progestin, while other agents have enjoyed popularity in Europe. Alternative agents have been used alone or in combined forms in the United States.

Combination hormone replacement therapy (HRT) became the standard therapy for women with an intact uterus. Hormone replacement therapy proved to be effective not only in relieving vasomotor symptoms[2] but also in preventing osteoporosis and fractures due to reduced bone mass in the hip and vertebrae.[3] Improvement in urogenital atrophy,[4] resulting in a reduction of urinary dysfunction,[5] urinary tract infection,[6] and sexual activity complaints;[7]

less sleep disturbance, with subsequently improved mood and cognitive function;[8] and beneficial effects on skin texture[9] and glucose metabolism[10] seemed to strengthen the case for HRT in all menopausal women. Furthermore, an apparent benefit with respect to coronary heart disease (CHD)[11] provided a strong argument for HRT as a health-promoting measure in aging women. This led to an active role for physicians, particularly obstetrician-gynecologists as primary providers for women's healthcare, in counseling perimeno-pausal and menopausal women for initiating and continuing HRT at the climacteric period and beyond.

Balanced against the benefits apparently derived from use of HRT in the menopause was the suspicion and accumulating evidence that estrogen therapy increased the incidence of breast cancer.[12] Data regarding use of combined oral contraceptives,[13] presence of estrogen receptors in breast cancers,[14] and observational epidemiologic reports[15,16] led to a growing concern about the role of HRT in development of cancer of the breast.

Multiple studies of various health end points have been performed in an effort to establish the preventive health benefits of HRT. The details of investigations into these multiple end points are beyond the scope of this chapter. We will, however, attempt to delineate the findings relevant to cardiovascular health, including CHD, venous thromboembolic disease, and stroke. Recommendations for management of the menopausal woman and the rationale for use of HRT in various settings will be provided.

CORONARY HEART DISEASE

Coronary heart disease is a major health concern regarding the life expectancy and quality of life among women in the United States. In 2002 it was the single leading cause of death in women and, when combined with other manifestations of cardiovascular disease (CVD), was more likely to lead to mortality than the combination of the next six causes of death.[17] Observation of disease and death rates among men and women over the last 50 years demonstrated that women suffered less than

men did from CHD during the premenopausal period. An acceleration of CHD rates among women after the menopause led to almost equivalent rates of heart disease in men and women after age of 50 years. Unfortunately, women were more likely than men to die in the first 12 months after an initial heart attack, meaning that developing CHD remains a threat for earlier demise.

Since women have a lower risk of CHD before menopause compared with men, it has been theorized that female reproductive hormones contribute to this effect. Surrogate markers for a lower risk of heart disease such as higher high-density lipoprotein (HDL) cholesterol levels and lower total and low-density lipoprotein (LDL) cholesterol are noted in premenopausal women, and can be maintained through appropriate HRT.[18] The apparent improved metabolic profile when using HRT after surgical or natural menopause offered expectations that progression of CHD could be reversed by creating and continuing the woman's reproductive hormonal milieu into the menopausal years. Initial attempts to understand the advantages of HRT were derived from observational studies of women across age ranges that described improved performance with respect to CHD.

The Nurses' Health Study provided the largest and most comprehensive report of outcomes for women utilizing HRT.[11,19,20] Begun in 1976, the Nurses' Health Study enrolled in excess of 120 000 women at age 30–55 years. Questionnaires inquired about medical history and postmenopausal hormone use. Continuing follow-up for up to 20 years allowed assessment of the relative benefits of HRT. Self-reporting suggested that 80% of these women began using HRT at the menopause or within 2 years. Relative risk (RR) for major coronary events was 0.61 (CI 0.52–0.71) among current users after adjusting for age and common CVD risk factors.

Randomized controlled trials (RCTs) to assess the effect of HRT on CVD were designed to identify cardiovascular end points. The first such large study was the Heart and Estrogen/progestin Replacement Study (HERS)[21] begun in January 1993, and initially reported in 1998. Elderly women, most of whom were over 65 years old and all of whom had CHD, were treated with 0.625 mg of Premarin (CEE), and 2.5 mg medroxyprogesterone acetate (MPA) for an average of 4.1 years. The investigators noted an increase in cardiovascular events in the first year of treatment, but this increase did not reach statistical significance when correction was made for treatment with statins or aspirin. Treatment appeared to reduce the CVD risks over time, but was not documented in follow-up reports.[22]

The Estrogen Replacement and Atherosclerosis (ERA) trial sought to demonstrate HRT arresting the progression of coronary artery atherosclerosis.[23] Patients with known CHD were assessed for disease status by angiography at baseline and repeated after treatment: CEE 0.625 mg + MPA 2.5 mg daily, CEE 0.625 mg alone, or a placebo were administered for 3.5 years. No significant difference in the progression of coronary artery atherosclerosis was identified among the groups.

Those seeking solutions to the question of HRT use as a primary preventive measure in reducing CVD were concerned about the difference in the outcome assessment for such studies. The Nurses' Health Study (NHS) represented a large observational assessment of HRT use and effects, but was flawed by the potential patient selection and the bias introduced by practicing physicians. Patients in the NHS who were generally healthier, more educated, trained in health care, and in a higher socioeconomic status were more likely to benefit from HRT. The results of this study could not be generalized to the whole female population. Both HERS and ERA demonstrated no benefit in the secondary prevention of progressive CVD. A properly designed RCT is needed to investigate HRT use for primary prevention of CVD.

WOMEN'S HEALTH INITIATIVE

In 1992, the Women's Health Initiative (WHI) was designed to investigate the impact of HRT on common morbidity and mortality issues in menopausal women,[24] Intervention arms included estrogen/progestin combinations, estrogen only, and placebo. Since it is well-established that taking estrogen alone in the presence of an intact uterus increases the risk for endometrial neoplasia, the estrogen-alone arm included only those women who had undergone hysterectomy. Investigators hoped to elucidate the impact of progestins on the outcome measure of CHD by studying a group of women who took estrogen replacement only.

Designed as an RCT for the evaluation of HRT in postmenopausal women, the WHI sought candidates in established menopause who would accept randomization to placebo or active hormone arms. This randomization led to withdrawal from or refusal to participate in the study by patients who were in the early menopause and suffered from significant climacteric symptoms, particularly vasomotor hot flushes. Consequently, the study population[25] was generally older (mean age 63 years, range 50–79 years) and remote from the onset of menopause when they entered the study. Participants were slightly obese – mean body mass index (BMI) 28.5 kg/m^2 – and many smoked or had smoked in the past. The study population was not comparable to many patients who take HRT as a primary intervention for climacteric symptoms.

Despite these objections to the selected patient population, the WHI has wrought a revolution in HRT management since its publication. The National Institutes of Health (NIH) stopped the combined estrogen/progestin arm short of its designed end point on advice of the Data and Safety Monitoring Board. After an average follow-up of 5.2 years (range 3.5–8.5 years), the risk of invasive breast cancer exceeded the previously established stopping boundaries,[25] and the NIH instructed combined HRT participants to discontinue the medications. Hormone replacement therapy was associated with increased CVD events compared with placebo (37 vs 30 per 10 000 patient years). This finding, contrary to previous observational reports of benefit for HRT in prevention of progressive CHD, received wide media airing. Additionally, several organizations, including the American College of Obstetricians and Gynecologists and the American Heart Association, revised their recommendations for HRT. Subsequently, many patients approached their physicians about the advisability of continuing HRT, or simply stopped therapy without consulting their physician.

The WHI has undergone wide scrutiny of its findings. A common criticism states that the information only applies to the specific agents studied – Premphase, Premarin 0.625 mg with Provera 2.5 mg administered daily (Wyeth Pharmaceuticals) – in the active arm. It is suggested that alternative regimens or different doses might change the outcome. Subsequently, many physicians counseled patients to change formulations or dosing schedule. Only additional studies with alternative arms will truly clarify this issue.

Other clinicians criticized WHI because patients were not representative of those who want to use HRT to reduce the risk of CVD at the earliest signs of the climacteric.[26] Women's Health Initiative patients were older at entry and generally did not suffer vasomotor symptoms requiring treatment because they would be screened out during a 'washout' period prior to study entry if symptoms were intolerable. Since the patients were more advanced into the perimenopause or menopause, they may have been at risk for atherosclerosis, silent CHD, or other manifestations of CVD when they began participation in the study. Thus, the finding that coronary events were higher in the first year of HRT was consistent with that in HERS.[21]

Subsequent to the initial publication of the WHI results, the data from the CEE-alone arm became available.[27] After an average follow-up of 6.8 years, the NIH terminated the CEE-only arm. The data suggested an increased risk for stroke (hazard ratio (HR) = 1.39, CI 1.10–1.77); no significant effect on CHD (HR = 0.91, CI 0.75–1.12); and reduced risk for breast cancer (HR = 0.77, CI 0.59–1.01). Confounding factors would make this conclusion invalid and contrary to the preponderance of existing data.

Work using animal models demonstrated that HRT worsened the progression of previously existing vascular disease. Clarkson et al used a cynomolgus monkey model to evaluate the progression of pre-existing atherosclerosis with or without exposure to HRT.[28] This female monkey shares 90% homology of DNA with humans and experiences a similar reproductive hormone profile. When monkeys were made surgically menopausal, 70% inhibition of progression in coronary artery atherosclerosis was noted if estrogen treatment was begun immediately following surgery and the monkey had little or no existing atherosclerosis.[29,30] If monkeys had moderate atherosclerotic disease prior to castration, estrogen replacement produced less inhibition of progression.[28] Moreover, if estrogen replacement was delayed following castration, no beneficial effect of estrogen replacement could be demonstrated.[31]

We may never see a primary prevention trial of HRT. A well-designed trial would require patients to be randomized at or before menopause to evaluate the benefits of early exposure to HRT in abating progression of coronary artery disease and/or reducing the morbidity and mortality from CHD. Since patients with severe menopausal symptoms would probably refuse randomization to a placebo arm, it will be difficult to accomplish a trial of treatment versus no treatment in the early menopause of women who clearly most benefit from HRT.

VENOUS THROMBOEMBOLIC DISEASE

Venous thromboembolic disease involves various vascular beds including the retina and deep veins of the upper or lower extremities. Included within this consideration are emboli, which break free from vascular attachments to lead to pulmonary embolism. This disease is debilitating and potentially lethal, especially among hospitalized patients or surgical patients. Additional risk factors for venous thromboembolic disease include obesity, smoking, cancer, or history of recent trauma including surgery. Venous thromboembolic disease leads to significant mortality each year.

The Postmenopausal Estrogen/Progestin Interventions (PEPI) trial assigned healthy menopausal women to CEE with or without progestins and followed them for 3 years to evaluate cardiovascular risk.[32] Cyclic or continuous MPA or cyclic micronized progesterone was used in conjunction with CEE in three arms of the study, while CEE alone or placebo constituted the fourth and fifth arms. Venous thromboembolic disease, ranging from superficial phlebitis to pulmonary emboli, was seen in each arm with active hormone administration, but not in the placebo arm. Despite a fivefold increase in relative risk for venous thromboembolic disease in the HRT groups, the absolute numbers did not reach statistical significance (calculated from raw data in PEPI, RR = 5.10, CI 0.3–86.7).[33]

Two subsequent trials exploring effects of HRT on intima-media thickness in carotid arteries failed to identify any venous thromboembolic disease reported as adverse events. The Postmenopausal HOrmone REplacement against Atherosclerosis (PHOREA) trial studied healthy women aged 40–70 years on placebo or oral 17β-estradiol with or without progestin (gestodene).[34] Patients were followed for only 1 year. The Estrogen in the Prevention of Atherosclerosis Trial (EPAT) followed patients for 2 years on placebo or unopposed 17β-estradiol.[35] No deep venous thrombosis or pulmonary embolus occurred in active treatment or placebo arms of this trial. Results may have been affected by small sample size (321 total participants in PHOREA and 222 in EPAT), alternate choice for estrogen replacement, or short follow-up time (although, as will be seen, venous thromboembolic disease tends to occur in the early years of treatment).

The WHI observed venous thromboembolic disease as a secondary end point. The data provided by WHI remain valuable, as this is the longest, largest RCT of HRT in otherwise-healthy women. In the combined CEE/MPA trial,[25] venous thromboembolic disease was more common on HRT (RR = 2.11, CI 1.26–3.55) when compared with the placebo arm. In the CEE-only arm (women with previous hysterectomy not requiring MPA), all venous thromboembolic disease occurred 33% more often on therapy than on placebo, but failed to reach significance (HR = 1.33, CI 0.99–1.79), although deep venous thrombosis demonstrated significance when examined separately.[27]

The HERS reported venous thromboembolic disease as a secondary end point in women with previously established CHD. Venous thromboembolic disease increased in patients on HRT and appeared to occur earlier in treatment in this group of patients followed for 4.1 years.[21] In HERS II, 2.7 years of additional follow-up was provided on the original subjects in HERS. The HR for venous thromboembolic disease was 1.40 compared with placebo (CI 0.64–3.05) for the additional 2.7 years,[36] a decrease from the earlier HR of 2.7 (CI 1.4–5.0) for the initial study period.[21,37]

Additional studies of venous thromboembolic disease occurrence in women treated for established heart disease either failed to show a difference in disease incidence or did not report on this outcome measure or adverse event. These studies are reviewed in summary in a review and treatment recommendation supplement from the American College of Obstetricians and Gynecologists.[38] The summary demonstrated a consistent twofold increase of venous thromboembolic disease for women using HRT. Venous thromboembolic disease appeared to be more likely to occur in the first year of therapy and in women with known risk factors for venous thromboembolic disease.

STROKE

Stroke refers to central nervous system injury as a result of changes in vascular perfusion of the brain and brainstem due to thrombosis, emboli, hemorrhage, or hypotension. More than 700 000 new strokes occur in the United States annually and at least 20% of these will be fatal.[39] Many non-fatal strokes result in paralysis, visual loss, and aphasias, with significant long-term morbidity. Many nursing home residents who recover from stroke require varying degrees of supportive care. Over 4.4 million stroke survivors live in the United States.

The health consequences of advancing age contribute to an increasing risk for stroke in the elderly, with more than 70% of strokes occurring in people over 65 years of age. Of the 25% of women less than 65 years of age who suffer stroke, many are in the perimenopause or early menopause. Thus, HRT usage in this population is a potential contributor to stroke.

Several RCTs have evaluated the risk of stroke among otherwise healthy women undergoing treatment with estrogen alone or combined estrogen/progestin versus placebo. The PHOREA and EPAT studies,[34,35] previously described, investigated carotid artery atherosclerosis progression by measuring the intima-media thickness via ultrasound, and classified CVD events as adverse events. A single death due to brain hemorrhage was reported in the HRT group taking progestin every 3 months, while no stroke occurred in the patient groups taking the placebo or monthly cyclic HRT. In the EPAT, two subjects suffered cerebrovascular events – one stroke and one transient ischemic attack (TIA) – among 111 participants who were on unopposed 17β-estradiol, while no subjects sustained cerebrovascular events among 111 participants who were on placebo. In the PEPI trial of healthy women with mean age 56.1 years, there was one stroke and one TIA in the combined group of 875 women on HRT compared with no cerebrovascular events in the placebo group.[32]

The WHI investigated stroke as a secondary end point in its study of cardiovascular events and breast cancer. Analysis of data after 5.6 years of follow-up showed an increased risk for those on HRT compared with placebo (HR = 1.31, CI 1.20–1.68).[40] In this study, ischemic strokes were most common, and were more common among HRT users (RR = 1.44, CI 1.09–1.90). Non-fatal strokes, while predominating in both groups (94/127 in HRT users, 59/85 in the placebo group), did not differ significantly (RR = 1.50, CI 0.83–2.70). The NIH stopped the intervention phase of the estrogen-only arm of the WHI study when data demonstrated no effect on CVD, but an increased risk for stroke similar to that recognized in the combined HRT arm (HR = 1.39, CI 1.10–1.77 (adjusted 95% CI 0.97–1.99)).[27] Two well-known, large observational studies also demonstrated an overall increase in stroke.[20,41]

Several RCTs have evaluated stroke in women with established heart disease when HRT was studied for secondary prevention of coronary events.[21–23,42–44] Although these studies vary as to medications, dose, route, and duration, no study could significantly demon-strate HRT preventing or causing cerebrovascular events (stroke or TIA).

The Women's Estrogen and Stroke Trial[45] investigated the impact of estrogen replacement (17β-estradiol) in women with a history of cerebrovascular disease in the secondary prevention of death from any cause or the occurrence of non-fatal stroke. In this study, 664 women were assigned to either oral 17β-estradiol (1 mg daily) or placebo within 90 days of an acute ischemic stroke or TIA. There was no significant difference between the two groups regarding non-fatal stroke or death within 3 years of the treatment. There was an increase in stroke in the first 6 months after the initiation of estrogen therapy (RR = 2.3, CI 1.1–5.0, p = 0.03). Overall, estrogen tends to worsen ischemic injury or fatal stroke.

SELECTIVE ESTROGEN RECEPTOR MODULATORS

Selective estrogen receptor modulators (SERMs) are synthetic compounds that bind to intracellular estrogen receptors and express variable results by altering the conformational shapes of the receptor. Different SERMs may act as either agonists or antagonists, or may have mixed activity. Tamoxifen is approved for use in the prevention or treatment of breast cancer in selected at-risk populations. Raloxifene has favorable effect on bone remodeling and lipids, while causing no proliferative effect in the endometrium. When these agents are used in patients who are not candidates for standard HRT, they may affect CVD risks.

Tamoxifen used for reducing the risk of recurrent breast cancer appeared to cause fewer hospitalizations for myocardial infarction in breast cancer survivors. Tamoxifen was associated with a 1.6–3-fold increased risk of venous thromboembolic disease when pulmonary embolus and deep vein thrombosis were evaluated in the Breast Cancer Prevention Trial.[46] In a subset of women using raloxifene in the Multiple Outcomes of Raloxifene Evaluation (MORE) trial, there was a reduction in cardiovascular events (RR = 0.60, CI 0.38–0.95) and a 62% reduction in stroke among the 1035 participants who were at increased risk for CVD.[47]

There was a trend toward increased risk for stroke in women over 50 years of age. The MORE trial demonstrated a twofold increased risk for venous thromboembolic disease, although the risk for cerebrovascular events was neither increased nor decreased in the total study population.

CONCURRENT MEDICATION

Among women with a history of CVD, venous thromboembolic disease, and cerebrovascular disease, a common pharmaceutical intervention involves anticoagulant therapy. Coronary thrombosis, atrial fibrillation, pulmonary embolus, deep vein thrombosis, and stroke may lead to anticoagulation as a secondary prevention method. Evaluation for possible heritable disorders of coagulation is indicated when patients suffer thrombotic events, especially when they are young or do not demonstrate predisposing risk factors. Healthcare providers must consider the altered risk for venous thromboembolic disease in women utilizing HRT when they develop new risks for venous thromboembolic disease such as cancer, fractures of the lower limbs, surgery, myocardial infarction, or immobilization due to debility or hospitalization. Warfarin (Coumadin), an antagonist of vitamin K metabolism, produces anticoagulation by reducing the synthesis of the clotting factors in the liver. Estrogen may significantly alter the therapeutic effect of a given dose of warfarin through hepatic enzyme activation. Combination oral contraceptives and raloxifene may act to decrease the prothrombin time (PT) and international normalized ratio (INR). Although estrogens typically used for postmenopausal HRT do not affect coagulation, it is prudent to consider the potential alteration of PT/INR and the therapeutic response to anticoagulation whenever estrogen doses are altered. When a patient on HRT begins Coumadin or vice versa, or when a patient stops or alters estrogen and/or estrogen/ progestin doses while taking Coumadin, laboratory evaluations are necessary to maintain Coumadin dosage in the therapeutic range.

SUMMARY AND RECOMMENDATIONS

At the beginning of the 21st century, the practicing physician faces a plethora of evidence to develop a reasonable management plan for HRT in the perimenopausal and postmenopausal woman. The pendulum has swung from treating all women except those with specific contraindications to therapy, to preferentially denying hormone therapy to most women. The earlier treatment goals of improving sense of well-being and reducing risks associated with aging have been supplanted by the concern for new risks. Early long-term observational trials supported the supposition that prolonging the reproductive hormonal environment would improve cardiovascular health. More recent prospective trials showed that HRT may not reduce CVD risk in all women, especially those with pre-existing risk factors. The WHI set out to be the definitive trial for HRT as an agent of primary prevention of CVD in the female population. Unfortunately, its study design was hampered not only by the limitation of a single agent used for HRT but also the introduction of HRT to seemingly healthy menopausal women who were remote from losing endogenous hormone production. Existing heart disease or atherosclerotic disease, even when silent in nature, serves as the underlying risk for progression of CVD. The results of the WHI are not surprising, but are consistent with those of previous studies examining HRT for the secondary prevention of CVD.

The reasonable question to ask with respect to HRT in the menopause is whether therapy begun at the time of initial perimenopausal or climacteric symptoms would provide a long-term benefit to the user. Certainly those patients who suffer significant disability due to vasomotor hot flushes, sleep disruption, or urogenital atrophy could find that HRT improves quality of life, including sense of well-being, even though WHI demonstrated that estrogen plus progestin therapy did not affect health-related quality of life in a clinically meaningful way.[48] It must be remembered that the participants in the WHI were menopausal, the majority for more than 10 years, and were recruited to the study as volunteers, not as patients with complaints or disability due to hormone withdrawal. Those women who were on HRT upon enrolling in the study had to undergo a 3-month washout period for hormone therapy. The investigators discouraged women who did not tolerate the return of symptoms during the washout period, because of concern these women might withdraw from the study at a later time. It is not surprising that women who were essentially asymptomatic for menopausal complaints during the washout period did not find a remarkable improvement in quality of life when placed on HRT.

Quality-adjusted life expectancy (QALE) based on measures of asymptomatic or mild-to-severe symptoms experienced in the menopause has been used in a decision model evaluating the burden of risk from HRT.[49] Based on the model, asymptomatic women beginning HRT would see net losses in life expectancy and QALE of 1–3 months from short-term hormone therapy, depending on pre-existing degree of CVD risk. Women with higher CVD risk needed to have more symptoms to justify the potential benefits of HRT. The model assumed that a 1-month trial of HRT would allow an individual patient to evaluate her improvement in quality of life. If symptoms improved, then short-term (2 years or more depending on the persistence of symptoms) HRT appeared to offer improved QALE over the life expectancy reduction due to associated risks.

The short-term hormone replacement seems to dovetail with the recommendations of the US Preventive Services Task Force (USPSTF) for using postmenopausal hormone replacement for primary prevention of chronic conditions.[50] The USPSTF recommended against the routine use of combined estrogen/progestin therapy for the prevention of chronic disease in postmenopausal patients. There was at least fair evidence that the intervention was ineffective or that harm caused by the intervention outweighed its benefits. The USPSTF gave a grade I recommendation regarding estrogen use. A grade I recommendation is given when:

- the evidence is insufficient to recommend for or against the routine use of an intervention

- the evidence of effective care is lacking, of poor quality, or conflicting
- the balance of benefits and harms cannot be determined.

The USPSTF recommended that a physician should discuss the risks and benefits of HRT with patients before initiating postmenopausal HRT and that HRT should be carried out with the lowest effective dose for a limited period of time to abate bothersome or significant symptoms.

The prudent physician needs to develop a plan for counseling patients regarding HRT based on the best-available scientific evidence, as discussed above, and specific symptoms, risks, and needs with which a woman presents.[38,51,52]

Recommendations

1. Hormone therapy used in the management of menopausal symptoms should be discussed with respect to risks and benefits to the individual patient and be maintained for the shortest possible time.

2. Women should pursue lifestyle modification for primary or secondary prevention of heart disease or its progression. Appropriate actions include smoking cessation as well as pursuing a healthy diet and adequate physical activity to effect weight reduction or maintenance.

3. Hormone therapy, whether combined estrogen/progestin or unopposed estrogen, should not be initiated for primary or secondary prevention of coronary heart disease.

4. Healthy women initiating HRT should carefully consider the small but increased risk for stroke and the twofold risk for venous thromboembolic disease before commencing treatment.

5. Women with active CHD or increased risk for development of disease should receive medical therapy as indicated with aspirin, ACE (angiotensin-converting enzyme) inhibitors, statins, and/or β-blockers, as discussed elsewhere in this book.

6. Women who have one of the following

conditions – history of spontaneous venous thromboembolic disease; a family history of venous thromboembolic disease; cancer; lower extremity fracture; myocardial infarction; or immobilization due to surgery, hospitalization, or disability – should carefully consider the increased risk for new or recurrent venous thromboembolic disease while on HRT. If a woman develops one of these conditions while receiving HRT, she should discontinue therapy at least temporarily. The therapy could be discontinued permanently or reinstituted when the recurrence risk lessens, 3 months after the episode of venous thromboembolic disease or return to full ambulation, or as indicated by other clinical considerations.

7. Practitioners should not offer use of HRT to women who have a prior history of stroke or TIA. Women who develop stroke or TIA while on HRT should discontinue therapy due to increased risk of recurrence and lack of evidence of preventing future strokes.

8. Current use or initiation of SERMs should be managed in a manner similar to traditional estrogen replacement therapy until further data are available.

REFERENCES

1. Gambrell RD Jr, Massey FM, Castaneda TA, et al. Use of the progestogen challenge test to reduce the risk of endometrial cancer. Obstet Gynecol 1980; 55:732.

2. MacLennan A, Lester S, Moore V. Oral estrogen replacement therapy versus placebo for hot flushes: a systematic review. Climacteric 2001; 4:58.

3. Wells G, Tugwell P, Shea B, et al. Meta-analyses of therapies for postmenopausal osteoporosis. V. Meta-analysis of the efficacy of hormone replacement therapy in treating and preventing osteoporosis in postmenopausal women. Endocr Rev 2002; 23:529.

4. Notelovitz M, Mattox JH. Suppression of vasomotor and vulvovaginal symptoms with continuous oral 17β-estradiol. Menopause 2000; 7:310.

5. Ishiko O, Hirai K, Sumi T, Tatsuta I, Ogita S. Hormone replacement therapy plus pelvic floor muscle exercise for postmenopausal stress incontinence: a randomized, controlled trial. J Reprod Med 2001; 46:213.

6. Cardozo L, Lose G, McClish D, Versi E, de Koning Gans H. A systematic review of estrogens for recurrent urinary tract infections: third report of the hormones and urogenital therapy (HUT) committee. Int Urogynecol J Pelvic Floor Dysfunct 2001; 12:15.

7. Cardozo L, Bachmann G, McClish D, Fonda D, Birgerson L. Meta-analysis of estrogen therapy in the management of urogenital atrophy in postmenopausal women: second report of the hormones and urogenital therapy committee. Obstet Gynecol 1998; 92:722.

8. Sherwin BB. Estrogen and/or androgen replacement therapy and cognitive functioning in surgically menopausal women. Psychoneuroendocrinology 1988; 13:345.

9. Creidi P, Faivre B, Agache P, et al. Effect of a conjugated oestrogen (Premarin®) cream on ageing facial skin. A comparative study with a placebo cream. Maturitas 1994; 19:211.

10. Cagnacci A, Soldani R, Carriero PL, et al. Effects of low doses of transdermal 17β-estradiol on carbohydrate metabolism in postmenopausal women. J Clin Endocrinol Metab 1992; 74:1396.

11. Stampfer MJ, Colditz GA, Willett WC, et al. Postmenopausal estrogen therapy and cardiovascular disease. Ten-year follow-up from the nurses' health study. N Engl J Med 1991; 325:756.

12. Collaborative Group on Hormonal Factors in Breast Cancer. Breast cancer and hormone therapy: collaborative reanalysis of data from 51 epidemiological studies of 52 705 women with breast cancer and 108 411 women without breast cancer. [published erratum appears in Lancet 1997; 350:1484]. Lancet 1997; 350:1047.

13. Rosenbeg L, Palmer JR, Rao RS, et al. Case-control study of oral contraceptive use and risk of breast cancer. Am J Epidemiol 1996; 143:25.

14. Khan SA, Rogers MAM, Obando JA, Tamsen A. Estrogen receptor expression of benign breast epithelium and its association with breast cancer. Cancer Res 1994; 54:993.

15. Colditz GA, Rosner B. Cumulative risk of breast cancer to age 70 years according to risk factor status: data from the Nurses' Health Study. Am J Epidemiol 2000; 152:950.

16. Ross RK, Paganini-Hill A, Wan PC, Pike MC. Effect of hormone replacement therapy on breast cancer risk: estrogen versus estrogen plus progestin. J Natl Cancer Inst 2000; 92:328.

17. American Heart Association. Heart Disease and Stroke Statistics – 2005 Update. Dallas: American Heart Association; 2005.

18. Bruschi F, Meschia M, Soma M, et al. Lipoprotein(a) and other lipids after oophorectomy and estrogen replacement therapy. Obstet Gynecol 1996; 88:950.

19. Stampfer MJ, Willett WC, Colditz GA, et al. A prospective study of postmenopausal estrogen therapy and coronary heart disease. N Engl J Med 1985; 313:1044.

20. Grodstein F, Manson JE, Colditz GA, et al. A prospective, observational study of postmenopausal hormone therapy and primary prevention of cardiovascular disease. Ann Intern Med 2000; 133:933.

21. Hulley S, Grady D, Bush T, et al. Randomized trial of estrogen plus progestin for secondary prevention of coronary heart disease in postmenopausal women. JAMA 1998; 280:605.

22. Grady D, Herrington D, Bittner V, et al. Cardiovascular disease outcomes during 6.8 years of hormone therapy: Heart and Estrogen/progestin Replacement Study follow-up (HERS II). JAMA 2002; 288:49.

23. Herrington DM, Reboussin DM, Brosnihan KB, et al. Effects of estrogen replacement on the progression of coronary-artery atherosclerosis. N Engl J Med 2000; 343:522.

24. The Women's Health Initiative Study Group. Design of the Women's Health Initiative clinical trial and observational study. Control Clin Trials 1998; 19:61.

25. Writing Group for the Women's Health Initiative Investigators. Risks and benefits of estrogen plus progestin in healthy postmenopausal women: principal results from the Women's Health Initiative randomized controlled trial. JAMA 2002; 288:321.

26. Mikkola TS, Clarkson TB, Notelovitz M. Postmenopausal hormone therapy before and after the women's health initiative study: what consequences? Ann Med 2004; 36:402.

27. The Women's Health Initiative Steering Committee. Effects of conjugated equine estrogen in postmenopausal women with hysterectomy: the Women's Health Initiative randomized controlled trial. JAMA 2004; 291:1701.

28. Clarkson TB, Anthony MS, Wagner JD. A comparison of tibolone and conjugated equine estrogens effects on coronary artery atherosclerosis and bone density of postmenopausal monkeys. J Clin Endocrinol Metab 2001; 86:5396.

29. Clarkson TB, Anthony MS, Jerome CP. Lack of effect of raloxifene on coronary artery atherosclerosis of postmenopausal monkeys. J Clin Endocrinol Metab 1998; 83:721.

30. Adams MR, Register TC, Golden DL, Wagner JD, Williams JK. Medroxyprogesterone acetate antagonizes inhibitory effects of conjugated equine estrogens on coronary artery atherosclerosis. Arterioscler Thromb Vasc Biol 1997; 17:217.

31. Williams JK, Anthony MS, Honore EK, et al. Regression of atherosclerosis in female monkeys. Arterioscler Thromb Vasc Biol 1995; 15:827.

32. The Writing Group for the PEPI Trial. Effects of estrogen or estrogen/progestin regimens on heart disease risk factors in postmenopausal women: the Post-menopausal Estrogen/Progestin Interventions (PEPI) Trial. JAMA 1995; 273:199.

33. Miller J, Chan BKS, Nelson HD. Postmenopausal estrogen replacement and risk for venous thromboembolism: a systematic review and meta-analysis for the US Preventive Services Task Force. Ann Intern Med 2002; 136:680.

34. Angerer P, Störk S, Kothny W, Schmitt P, von Schacky C. Effect of oral postmenopausal hormone replacement on progression of atherosclerosis: a randomized, controlled trial. Arterioscler Thromb Vasc Biol 2001; 21:262.

35. Hodis HN, Mack WJ, Lobo RA, et al. Estrogen in the prevention of atherosclerosis: a randomized, double-blind, placebo-controlled trial. Ann Intern Med 2001; 135:939.

36. Hulley S, Furberg C, Barrett-Connor E, et al. Non-cardiovascular disease outcomes during 6.8 years of hormone therapy: Heart and Estrogen/progestin Replacement Study follow-up (HERS II). JAMA 2002; 288:58.

37. Grady D, Wenger NK, Herrington D, et al. Postmenopausal hormone therapy increases risk for venous thromboembolic disease: the Heart and Estrogen/progestin Replacement Study. Ann Intern Med 2000; 132:689.

38. American College of Obstetricians and Gynecologists Women's Health Care Physicians. Venous thromboembolic disease. Obstet Gynecol 2004; 104(Suppl): 118S.

39. Goldstein LB, Adams R, Becker K, et al. Primary prevention of ischemic stroke: a statement for healthcare professionals from the Stroke Council of the American Heart Association. Circulation 2001; 103:163.

40. Wassertheil-Smoller S, Hendrix SL, Limacher M, et al. Effect of estrogen plus progestin on stroke in postmenopausal women: the Women's Health Initiative: a randomized trial. JAMA 2003; 289:2673.

41. Wilson PWF, Garrison RJ, Castelli WP. Postmenopausal estrogen use, cigarette smoking, and cardiovascular morbidity in women over 50: the Framingham Study. N Engl J Med 1985; 313:1038.

42. Simon JA, Hsai J, Cauley JA, et al. Postmenopausal hormone therapy and risk of stroke: the Heart and Estrogen-progestin Replacement Study (HERS). Circulation 2001; 103:638.

43. The ESPIRIT Team. Oestrogen therapy for prevention of reinfarction in postmenopausal women: a randomised placebo controlled trial. Lancet 2002; 360:2001.

44. Waters DD, Alderman EL, Hsia J, et al. Effects of hormone replacement therapy and antioxidant vitamin supplements on coronary atherosclerosis in postmenopausal women: a randomized controlled trial. JAMA 2002; 288:2432.

45. Viscoli CM, Brass LM, Kernan WN, et al. A clinical trial of estrogen-replacement therapy after ischemic stroke. N Engl J Med 2001; 345:1243.

46. Fisher B, Costantino JP, Wickerham DL, et al. Tamoxifen for prevention of breast cancer: report of the National Surgical Adjuvant Breast and Bowel Project P-1 Study. J Natl Cancer Inst 1998; 90:1371.

47. Barrett-Connor E, Grady D, Sashegyi A, et al. Raloxifene and cardiovascular events in osteoporotic postmenopausal women: four-year results from the MORE (Multiple Outcomes of Raloxifene Evaluation) randomized trial. JAMA 2002; 287:847.

48. Hays J, Ockene JK, Brunner RL, et al. Effects of estrogen plus progestin on health-related quality of life. N Engl J Med 2003; 348:1839.

49. Col NF, Weber G, Stiggelbout A, et al. Short-term menopausal hormone therapy for symptom relief: an updated decision model. Arch Intern Med 2004; 164:1634.

50. US Preventive Services Task Force. Postmenopausal hormone replacement therapy for primary prevention of chronic conditions: recommendations and rationale. Ann Intern Med 2002; 137:834.

51. American College of Obstetricians and Gynecologists Women's Health Care Physicians. Coronary heart disease. Obstet Gynecol 2004; 104(4 Suppl):41S.

52. American College of Obstetricians and Gynecologists Women's Health Care Physicians. Stroke. Obstet Gynecol 2004;104(4 Suppl):97S.

12

Nutrition

Laura S Hillman, Pamela S Hinton, Catherine A Peterson, Tom R Thomas, Grace Y Sun, Richard Hillman and Maurine D Raedeke

Introduction • **Metabolic syndrome and lifestyle diseases** • **Saturated and *trans* fatty acids** • **Polyunsaturated fatty acids: dietary ω-3 fatty acids** • **Carbohydrates** • **Protein** • **Minerals** • **Water-soluble vitamins** • **Fat-soluble vitamins** • **Antioxidants, oxidative stress, and cardiovascular diseases** • **Summary: the sensible diet**

INTRODUCTION

Although most heart disease presents later in life, even later in women than in men, the roots of the problems begin in childhood. Because this is true for many other health problems women face, such as osteoporosis, good nutrition habits and a healthy, active lifestyle must begin early. Pregnancy and lactation present special nutritional needs that should influence women's lifelong diet habits.

METABOLIC SYNDROME AND LIFESTYLE DISEASES

Americans are gaining weight at unprecedented rates, and markers of the metabolic syndrome and type 2 diabetes are accompanying this trend.[1] The National Health and Nutrition Examination Survey (NHANES) found obesity rates in US adults increased from 13.4% in 1960–62 to 30.9% in 1999–2000. The prevalence of overweight increased from 55.9% in 1988–94 to 64.5% in 1999–2000. Eighty percent of African-American women aged 40 and older were overweight, but this dramatic increase affected virtually every age, ethnic, and socioeconomic group. Whereas NHANES categorized only 4.6% of youths (aged 12–19) as overweight in 1966–70, by 1999–2000 the figure was 15.5%, and most of the increase occurred since 1980. In a recent study, scientists estimated overweight/obesity in young adulthood may double healthcare costs in older age.

Although overweight itself is a risk factor for chronic diseases, most of the increased risk may be associated with aberrations in metabolism that accompany overweight. Recently, epidemiologic studies suggest increased prevalence of CHD and type 2 diabetes in individuals with the metabolic syndrome.[2] The third report of the National Cholesterol Education Program (NCEP) defined the metabolic syndrome as the presence of three of the following metabolic abnormalities:

- waist circumference >102 cm in men, >88 cm in women
- serum triglyceride (TG) concentration >150 mg/dl
- high-density lipoprotein cholesterol (HDL-C) concentration <40 mg/dl in men, <50 mg/dl in women
- blood pressure >130/85 mmHg
- fasting glucose 110–125 mg/dl.

Ford et al[1] estimated the metabolic syndrome is present in 24% of men and 23% of women, for a total of about 47 million Americans, and the number is expected to grow rapidly. Overall, elevated waist circumference is the most prevalent metabolic syndrome risk factor for women, but high blood pressure is the most prevalent risk factor after age 65.

Weight loss, whether by restricting energy intake, increasing energy output, or both, improves metabolic fitness, as demonstrated by beneficial changes in insulin sensitivity, abdominal adiposity, blood lipid profile, markers of inflammation, and blood pressure. Thus, the impact of weight loss is clear.

Professional groups have increasingly recognized exercise as a primary tool in the battle against obesity and associated metabolic disorders. Yet 60% of US adults do not participate in regular physical activity, with women of all age groups slightly less active than men. Hill et al[3] calculated the average adult American gains almost 1 kg annually and estimated weight stabilization would require an energy deficit from diet and exercise combined of only 100 kcal/day. In spite of such encouraging findings and the consistent recommendations of health agencies, the national trend toward an increasingly sedentary lifestyle continues.

Exercise training without weight loss has been shown to affect each variable of the metabolic syndrome, including insulin sensitivity, apparently by increasing glucose transporter GLUT4 protein expression, abdominal obesity, the lipoprotein profile, C-reactive protein, and blood pressure. Epidemiologic studies suggest being overweight does not increase the risk of death for fit men, although this finding is not unanimous. Taken together, these data suggest many of the benefits from exercise training may not require weight loss.

An area of important health consequences that the obesity literature has not resolved is maintaining body weight after weight loss. Although millions of Americans lose weight each year, only a small percentage sustain the reduction. The cause is unknown, but reduced physical activity, ingestion of high glycemic index foods, and system response to insulin and/or leptin concentrations have been suggested.

Data from the National Weight Control Registry offer a more positive picture of weight maintenance success.[4] In that registry, over 3000 men and women have maintained a 13.6 kg weight loss for at least 1 year, and a subgroup maintained the same loss for 5 years. These successful individuals used a variety of strategies to control weight, including energy (1444 kcal/day) and fat (20% kcal) restriction and considerable daily exercise (3000 kcal/week). Over 91% of registrants reported using exercise to maintain weight loss, indicating the importance of exercise in weight maintenance.

The epidemiologic literature provides evidence that repeated weight loss may be unhealthy,[5] but the mechanism of this effect has not been well studied. Results from recent cross-sectional follow-up studies indicated weight cycling was not consistently associated with adverse effects on body composition, lipoproteins, or blood pressure.[5,6]

SATURATED AND *TRANS* FATTY ACIDS

Blood lipids have been linked to a variety of lifestyle-related diseases. The key lipid aspects of the increased risk are elevated cholesterol and low-density lipoprotein cholesterol (LDL-C), and reduced HDL-C. Dietary fatty acids are the primary determinants of alterations in lipids and lipoproteins. In general, unsaturated fatty acids reduce cholesterol in all lipoproteins, primarily by upregulating the LDL receptors and increasing cholesterol uptake by cells.[7] On the other hand, saturated fatty acids and *trans* fatty acids elevate plasma cholesterol primarily by down-regulating LDL receptors and decreasing uptake of cholesterol by cells, especially the liver, and LDL accumulates in plasma.[8] Saturated fatty acids may also interfere with the cholesterol-esterifying enzyme acyl-CoA cholesterol acyl transferase (ACAT).[8] *Trans* fatty acids also increase postprandial lipemia and increase the activity of cholesteryl ester transfer protein (CETP), which may increase LDL-C concentrations and promote the formation of small, dense LDL, a risk for atherosclerosis.[9] Monounsaturated fatty acids appear to reduce plasma cholesterol and LDL-C while maintaining HDL-C.[10]

POLYUNSATURATED FATTY ACIDS; DIETARY ω-3 FATTY ACIDS

The last two decades have seen a marked rise in scientific inquiry and public interest in dietary ω-3 (n-3) and ω-6 (n-6) fatty acids and their influence on health. The current Western diet is very high in n-6 fatty acids (n-6:n-3 ratio = 20–30:1), purportedly because of the indiscriminate recommendation to substitute n-6 fatty acids for saturated fats to lower serum cholesterol concentrations. Conversely, compared with the diets of humans >150 years ago (estimated n-6:n-3 ratio = 1–4:1), the consumption of n-3 fatty acids is dwindling, owing to decreased fish consumption and the use of animal feeds abundant in grains containing n-6 fatty acids, leading to production of meat rich in n-6 and poor in n-3 fatty acids. Both the absolute intake of n-3 fatty acids and the ratio of dietary n-6:n-3 must be considered in the prevention or treatment of cardiovascular disease.

Sources and metabolism

The polyunsaturated fatty acids (PUFAs) of the n-3 and n-6 series are deemed essential because they are not synthesized by the body and must be obtained from the diet or supplementation. α-Linolenic acid (ALA, 18:3 n-3) represents the basis of the n-3 family, and linoleic acid (LA, 18:2 n-6) represents the basis of the n-6 family. Through a rather inefficient enzymatic process of desaturation, ALA produces eicosapentaenoic acid (EPA, 20:5 n-3) and docosahexaenoic acid (DHA, 22:6 n-3), precursors to a group of anti-inflammatory, antiarrhythmic, antithrombotic, vasodilatory eicosanoids (prostaglandins, thromboxanes, and leukotrienes). The longer-chain fatty acid derivative of LA is arachidonic acid (AA, 20:4 n-6), a precursor to a different group of proinflammatory, prothrombotic eicosanoids (Figure 12.1).

The n-3 and n-6 fatty acids compete during eicosanoid formation as the same enzymes are

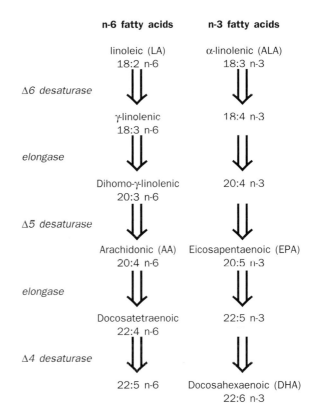

Figure 12.1 Production of long-chain polyunsaturated fatty acids (PUFAs) of the n-6 and n-3 series from their dietary precursors, linoleic and α-linolenic acid, respectively. The n-6 and n-3 fatty acids compete for the same enzymes along desaturation and elongation pathways.

Table 12.1 Dietary and supplemental sources of n-3 and n-6 fatty acids		
ω-3 fatty acids		*ω-6 fatty acids*
α-linolenic acid (ALA)	*Docosahexaenoic acid (DHA) + eicosapentaenoic acid (EPA)*	*Linoleic acid (LA)*
Canola oil	Fish – fattier fish (salmon, sardines, trout) are richer sources	Corn oil
Flaxseed oil	Fish oil – most 1 g capsules contain 120 mg DHA and 180 mg EPA	Cottonseed oil
Soybean oil (also high in n-6)	DHA-only supplements (made from algae) – most capsules contain 100 mg DHA	Margarine
Walnut oil		Peanut oil
Designer eggs (hens are fed flaxseed, fish oil, or algae derived DHA) – one egg can contain 50–150 mg of DHA		Sesame oil
		Soybean oil
		Sunflower oil

involved in their synthesis. Common food-grade vegetable oils such as corn, peanut, safflower, sunflower, and cottonseed oils are rich in LA, but dietary sources of ALA are relatively few (Table 12.1). Fish and fish oil uniquely provide EPA and DHA directly, avoiding the need and therefore the competition (with n-6 fatty acids) for enzymes to convert ALA to EPA and/or DHA.

Biologic effects

The ω-6 and ω-3 fatty acids exert many biologic effects on cardiovascular risk factors across a wide range of intakes.[11] LA has been shown to lower both total and LDL-C, and to increase, decrease, or have no effect on HDL-C. ALA is known to decrease or have no effect on LDL-C and HDL-C and to decrease arrhythmia and thrombosis. DHA + EPA have been demonstrated to lower serum TGs but increase LDL-C. Moreover, these two long-chain n-3 PUFAs have also been shown to decrease arrhythmia, blood pressure, and proinflammatory factors, and to improve vascular endothelial function.

Randomized controlled trials

In the Diet and Reinfarction Trial (DART) 2-year follow-up, men who had been advised to consume two fish servings weekly had a 29% reduction in all-cause mortality but no reduction in the incidence of myocardial infarction.[12] The GISSI-Prevenzione Trial[13] tested the effects of two types of supplements (850 mg DHA + EPA and 300 mg vitamin E), taken alone or in combination, in >11 000 patients with a previous history of myocardial infarction. After 42 months, the group given the DHA + EPA alone had a 45% reduction in sudden death and a 20% reduction in all-cause mortality. Little research has been conducted in individuals without pre-existing cardiovascular disease.

There is only one study to date on the effect of DHA (free of EPA) supplementation on selected cardiovascular risk factors in postmenopausal women:[14] 18 women receiving and 14 women not receiving hormone replacement therapy (HRT) completed a randomized,

double-blind, placebo-controlled, cross-over trial with a daily dose of 2.8 mg of an algal source of DHA for 28 days. In all women, DHA supplementation was associated with several significant changes in cardiovascular disease risk factors, including 20% lower serum TG concentrations, 8% higher HDL-C concentrations, and a 7% decrease in resting heart rate.

Omega-3 index as a novel risk factor

An omega-3 index, recently described for consideration as a new risk factor for death from coronary heart disease (CHD), may prove to have significant clinical utility.[15] Since red blood cell (RBC) fatty acid composition reflects long-term fatty acid intake, it was proposed that the RBC EPA + DHA content (named the omega-3 index) be used as a CHD risk predictor. Data from clinical and laboratory experiments have been used to validate this index; results showed an omega-3 index of ≥8% was associated with the greatest cardioprotection, whereas an index of ≤4% was associated with the least.

Recommended dietary intake and supplement dosages

The American Heart Association published a set of recommendations for n-3 fatty acid intake based on health status. Individuals with no documented CHD are encouraged to eat a variety of oily fish at least twice weekly and to include oils and foods rich in ALA.[16] Those with documented CHD are recommended to consume ~1 g of EPA + DHA daily, preferably from oily fish, with supplements considered in consultation with a physician. In patients requiring a lowering of serum TG levels, 2–4 g of EPA + DHA daily, provided as capsules under a physician's care, are suggested.

DHA is very important for infant brain and eye development and is actively transported across the placenta during pregnancy and into the milk during lactation. Infants fed breast milk containing higher levels of DHA have better visual acuity and cognitive function. Consumption of low-mercury-containing fish is especially recommended during pregnancy and lactation. Supplements may also be considered. Although there is not yet a DRI (dietary reference intake) established for DHA, recommendations for pregnant and lactating women that came out of the 1999 NIH (National Institutes of Health)-sponsored 'Workshop on the essentiality of and recommended dietary intakes for omega-6 and omega-3 fatty acids' include ensuring at least 300 mg of DHA per day.[17]

CARBOHYDRATES

Since type 2 diabetes is a leading risk factor for coronary artery disease, carbohydrates deserve as much attention as fats. Inflammation is also believed to play a role in cardiovascular disease, with hyperinsulinism playing a large part.

It is still recommended that 45–65% of total *required* calories for activity level come from carbohydrates, but the type of carbohydrates has assumed greater importance. To reduce rapid rises in blood glucose, which stimulate increases in insulin release, many sources recommend consuming intact fruits, vegetables, and whole grains, and avoiding simple sugars, corn syrup, and other sweeteners used in processed foods. The fiber in fruits, vegetables, and whole grains has the advantage of slowing the absorption of sugars from the intestine as well as stimulating intestinal activity. Soluble fiber can also bind cholesterol and thus reduce its absorption. Consuming 30 g of fiber/day, which both the USDA (US Department of Agriculture) Food Guide and the DASH (Dietary Approaches to Stop Hypertension) diet recommend at 2000 calories/day, requires considerable amounts of fruits, vegetables, and whole grains. According to the USDA Food Guide, this translates into four servings of fruits, five servings of vegetables, and three servings of whole grains a day. DASH recommends four–five servings of fruit, four–five servings of vegetables, and seven–eight servings of grains, of which the majority are whole grain. DASH emphasizes nuts, seeds, and legumes as a rich source of energy, magnesium, potassium, protein, and fiber. Avoiding processed foods containing corn sweeteners, corn syrup, dextrose, fructose, fruit juice concentrate, high fructose corn syrup, maltose,

malt syrup, molasses, and other forms of sugar is crucial.

The glycemic index (GI), the area under the serum glucose curve a food generates, is attracting increasing attention. A prospective case-controlled study found that the relative risk of developing type 2 diabetes was significantly related to the GI of the diet and inversely related to intake of cereal (but not vegetable) fiber. Glycemic load (GI × amount of carbohydrate) was not related.[18] Cross-sectional studies have also shown a higher likelihood of developing the metabolic syndrome in subjects whose diet had a high GI and low cereal fiber. However, a meta-analysis of 15 randomized, relatively short-term treatment trials on low-GI diets with cardiovascular disease end points showed only weak evidence of benefit.[19] Focusing on low-GI foods for weight reduction is increasingly popular, especially in childhood obesity. The overall increase in the GI of food (as opposed to total calories, total carbohydrates, fats, etc.) has been suggested as a potential cause of the obesity epidemic.[20]

PROTEIN

As with carbohydrates, the daily amount of protein recommended has not changed, but the recommended source has: USDA (Dietary Guidelines for America 2005) recommends 18% of required calories (91 g at 2000 calories). DASH (Dietary Approaches to Stop Hypertension, from the National Heart, Lung, and Blood Institute) recommends 21% of calories (108 g). USDA recommends 5.5 oz equivalents of lean meat and beans together as a protein source. DASH recommends two or fewer servings of meat, poultry, or fish, and four–five servings of nuts, seeds, or legumes. However, many sources recommend increasing consumption of fish to increase ω-3 fatty acids, especially DHA, as described earlier. Low-fat milk is an increasingly recognized important source of protein as well as minerals, and recommendations have been increased to three servings a day.

A health claim has been allowed for 25 g of soy protein to reduce heart disease by reducing cholesterol. How this works is unclear, but it does not require the presence of phytoestrogens and cannot be reproduced by equivalent amounts of phytoestrogens.[21]

MINERALS

Sodium

Minerals play an important role in heart health, primarily through their effect on blood pressure. Sodium has for many years been known to increase blood pressure – in some people. It is still unclear how or why 'salt-sensitive' individuals differ from others. Reducing sodium intake can have an impressive effect in salt-sensitive hypertensives. Current guidelines recommend limiting salt intake to 1.5 g for those with risk factors for hypertension and cardiovascular disease and 2.5 g for others. Most natural foods contain little salt. Table salt contributes significant and highly variable amounts, but the major source is processed foods. The sodium content of foods from different manufacturers varies markedly; consumers should read labels carefully and purchase foods lower in salt.

Potassium

Increasing potassium intake is important for most people. The National Academy of Sciences reported US women consume 2500 mg/day and men 3000 mg/day.[22] It recommended to increase intake to 4700 mg/day from fruits and vegetables (about 10 portions/day). Potassium is more available from vegetables than from other sources, such as meat and milk. Thirty-one potassium supplementation studies showed significant drops in blood pressure, and the higher the blood pressure the greater the drop.[23] Potassium makes the kidneys excrete more sodium. Potassium citrate, the form found in fruits and vegetables, can reduce the body's acid load and the calcium carbonate pulled from the bone to neutralize the acid load.[24] Potatoes, lima beans, bananas, squash, and spinach have about 500 mg/serving.

Calcium

Although calcium has been shown to reduce blood pressure in animal models,[25] clinical trials of calcium supplements have had mixed and unimpressive results.[26] Additional calcium supplementation for the general public has not been recommended, although identifying and correcting exceptionally low intakes seems advisable and may benefit certain subgroups of the population. It had been hoped that additional calcium would reduce the incidence of preeclampsia during pregnancy; however, a large randomized, multicenter trial of calcium supplementation failed to reduce the incidence.[27]

However, calcium intake is particularly important for women because of the eventual risk of osteoporosis. Adequate calcium intake is particularly important in prepuberty and puberty, when peak bone mass is accreting. Failure to maximize peak bone mass puts women at increased risk of fractures and osteoporosis postmenopause. Although percent calcium absorption increases during pregnancy to provide additional calcium for the fetus, adequate intake is important for the mother's bone mineralization.[28] During lactation, calcium absorption is not increased, and calcium for milk production is removed from the maternal skeleton.[28] Fortunately, mineral is returned to the skeleton postweaning.[28] Intakes of about 1000 mg are recommended, but further increases will not prevent bone resorption during lactation.[29] Adequate calcium intake (1200 mg) is important around menopause but will not in itself prevent bone loss. Starting at least three servings of fat-free dairy products daily during childhood increases calcium intake and provides protein, potassium, and magnesium. Furthermore, findings from a recent study involving >2500 subjects suggest the treatment of postmenopausal osteoporosis should include consideration of measures to prevent cardiovascular outcomes. After adjustment for potential confounders, women with osteoporosis had a 3.9-fold increased risk for cardiovascular events compared with women with normal bone mass; the risk of cardiovascular events increased incrementally with the number and severity of baseline vertebral fractures.[30]

Magnesium

Magnesium, like calcium, lowers blood pressure in animal models,[31] and low magnesium in the diet is associated with high blood pressure. However, limited treatment trials in humans have not demonstrated significant results. Fruits and vegetables that are high in potassium are also high in magnesium.

More important are magnesium's probable effects on insulin resistance and the metabolic syndrome. Diabetics have been known to have lower serum magnesium levels for many years; more recent studies suggest that magnesium deficiency may lead to insulin resistance before the onset of diabetes. An 18-year follow-up study showed a relative risk (RR) of developing diabetes of 0.66 for the highest quintile of magnesium intake versus the lowest quintile.[32] In a case-controlled study, subjects with the metabolic syndrome had significantly lower serum magnesium levels, and a much higher percentage had values below the normal range.[33] Hypertension and hyperlipidemia were the most strongly associated components of the metabolic syndrome.

Limited treatment trials of magnesium supplementation in diabetes yielded conflicting results. Prevention trials have not yet been carried out. Increasing the consumption of magnesium is relatively simple – more fruits, vegetables, and milk – and is recommended.

Iron

In women of reproductive age, the normal iron content of the body is 40 mg/kg of body weight. The iron content of the body is regulated by duodenal absorption; the body cannot actively excrete iron. The typical US diet is 10–15% heme iron and 85–90% non-heme iron. Non-heme dietary iron, or ferric iron (Fe^{3+}), requires the acidic environment of the stomach to be solubilized. Ferric reductase of the duodenal mucosa reduces ferric iron to ferrous iron, which is transported across the apical membrane via divalent metal transporter-1 (DMT-1). Iron available during mucosal cell development regulates the amount of DMT-1 expressed by enterocytes. Iron export across the basolateral membrane requires oxidation to the ferric state by ferric oxidase activity of copper-containing ceruloplasmin for binding to transferrin. Iron not transported across the basolateral membrane is lost when cells are sloughed every 48–72 hours.

Absorption of non-heme iron is inhibited when the gastric pH increases and in the presence of phytates, polyphenols, and calcium. The bioavailability of non-heme iron from a mixed diet decreases twofold in the presence of these inhibitors. Ascorbic acid and an unidentified compound (or compounds), probably short peptides, in meat, increase non-heme iron absorption. Heme iron is absorbed via a mechanism independent of that for non-heme iron. Heme iron binds to a receptor (unidentified, in humans), is internalized, and is degraded by heme oxygenase. The iron released from heme degradation enters the intracellular pool and is exported via transferrin, as described for non-heme iron. About 25% of heme iron is absorbed; absorption of non-heme iron varies from 10% in a mixed diet to 5% in a vegetarian diet. The estimated overall bioavailability of iron from a typical US diet is 18%.

Iron is transported in the blood bound to the protein transferrin. Cellular iron uptake is mediated by binding to a cell surface receptor for transferrin. The iron–transferrin complex is internalized, and the iron is released from the protein upon acidification in an endosome. The free iron can be stored in the cell bound to ferritin or hemosiderin or exported from the cell via DMT-1 or SFT (stimulator of Fe transport). Iron is stored primarily in the liver, spleen, and bone marrow. Cellular iron status influences further storage and uptake of iron via regulating the translation of ferritin and transferrin receptor mRNA by the iron-responsive element binding protein (IRE-BP).[34]

Iron losses and dietary requirements

Daily basal iron losses are small compared with total body iron (0.9–1.2 mg iron/day): 0.6 mg/day from the gastrointestinal tract, mostly in sloughed mucosal cells; 0.08 mg/day in urine; and 0.2–0.3 mg/day in skin. Menstruating women require an additional 0.6–0.7 mg/day to account for menstrual blood loss. Women with high menstrual blood flow and women who use intrauterine devices lose more iron; oral contraceptive agents reduce menstrual bleeding. The

Table 12.2 EARs and RDAs of adult women (mg iron daily)

	EAR	RDA
Non-pregnant, non-lactating:		
19–30 years old	8.1	18
31–50 years old	8.1	18
50–70 years old	5	8
>70 years old	5	8
Pregnant:		
19–30 years old	22	27
31–50 years old	22	27
Lactating:		
19–30 years old	6.5	9
30–50 years old	6.5	9

EARs, estimated average requirements;
RDAs, recommended daily allowances.

Table 12.3 Laboratory measurements commonly used to evaluate iron status

Stage of iron deficiency	Indicator	Diagnostic range
Depleted stores	Stainable bone marrow iron	Absent
	Total iron-binding capacity	>400 µg/dl
	Serum ferritin concentration	<12 µg/l
Early functional iron deficiency	Transferrin saturation	<16%
	Free erythrocyte protoporphyrin	>70 µg/dl
	Serum transferrin receptor	>8.5 mg/l
Iron-deficiency anemia	Hemoglobin concentration	<130 g/l male
		<120 g/l female
	Mean cell volume	<80 fl

From NAS.[38]

EARs (estimated average requirements) and RDAs (recommended daily allowances) for adult women are shown in Table 12.2.

Iron deficiency

Iron deficiency is a degenerative condition that progresses through three stages:

- iron stores depleted, but functional iron unchanged
- early functional iron deficiency without anemia
- iron-deficiency anemia.

Table 12.3 shows the clinical indicators used to assess each stage of iron deficiency. The clinical signs and symptoms of iron depletion reflect the severity of the deficiency. Early functional iron deficiency reduces endurance capacity and energetic efficiency during submaximal work in young women.[35,36] Animal studies suggest this deficit is due to decreased activity of iron-containing oxidative enzymes and cytochromes.

The hallmark symptoms of anemia are fatigue, lack of energy, and apathy. Anemia impairs maximal work performance (maximal oxygen consumption, VO_2max) by reducing oxygen delivery to the body.[37] Iron-deficiency anemia during pregnancy increases maternal morbidity and perinatal morbidity and mortality. Iron deficiency impairs non-specific immunity by decreasing the ability of macrophages and neutrophils to kill pathogens.[39] Recently, iron-deficiency anemia has been associated with postpartum depression and impaired cognition in women.[40]

Iron overload

When body iron exceeds the storage and transport capacity of ferritin and transferrin, respectively, the excess iron remains unbound to proteins. This free iron causes lipid peroxidation and free radical production, processes that damage the cardiovascular system, kidneys, liver, and central nervous system. Although a positive association between serum ferritin and risk of heart attack in an epidemiologic study of Finnish men[41] led to the hypothesis that body iron excess contributed to cardiovascular disease, prospective cohort studies suggested that iron status neither caused coronary heart disease[42] nor increased all-causes mortality risk.[43] Recent epidemiologic studies suggest ferritin may be a marker of inflammation, rather than a causative factor in cardiovascular disease.[44] Iron status had no effect on LDL oxidation in controlled feeding studies of healthy men and women.[45] Likewise, iron supplementation of women with low-iron status did not increase susceptibility of LDL to oxidation.[46] There is no conclusive evidence that dietary iron causes liver or colon cancer in healthy populations.

In summary, women have increased iron requirements due to menstrual losses and pregnancy. Although absorption of iron increases during pregnancy, the high incidence of iron-deficiency anemia during pregnancy has prompted the recommendation of iron supplementation in the form of prenatal vitamins. During other periods, adequate iron should be available from the diet as non-heme and heme iron. Because heme iron is more easily absorbed, and other meat proteins facilitate absorption of non-heme iron, some red meat in the diet will assure adequate iron status. Strict vegetarians are at increased risk of iron deficiency and should be monitored. Normal individuals do not appear to be at significant risk of iron overload from meat consumption, and increased risk of cardiovascular disease has not been related to iron stores. Anemia increases the cardiovascular stress imposed by pregnancy and may contribute to postpartum depression.[40]

WATER-SOLUBLE VITAMINS

Water-soluble vitamins function mostly as cofactors for enzymes. They are necessary either for the conformational shape of the functioning enzyme or as participants in the chemical reaction catalyzed by the enzyme protein(s). Deficiencies of the water-soluble vitamins can lead to classical deficiency diseases, which space does not allow to be reviewed in this chapter. These deficiencies in Western diets are usually found only in people receiving unbalanced diets (usually vegetarian) or in people with inherited diseases of the absorption or processing of the substances. Instead, this section will concentrate on two important metabolic defects that do not result primarily from nutritional deficiency but can be corrected with pharmacologic (relatively large) doses of water-soluble vitamins.

In the 1980s and 1990s, several studies demonstrated that B-complex vitamins, and specifically folic acid, could reduce (by as much as 80%) the risk of neural tube defects (NTD: open spine defects and anencephaly) in families in which a previous child had one of these conditions. The biochemical mechanisms for these findings have been well studied. Mills et al[47] noted that homocysteine metabolism seemed to be the critical pathway affected by folic acid. They and others demonstrated that defects or polymorphisms in several different genes in the pathway from homocysteine to methionine could be associated with NTD. In particular, Frosst et al[48] had reported that persons with a specific mutation in MTHFR (5,10 methylenetetrahydrofolate reductase) were at a 7.2-fold increased risk of having children with NTD. These and later studies demonstrated that the mutant enzyme was thermolabile and that folic acid could stabilize the protein. This mutation in MTHFR is only a partial answer to the response to folic acid. Defects in at least three other enzymes in this pathway are also associated with NTD. Because of these findings, folic acid has now been added to flour, and it is recommended that all women of childbearing age receive additional folic acid (1 mg daily).

Changes in this same pathway, associated with increases in homocysteine concentrations, have also been associated with increased evidence of ischemic heart disease. In most cases, when mutations have been detected, the patients seem to be heterozygotes for mutations in one of the same enzymes (usually cystathione β-synthase) involved in NTD. Chao et al[49] found that treatment with a combination of folic acid, vitamin B_{12}, and pyridoxine (the three B-complex vitamins involved in this pathway) significantly reduced homocysteine levels and improved the outcome in patients who had required coronary angioplasty. Although women have a lower risk than men of coronary stenosis until postmenopausal years, these studies strongly suggest women as well as men should receive extra folic acid (the usual recommendation for men) or all three B vitamins because of the risk of vitamin B_{12} malabsorption with increasing age.

FAT-SOLUBLE VITAMINS

Vitamin D

Vitamin D is particularly important in women because of the risks of osteoporosis, but has more general potential benefits because of its emerging anti-inflammatory properties, which may reduce risks of cardiovascular disease and some cancers.

Vitamin D_3 is meant to be obtained by synthesis in the skin from UV rays acting on 7–dehydrocholesterol. Naturally occurring vitamin D_2 in foods is very rare, and most vitamin D in foods has been added either as vitamin D_2 or D_3, increasingly vitamin D_3. Fish oils, including cod liver oil, have remained the primary natural source of vitamin D_2 for centuries in many countries. In the United States, all milk is supplemented, usually with vitamin D_3, at 400 IU per quart, and many other cereals and food products are also supplemented. Because vitamin D is fat-soluble, its toxicity, primarily hypercalcemia, can occur orally. Fear of intoxication has limited the content of all multivitamin tablets to 400 IU. In fact, there are very few data to establish 'requirements' or toxic levels for adults. Most of the work establishing 'requirements' was done in infants over half a century ago. Because nutritional 'requirements' depend on what has not been obtained by sun exposure and skin synthesis, this is a difficult task. Effective sun exposure depends on the time spent in the sun, the cloud/pollution conditions, latitude of location, and, importantly, the season of the year. Seasonal differences in serum 25–hydroxyvitamin D (25–OHD), the liver metabolite of vitamin D, can easily be shown in most parts of the United States and other countries, especially those at very northern latitudes. Serum 25–OHD does not change during pregnancy or lactation and is subject to the same seasonal, sun exposure, skin pigmentation, and intake effects.[28,50] 25-OHD is transferred across the placenta to the fetus only passively, so that infants of deficient mothers are born deficient.[51] Because passage of both vitamin D and 25-OHD into milk is passive, milk with reduced amounts of both vitamin D and 25-OHD may be produced, especially in highly pigmented populations.[52] The classical case of vitamin D deficiency rickets in infants is an African-American infant born in late winter and exclusively breast-fed presenting in the next winter with clinical rickets. With the increased use of sun screens, avoidance of sun, and other cultural changes, more rickets cases have appeared in exclusively breast-fed Caucasian infants from all latitudes and seasons, prompting the American Academy of Pediatrics to recommend 200 IU vitamin D supplementation for all breast-fed infants. Official recommended vitamin D intakes for pregnancy and lactation have been set at 800 IU, with 400 IU coming from a prenatal vitamin during both pregnancy and lactation. For maximal recovery of the skeleton postweaning and the return of menses, adequate vitamin D should be assured for about another 6 months. Because of decreased sun exposure and dietary intakes, and because vitamin D absorption may decrease with age, intakes of 800 IU have also been recommended for the elderly. Also, because vitamin D has beneficial effects on muscle function, it has been postulated that decreased fracture rates are related to both improved muscle and bone strength.

The anti-inflammatory and immunoregulating effects of vitamin D could have implications for type 2 diabetes and cardiovascular disease. Several human and animal studies suggest that vitamin D affects insulin sensitivity and the development of type 2 diabetes and the metabolic syndrome. In a recent study of disease-free adults, serum 25-OHD was positively correlated with insulin sensitivity and inversely correlated with serum glucose at 60, 90, and 120 minutes. Subjects with low 25-OHD were more likely to have the metabolic syndrome.[53]

Campaigns are underway to increase sun exposure in multiple limited doses – e.g. by walking to the beach without sunscreen and applying it only after arriving. Fortunately, a lot of vitamin D can be made in periods of 10–15 minutes. UV exposure from special lighting sources has been recommended for the elderly.

Vitamin K

Vitamin K may offer some osteoporosis protection.[54] Osteocalcin, a protein produced by osteoblasts and secreted into the matrix, is a vitamin K-dependent protein. Serum levels of osteocalcin have been used as markers of bone formation, and osteocalcin plays a role in mineralization. Compared with placebo, a combination of calcium, magnesium, zinc, and vitamin D reduced bone loss in post-menopausal women by 1.7%. Adding vitamin K to this mixture reduced loss by an additional 1.3%.[55] However, excessive vitamin K might increase the hypercoagulation risks already associated with cardiovascular diseases, and supplements are not recommended.[56] There is some thought that vitamin K is important for arterial health and that deficiency could lead to increased arteriosclerosis.[57]

Vitamin A

Vitamin A is important for visual acuity. It was once believed to have important antioxidant effects, but trials using β-carotene to decrease cardiovascular disease had the opposite effect. In eight studies, 138 000 men and women who took 15–50 mg β-carotene were 10% likelier to die from heart disease.[58]

Vitamin E

Vitamin E is a powerful antioxidant, protecting cell membrane PUFAs, thiol-rich proteins, and nucleic acids from oxidative damage initiated by free radical reactions. It is essential for maintaining the nervous system, retina, and skeletal muscle. Toxicity is less evident in vitamin E, leading to significant abuses of the vitamin to 'prolong life,' 'increase sexual potency,' and 'prevent cancer.' Early data suggested vitamin E might reduce cardiovascular disease.[59] However, several large clinical trials have failed to show efficacy.[60] Seven major studies supplementing 50–800 IU of vitamin E

did not reduce the risk of dying from heart disease.[58]

Vitamin C

Vitamin C is important for iron absorption and bone formation. However, the hope that its antioxidant properties would reduce cardiovascular disease has so far not been supported.[61]

ANTIOXIDANTS, OXIDATIVE STRESS, AND CARDIOVASCULAR DISEASES

There is strong evidence supporting the involvement of oxidative stress in the pathophysiology of a number of vascular and cardiovascular diseases, including atherosclerosis, diabetes, hypertension, and hyperlipidemia.[62–64] In the living cell, oxidative and antioxidative pathways are present to mediate cell function. Under normal conditions, intracellular ROS (reactive oxygen species) production can be balanced by antioxidant enzymes such as superoxide dismutase, glutathione peroxidase, and catalase. Many factors can upset the oxidative–antioxidative balance, resulting in disease states.

In the endothelium, production of nitric oxide (NO) through the endothelial nitric oxide synthase (eNOS) enzyme is considered a major factor for regulating endothelial function. ROS are detrimental to vascular cells (endothelial cells, vascular smooth muscle cells, and adventitial fibroblasts), causing lipid peroxidation and membrane damage, leading to increased Ca^{2+} influx, perturbation of intracellular signaling pathways, and subsequent alteration of cellular functions (proliferation, migration, inflammation and apoptosis). In endothelial cells, production of ROS from NAD(P)H oxidase can lead to stimulation of vascular endothelial growth factor (VEGF) and angiogenesis.[65]

Markers

Markers for assessment of oxidative stress in the cardiovascular system include measurement of C-reactive proteins, lipoproteins (LDL and HDL), platelet aggregation, and lipid peroxidation. Recently, measurement of 8-isoprostane (8-epiPGF2α) has been regarded a good marker of lipid peroxidation. Several studies have indicated increased plasma levels of 8-isoprostane in subjects with coronary artery disease (CAD), and the increase in this marker correlates well with the severity of the disease.[62]

Prevention

The involvement of oxidative stress and upset of the oxidant–antioxidant system in cardiovascular diseases have generated considerable interest in antioxidants as therapeutic measures for prevention of these and other chronic diseases. However, studies to evaluate the effectiveness of α-tocopherol, ascorbic acid, and β-carotene in reducing cardiovascular diseases have not provided conclusive results.[61,66] There is increasing interest in investigating effects of polyphenol antioxidants from fruits and vegetables.[67] In particular, many studies have focused on resveratrol from grapes and red wine.[68] Future intervention studies should include developing more biomarkers for assessing cell damage due to oxidative stress and information regarding bioavailability and metabolism of these compounds.[69]

SUMMARY: THE SENSIBLE DIET

Numerous guidelines and eating plans that emphasize low-fat and low-sodium food choices are available. The Dietary Guidelines for Americans, 2005, a report from the US Department of Health and Human Services and the US Department of Agriculture (www.healthierus.gov/dietaryguidelines), provide suggestions on dietary intake for healthy individuals. The American Heart Association (AHA, www.americanheart.org) also lists dietary guidelines. The National Cholesterol Education Program (NCEP), started by the National Heart, Lung and Blood Institute (www.nhlbi.nih.gov), focuses on lowering blood cholesterol levels through the Therapeutic Lifestyle Changes (TLC) diet. The Institute also supports the Dietary Approaches to Stop Hypertension (DASH) diet. These guidelines and eating plans control intake through appropriate food choices (discussed below) and regulation of serving size and number. Accurately determining serving sizes is important not only for following the plans but also for reading food labels and understanding the nutritional content of foods, including convenience and fast foods.

Although slight variations occur, these guidelines and eating plans typically emphasize a diet rich in fruits, vegetables, nuts, legumes, and whole grains. The newly revised Dietary Guidelines for Americans, 2005, recommend nine servings (4½ cups) of fruits and vegetables daily for someone requiring 2000 kcal daily. They emphasize consuming a wide variety of fruits and vegetables of all colors. Most fruits and vegetables have significant levels of potassium (and are thus probably important for blood pressure control) and significant amounts of vitamins and other antioxidants that may be important for cardiovascular disease prevention.

Fruits and vegetables also have significant amounts of fiber. However, consuming adequate fiber intake also requires adding whole grains, nuts, and legumes to the diet. Soluble fiber – found in oatmeal, psyllium seeds, legumes, and some fruits and vegetables – can help lower blood cholesterol. Dietary fiber typically increases satiety, reducing the desire to eat low-nutrient foods.

Dietary fat and cholesterol intake must also be considered. The dietary reference intake for fat consumption is 20–35% of total kilocalories (www.nap.edu). The Dietary Guidelines for Americans, 2005, recommend <10% and the TLC diet <7% of total kilocalories from saturated fat. Fat selection should emphasize sources of monounsaturated and polyunsaturated fatty acids. At least two servings of fish weekly are recommended for additional longchain ω-3 fatty acids. Intake of *trans* fatty acids, found in baked goods containing partially hydrogenated vegetable oils, commercially fried foods, and some margarines, should be limited. Dietary cholesterol is found exclusively in animal products and should be limited to <300 mg daily for the general population (Dietary Guidelines for Americans, 2005) and <200 mg daily for those following the TLC diet.

The Dietary Guidelines for Americans, 2005, recommend sodium intake of <2300 mg daily.

This is approximately one teaspoon of table salt. Processed foods and salt used for seasoning are significant sources of sodium in the diet. A blend of herbs and spices or pepper can be used in place of table salt for seasoning.

Low-fat and fat-free dairy products provide protein, potassium, magnesium, and especially calcium and phosphorus in the diet. The Dietary Guidelines for Americans, 2005, recommend three cups of fat-free or low-fat milk or equivalent milk products daily. Research with the DASH diet has shown that drinking three glasses of skim milk daily further lowers blood pressure.[70] Whether low-fat dairy also helps control weight remains controversial. It certainly contributes toward adequate bone formation in youth and maintaining bone through pregnancy, lactation, and the postmenopausal period.

Along with adequate physical activity, these recommendations will help individuals to maintain or achieve a healthful weight and provide a foundation for sensible eating for cardiovascular health.

REFERENCES

1. Ford ES, Giles WH, Dietz WH. Prevalence of the metabolic syndrome among US adults: findings from the third National Health and Nutrition Examination Survey. JAMA 2002; 287:356.

2. Knowler WC, Barrett-Connor E, Fowler SE, et al. Reduction in the incidence of type 2 diabetes with lifestyle intervention or metformin. N Engl J Med 2002; 346:393.

3. Hill JO, Wyatt HR, Reed GW, Peters JC. Obesity and the environment: where do we go from here? Science 2003; 299:853.

4. Klem ML, Wing RR, McGuire MT, Seagle HM, Hill JO. A descriptive study of individuals successful at long-term maintenance of substantial weight loss. Am J Clin Nutr 1997; 66:239.

5. Graci S, Izzo G, Savino S, et al. Weight cycling and cardiovascular risk factors in obesity. Int J Obes Relat Metab Disord 2004; 28:65.

6. Petersmarck KA, Teitelbaum HS, Bond JT, et al. The effect of weight cycling on blood lipids and blood pressure in the Multiple Risk Factor Intervention Trial Special Intervention Group. Int J Obes Relat Metab Disord 1999; 23:1246.

7. Nicolosi RJ, Rogers EJ. Regulation of plasma lipoprotein levels by dietary triglycerides enriched with different fatty acids. Med Sci Sports Exerc 1997; 29:1422.

8. Grundy GM. Nutrition and diet in the management of hyperlipidemia and atherosclerosis. In: Shils ME, Olson JA, Shike M, Ross AC, eds. Modern Nutrition in Health and Disease. Baltimore: Lippincott, Williams and Wilkins; 1999.

9. Gatto LM, Sullivan DR, Samman S. Postprandial effects of dietary trans fatty acids on apolipoprotein(a) and cholesteryl ester transfer. Am J Clin Nutr 2003; 77:1119.

10. Kris-Etherton PM, Pearson TA, Wan Y, et al. High-monounsaturated fatty acid diets lower both plasma cholesterol and triacylglycerol concentrations. Am J Clin Nutr 1999; 70:1009.

11. Wijendran V, Hayes KC. Dietary n-6 and n-3 fatty acid balance and cardiovascular health. Annu Rev Nutr 2004; 24:597.

12. Burr ML, Fehily AM, Gilbert JF, et al. Effects of changes in fat, fish, and fibre intakes on death and myocardial reinfarction: diet and reinfarction trial (DART). Lancet 1989; 2(8666):757.

13. Gruppo Italiano per lo Studio della Sopravvivenza nell'Infarto Miocardico. Dietary supplementation with n-3 polyunsaturated fatty acids and vitamin E after myocardial infarction: results of the GISSI-Prevenzione trial. Lancet 1999; 354(9177):447.

14. Stark KD, Holub BJ. Differential eicosapentaenoic acid elevations and altered cardiovascular disease risk factor responses after supplementation with docosahexaenoic acid in postmenopausal women receiving and not receiving hormone replacement therapy. Am J Clin Nutr 2004 79(5):765.

15. Harris WS, Von Schacky C. The Omega-3 Index: a new risk factor for death from coronary heart disease? Prev Med 2004; 39(1):212.

16. Kris-Etherton PM, Harris WS, Appel LJ, for the American Heart Association Nutrition Committee. Fish consumption, fish oil, omega-3 fatty acids, and cardiovascular disease. Circulation 2002; 106(21):2747.

17. Simopoulos AP, Leaf A, Salem N Jr. Workshop on the essentiality of and recommended dietary intakes for omega-6 and omega-3 fatty acids. The Cloisters, National Institutes of Health (NIH), Bethesda, Maryland, USA, April 1999. Available HTTP: http://www.issfal.org.uk/adequateintakes.htm (accessed 26 October 2005).

18. Schulze MB, Liu S, Rimm EB, et al. Glycemic index, glycemic load, and dietary fiber intake and incidence of type 2 diabetes in younger and middle-aged women. Am J Clin Nutr 2004; 80(2):348.

19. Kelly S, Frost G, Whittaker V, Summerbell C. Low glycaemic index diets for coronary heart disease. Cochrane Database Syst Rev 2004; 18(4):CD004467.

20. Slyper AH. The pediatric obesity epidemic: causes and controversies. J Clin Endocrinol Metab 2004; 89(6):2540.

21. Weggemans RM, Trautwein EA. Relation between soy-associated isoflavones and LDL and HDL cholesterol concentrations in humans: a meta-analysis. Eur J Clin Nutr 2003; 57:940.

22. Dietary Reference Intakes for Water, Potassium, Sodium, Chloride and Sulfate. Washington, DC: The National Academies Press; 2004.

23. Whelton PK, He J, Cutler JA, et al. Effects of oral potassium on blood pressure: meta-analysis of randomized controlled clinical trials. JAMA 1997; 277:1624.

24. Sakhaee K, Poindexter JR, Griffith CS, Pak CY. Stone forming risk of calcium citrate supplementation in healthy postmenopausal women. J Urol 2004; 172:958.

25. Hatton DC, McCarron DA. Dietary calcium and blood pressure in experimental models of hypertension: a review. Hypertension 1994; 23(4):513.

26. Allender PS, Cutler JA, Follmann D, et al. Dietary calcium and blood pressure: a meta-analysis of randomized clinical trials. Ann Intern Med 1996; 124:825.

27. Levine RJ, Hauth JC, Curet LB, et al. Trial of calcium to prevent preeclampsia. N Engl J Med 1997; 337:69.

28. Cross NA, Hillman LS, Allen SH, Krause GF, Vieira NE. Calcium homeostasis and bone metabolism during pregnancy, lactation, and postweaning: a longitudinal study. Am J Clin Nutr 1995; 61:514.

29. Cross NA, Hillman LS, Allen SH, Krause GF. Changes in bone mineral density and markers of bone remodeling during lactation and postweaning in women consuming high amounts of calcium. J Bone Min Res 1995; 10:1312.

30. Tanko LB, Christiansen C, Cox DA, et al. Relationship between osteoporosis and cardiovascular disease in postmenopausal women. J Bone Miner Res 2005; 20(11):1912.

31. Summanen JO, Vuorela HJ, Hiltunen RK. Does potassium and magnesium supplementation lower the blood pressure of spontaneously hypertensive rats? J Pharm Sci 1994; 83:249.

32. Lopez-Ridaura R, Willett WC, Rimm EB, et al. Magnesium intake and risk of type 2 diabetes in men and women. Diabetes Care 2004; 27(1):134.

33. Guerrero-Romero F, Rodriguez-Moran M. Low serum magnesium levels and metabolic syndrome. Acta Diabetol 2002; 39(4):209.

34. Eisenstein RS. Iron regulatory proteins and the molecular control of mammalian iron metabolism. Annu Rev Nutr 2000; 20:627.

35. Hinton PS, Giordano CG, Brownlie T, Hass JD. Iron supplementation improves endurance after training in iron-depleted, nonanemic women. J Appl Physiol 2000; 88(3):1103.

36. Brownlie T 4th, Utermohlen V, Hinton PS, Haas JD. Tissue iron deficiency without anemia impairs adaptation in endurance capacity after aerobic training in previously untrained women. Am J Clin Nutr 2004; 79(3):437.

37. Celsing F, Blomstrand E, Werner B, Pihlstedt P, Ekblom B. Effects of iron deficiency on endurance and muscle enzyme activity in man. Med Sci Sports Exerc 1986; 18:156.

38. Food and Nutrition Board, Institute of Medicine. Dietary reference intakes for vitamin A, vitamin K, arsenic, boron, chromium, copper, iodine, iron, manganese, nickel, silicon, vanadium, zinc. Washington, D.C.: National Academy of Sciences, 2001; 157.

39. Beard JL. Iron biology in immune function, muscle metabolism and neuronal functioning. J Nutr 2001; 131(2S-2):568S.

40. Beard JL, Hendricks MK, Perez EM, et al. Maternal iron deficiency anemia affects postpartum emotions and cognition. J Nutr 2005; 135(2):267.

41. Salonen JT, Nyyssonen K, Korpela H, et al. High stored iron levels are associated with excess risk of myocardial infarction in eastern Finnish men. Circulation 1992; 86(3):803.

42. Danesh J, Appleby P. Coronary heart disease and iron status: meta-analyses of prospective studies. Circulation 1999; 99(7):852.

43. Sempos CT, Looker AC, Gillum RE, et al. Serum ferritin and death from all causes and cardiovascular disease. The NHANES II Mortality Study. Ann Epidemiol 2000; 10(7):441.

44. Williams MJ, Poulton R, Williams S. Relationship of serum ferritin with cardiovascular risk factors and inflammation in young men and women. Atherosclerosis 2002; 165(1):179.

45. Derstine JL, Murray-Kolb LE, Yu-Poth S, et al. Iron status in association with cardiovascular disease risk in 3 controlled feeding studies. Am J Clin Nutr 2003; 77(1):56.

46. Binkoski AE, Kris-Etherton PM, Beard JL. Iron supplementation does not affect the susceptibility of LDL to oxidative modification in women with low iron status. J Nutr 2004; 134(1):99.

47. Mills JL, Scott JM, Kirke PN, et al. Homocysteine and neural tube defects. J Nutr 1996; 126:756S.

48. Frosst P, Blom HJ, Milos R, et al. A candidate genetic risk factor for vascular disease: a common mutation in methylenetetrahydrofolate reductase. Nat Genet 1995; 10:111.

49. Chao C-L, Tsai HH, Lee CM, et al. The graded effect of hyperhomocysteinemia on the severity and extent of coronary atherosclerosis. Atherosclerosis 1999; 147:379.

50. Hillman L, Sateesha S, Haussler M, et al. Control of mineral homeostasis during lactation: interrelationships of 25-hydroxyvitamin D, 24,25-dihydroxyvitamin D, 1,25-dihydroxyvitamin D, parathyroid hormone, calcitonin, prolactin, and estradiol. Am J Obst Gynecol 1981; 139:471.

51. Hillman LS, Haddad JG. Human perinatal vitamin D metabolism I: 25–hydroxyvitamin D in maternal and cord blood. J Pediatr 1974; 84:742.

52. Specker BL, Tsang RC, Hollis BW. Effect of race and diet on human-milk vitamin D and 25–hydroxyvitamin D. Am J Dis Child 1985; 139:1134.

53. Chiu KC, Chu A, Go VL, Saad MF. Hypovitaminosis D is associated with insulin resistance and β cell dysfunction. Am J Clin Nutr 2004; 79(5):820.

54. Bugel S. Vitamin K and bone health. Proc Nutr Soc 2003; 62(4):839.

55. Braam LA, Knapen MH, Geusens P, et al. Vitamin K1 supplementation retards bone loss in postmenopausal women between 50 and 60 years of age. Calcif Tissue Int 2003; 73(1):21.

56. Brown JP, Josse RG, and Scientific Advisory Council of the Osteoporosis Society of Canada. 2002 clinical practice guidelines for the diagnosis and management of osteoporosis in Canada. Can Med Assoc J 2002; 167(10 Suppl):S1.

57. Vermeer C, Schurgers LJ. A comprehensive review of vitamin K and vitamin K antagonists. Hematol Oncol Clin North Am 2000; 14(2):339.

58. Vivekananthan DP, Penn MS, Sapp SK, Hsu A, Topol EJ. Use of antioxidant vitamins for the prevention of cardiovascular disease: meta-analysis of randomised trials. Lancet 2003; 361:2017.

59. Pryor WA. Vitamin E and heart disease; basic science to clinical intervention trials. Free Radical Biol Med 2000; 28:141.

60. Clarke R, Armitage J. Antioxidant vitamins and risk of cardiovascular disease. Review of large-scale randomized trials. Cardiovasc Drugs Ther 2002; 16:411.

61. Blomhoff R. Dietary antioxidants and cardiovascular disease. Curr Opin Lipidol 2005; 16:47.

62. Vassalle C, Petrozzi L, Botto N, Andreassi MG, Zucchelli GC. Oxidative stress and its association with coronary artery disease and different atherogenic risk factors. J Intern Med 2004; 256:308.

63. Abrescia P, Golino P. Free radicals and antioxidants in cardiovascular diseases. Expert Rev Cardiovasc Ther 2005; 3:159.

64. Madamanchi NR, Vendrov A, Runge MS. Oxidative stress and vascular disease. Arterioscler Thromb Vasc Biol 2005; 25:29.

65. Ushio-Fukai M, Alexander RW. Reactive oxygen species as mediators of angiogenesis signaling: role of NAD(P)H oxidase. Mol Cell Biochem 2004; 264:85.

66. Gaziano JM. Vitamin E and cardiovascular disease: observational studies. Ann NY Acad Sci 2004; 1031:280.

67. Scalbert A, Johnson IT, Saltmarsh M. Polyphenols: antioxidants and beyond. Am J Clin Nutr 2005; 81:215S.

68. Araim O, Ballantyne J, Waterhouse AL, Sumpio BE. Inhibition of vascular smooth muscle cell proliferation with red wine and red wine polyphenols. J Vasc Surg 2002; 35:1226.

69. Manach C, Mazur A, Scalbert A. Polyphenols and prevention of cardiovascular diseases. Curr Opin Lipidol 2005; 16:77.

70. Sacks FM, Svetkey LP, Vollmer WM, et al, DASH–Sodium Collaborative Research Group. Effects on blood pressure of reduced dietary sodium and the Dietary Approaches to Stop Hypertension (DASH) diet. DASH–Sodium Collaborative Research Group. N Engl J Med 2001; 344(1):3.

Index